Neurophilosophy of Free Will

Neurophilosophy of Free Will
From Libertarian Illusions to a Concept of Natural Autonomy

Henrik Walter
Translated from German by Cynthia Klohr

A Bradford Book
The MIT Press
Cambridge, Massachusetts
London, England

First MIT Press paperback edition, 2009
© 2001 The Massachusetts Institute of Technology
This work originally appeared in German under the title *Neurophilosophie der Willensfreiheit*
© 1999 by Mentis Verlag, Paderborn, 2nd ed.

This book was set in Sabon by Best-set Typesetter Ltd., Hong Kong

Library of Congress Cataloging-in-Publication Data
Walter, Henrik.
    [Neurophilosophie der Willensfreiheit. English]
    Neurophilosophy of free will : from libertarian illusions to a concept of natural autonomy / Henrik Walter ; translated from German by Cynthia Klohr.
        p.   cm.
    "A Bradford book."
    Includes bibliographical references (p.) and index.
    ISBN 978-0-262-23214-2 (hc.: alk. paper)—978-0-262-51265-7 (pb.: alk. paper)
        1. Free will and determinism.   2. Neurosciences.   I. Title.
    BJ1463 .W3413 2001
    123'.5–dc21
                                                                    00-046579

10 9 8 7 6 5 4 3 2

For Sven

Contents

Preface

Beyond a doubt, neuroscience has become as important to contemporary philosophy as physics and evolutionary theory were to past modern philosophy. This development questions the general liaison of science and philosophy. It requires that we first outline our concept of philosophy before we carefully explore neurophilosophy's research ventures. Anyone defining philosophy as a discipline dealing with issues irrelevant to empirical science is likely to reject or oppose the endeavors of neurophilosophy. My experience and opinion is that philosophical questions inevitably arise at a certain stage within scientific work in progress, unintentionally and in spite of the fact that the scientists involved might themselves prefer to ignore them. This is decidedly true for any science investigating the "soul's organ." Neuroscience already investigates such classical philosophical topics as consciousness, thought, meaning, language, aesthetics, and death—just to mention a few. Philosophers in tune with the state of the art should, in turn, reach out and embrace the wealth of research findings and ideas provided by neuroscience.

Why? Philosophy's primary concern, writes Thomas Nagel, is "to question and understand very common ideas that all of us use every day without thinking about them" (Nagel 1987, p. 5). Science also questions and reconsiders these general pet notions in light of new empirical findings. Philosophical fantasy frequently sails past the real data, but it also tends to assimilate recent empirical findings to our commonplace experience. Good philosophy needs a dab of speculation, which, however, should be firmly anchored in historical and empirical knowledge. We may inquire at length whether plants have souls; our pondering of the microcosm and macrocosm may be roused by observing the structural similarities of the solar system and atoms. But serious philosophy must liken and link such musings with our knowledge of the world. Our knowledge no longer is drawn solely from ordinary experience or the Holy Scriptures: Most of it results from scientific endeavor. Speculative philosophy should not—out of ignorance—be inconsistent with reliable scientific findings. If today we were to found a philosophical theory about a *vis vitalis* on the wonder of how plants adjust themselves to the position of the sun, without noticing that this phenomenon can be well explained in terms of physiological mechanisms, or if we were to wonder about the significance of star constellations in the heavens without using any knowledge of our universe, our theories would have very little philosophical impact. And this is equally true for our inner, mental world: The mental does not exist in a theoretical vacuum, it is real and it is seated in the brain.

Consequently, philosophy is *not* on the retreat, as some believe it to be.[1] On the contrary, new scientific findings increase our need for philosophical reflection. Sciences and scientists themselves are involved in philosophical debates, sometimes quite unintentionally, drawn in through the very nature of their own quests and topics. Unfortunately, they are seldom good philosophers, because they are simply unaware of the numerous pitfalls and perils in arguments accumulated throughout the history of philosophy. And often scientists fail to notice that their theories inherently make certain metaphysical assumptions of questionable validity. So what marks philosophy as opposed to science? Method. Doing philosophy means "asking questions, arguing, trying out ideas and thinking of possible arguments against them, and wondering how our concepts really work" (Nagel 1987, p. 4). This kind of debate should be sufficiently scientifically informed, if our aim is to "push our understanding of the world and ourselves a bit deeper" (Nagel 1987, p. 5). In philosophy we strive to comprehend ourselves, our world, and our concepts. Using contemporary knowledge as the backdrop, our strategy is to examine arguments pro and con philosophical standpoints. That is the interpretation of philosophy that inspired this book.

I once held a lecture on the topic of this book and afterward a member of the audience confided that he felt he had heard two distinct speeches: One on free will and another on neurophilosophy. Chapters 1 and 2 of this book likewise cover the two topics separately and can be read as independent essays. Chapter 3 brings them together by applying the *method* of neurophilosophy to the *issue* of the freedom of will.

The controversy over free will is one of philosophy's perpetual challenges. Thematically, it is associated with two different philosophical topics: the question of whether and how our self-determined action ties in with the rest of nature's causal order, and the fact that free will traditionally has been considered either a matter of natural philosophy or an ethical issue. I myself view it as a challenge to natural philosophy, but I am careful not to lose sight of its ethical relevance. I ask whether or not there is free will, and my answer is, it depends. As in most cases the existence of something depends on exactly what it is to which we are attributing or questioning its existence. We cannot get by without defining free will. Struggling with it takes us right to the heart of philosophical debate. Many philosophers regard the definition of free will as the most urgent challenge of the controversy. Settling for a specific definition is almost equivalent to taking sides.

I try to avoid that complication by utilizing a component theory to characterize free will. It is designed to accommodate the expression of each important theory of the free will by varying degrees of interpretation and by combining components. The three components relate to (1) whether we are able to choose other than we actually do, (2) whether our choices are made intelligibly, and (3) whether we are really the originators of our choices. I discuss arguments pro and con of some versions of varying strength and conclude that free will is an illusion, if by it we mean that under *identical* conditions we would be able to do or decide otherwise, while simultaneously acting only for reasons and considering ourselves the *true originators* of our actions.

Chapter 2 discusses the development and basic concepts of neurophilosophy and the difficulties it encounters. Calling my approach *minimal neurophilosophy*, I purposively neglect the Weltanschauung-aspect of this science. All neurophilosophy, however, rests on three principles: Mental processes are due to brain processes; statements about mental processes should not contradict our operative knowledge about the brain; and by studying the dynamics of brain functioning we can learn about mental processes—including free will.

Chapter 3 modifies all three components of free will in such a way that these become plausible in terms of neurophilosophy. That is, we modify them such that we have respectable reasons to believe that a moderate version of free will is compatible with scientific findings. In each case this weakens the interpretations of the components. The result is what I call *natural autonomy*. Natural autonomy as self-determination unaided by supernatural powers could exist even in an entirely determined universe. But since natural autonomy is not the same as the free will in the strong sense mentioned above, part of that interpretation *is* lost. Natural autonomy can sustain neither our traditional concept of guilt, for example, nor certain attitudes and hopes about ourselves and our lives. But we are also not marionettes, mere puppets without thoughts and ideas that influence events happening to us. The lack of a strong version of free will does not imply that all moral order collapses or that we need abandon every concept of responsibility. We do, however, have to give up some cherished illusions about ourselves.

Three people accompanied the genesis of this book and to them I owe special thanks. Gerhard Vollmer not only contributed to its origin, but also to my decision to devote part of my life to philosophy. He taught me that science and philosophy can coincide in *one and the same* culture. He himself covers several fields. Trained initially in physics, he gained renown for evolutionary epistemology and he teaches philosophy. At heart, however, he is a mathematician, the kind who unites mathematics and philosophy: clear, precise, and consistent! Philosophizing with him is as fun as it is informative.

For professional and personal support I also thank Wolfgang Buschlinger. The Department of Philosophy at Braunschweig owes its vibrant life more to his presence, his initiatives, his refreshingly candid opinions, and his Dionysian laughter than to anything else. I had abundant intellectual qualia flashes during our extensive experimental studies and sessions on consciousness. Neither before nor after (yet) have I had such pleasure combining ideas and emotions, arguments and jokes, in short: joining pensiveness and nonsense with such prolific intensity.

Last, but not—really not—least, I thank my dear wife, Bettina, who suffered the making of this book the greatest. PC keys clicking away became her most familiar lullaby. She was the *sine qua non* of this work.

Without her love and enduring patience this work would have gathered dust in an early version stored away in an apathetic notebook.

I would also like to mention the Heidelberg Mind-Corpo-Ration (Hans-Peter Schütt, Achim Stephan, Cynthia Klohr, and occasionally Christian Nimtz). Our discussion sessions were tough but always pleasant. I learned immensely from them and they helped me to correct some misconceptions. Thanks also to Matthias Behne, who proofread most of the first version, and to Mehdi Parvizian, who patiently fulfilled my urgent need for diagrams.

Finally, my editor, Thomas Metzinger, advised me not to print some things prematurely. Thanks for that. But not only that. He encouraged me and other young philosophers in Germany not to quit the balance act between empirical science and philosophy. And that is good, because once you swerve off the tightrope to one side, you lose sight of what is happening on the other. And once you have landed on one side or the other, its difficult to climb back up onto the wire.

Ulm, 1997

Let those who call themselves philosophers bear the risk to their mental health that comes from thinking too much about free will.

—John Earman

1

Free Will: Challenges, Arguments, and Theories

Synopsis

After turning briefly to Kant, I introduce a concept of free will that addresses three essential constituents of philosophical and commonplace discourse on the subject: These are alternativism, intelligibility, and origination (section 1). Examples are provided to demonstrate these components (sections 2–4). Each of them is closely tied to an underlying philosophical challenge (such as determinism, intentionality, and personal ascription). Determinism is directly and indirectly relevant to all three components; therefore I deal with it separately (section 2.3). Although our world probably is undetermined, determinism does remain a challenge for free will. A three-component model of free will is laid out in section 5 and applied to pivotal philosophical positions. I address some matters in terminology and cast light on related topics. Section 6 gathers and organizes important arguments for both parties in the case of free will. It shows how they relate to the aforementioned components when they are interpreted more or less strictly. An evaluation of those arguments shows that there is no concept for free will that satisfies all three demands in the strictest sense. Philosophical theories either tend to describe how the world would need to be if it were to allow for a strong free will, or how strong versions of free will require modification in order to accommodate what we usually consider to be free will. Section 7 takes us on an excursion to the current scene of philosophical theory and shows how the three-component model is useful for understanding topics discussed there.

1   The Three Components of Free Will

1.1   The Challenge

The question of free will undoubtedly belongs to the perennial matters of philosophy. Equally stubborn is the meta-difficulty of defining free will itself. Some theorists claim that finding a definition for free will is the real problem, because such a definition would, per se, answer many of the pressing questions. Among the questions, which taken together with others comprise the problem of free will, are these: In a determined world, can we establish a concept of possibility, which does not coincide with what actually exists? How does a real instance of it look *sub species aeternitatis*? Can reason-guided action be undetermined? How can we say that a material thing acts for reasons? How can a person be the author of his decisions and not merely a locus where extraneous influences add up? How are we to understand our intuition that we are only responsible for our actions in cases where we *could have* done otherwise? How do free will and moral responsibility depend on each other? Can we justify personal responsibility? How can we reasonably tell the relevant mental history of a truly guilty person, for whom no apologies are acceptable? Can a person knowingly do evil? What are willed acts? What is self control? How can a weak will be possible? What would the consequences be, if there were no such thing as free will?[1]

I do not claim to provide exhaustive expositions on all of these issues, although I will touch upon most of them at one place or another. I am essentially concerned with the question of whether or not free will actually exists. Naturally, this question cannot be answered before we determine which kind of free will we are considering. We need a clear concept that will support our studies. Our strategy will be to begin with a fairly sophisticated working concept for free will, while leaving its explication as open as possible, so that if necessary we can correct and modify it. We can gain a first impression by observing an example by the renowned Libertarian[2] Isaiah Berlin:

> I wish my life and my decisions to depend on myself, not on external forces of whatever kind. I wish to be the instrument of my own, not of other men's acts of will. I wish to be a subject, not an object; to be moved by reasons, by conscious purposes, which are my own, not by causes that affect me, as it were, from outside. . . . I wish, above all, to be conscious of myself as a thinking, willing, active being, bearing responsibility for my choices and able to explain them by reference to my own ideas and purposes. (Isiaah Berlin, quoted from Double 1991, p. 12)

This almost incantatorily expressed desire is certainly familiar to most of us. It is one of our deeply rooted cultural ideals and corresponds to the historical development in western societies of marked individualism in an environment of political freedom. However, we should not be so taken in by Berlin's thoroughly praiseworthy intuitions and aims as to readily agree that this is really the concept of free will used by *everyone* talking about free will; or that it is undoubtedly clear that we actually possess a will of that kind. It depends very much on which significance we lend to crucial phrases such as "by myself," "for reasons, not due to causes," "to bear responsibility," and so on. For our answer to the question of whether free will exists depends on the interpretation of just such expressions. I want to discover *what really exists*, not merely what could exist or whether a particular interpretation of the free will is true. For this purpose it will be necessary to introduce a concept of free will wide enough to capture essential ordinary and philosophical intuitions on the subject while simultaneously not prematurely answering the question "Does free will exist?" per definitionem.

Using a three-part model which allows us to combine and interpret its components in varying degrees we can grasp the cardinal theories of free will, without resolving the question of the existence of free will from the start by making it part of our concept.

1.2   Kant and Free Will

People have divergent ideas and intuitions about free will. How can we isolate the essential notions? One way would be to analyze ordinary language. But because everyday language is not as homogeneous as some philosophers suppose and because it is also a poor advisor in some instances, I do not consider it the best route to take. Another method would be to examine what important philosophers have said on the topic. But that would mean writing a comprehensive history of philosophy, for almost every important philosopher has had something to say about free will (see Adler 1958; Steinvorth 1987; Dihle 1985). What we are interested in is the common denominator of those philosophical efforts relating to the free will: their argument value. Instead of laying out the challenge in terms of philosophical history, I intend to concentrate on the arguments in the form in which they are discussed in current relevant philosophical literature. First we need to know just what these arguments refer to. We must start somewhere. But where?

The English mathematician and philosopher Whitehead once said that the entire history of philosophy is merely a footnote to Plato. Slightly altering this bon mot—not too seriously—we can say that for German speaking countries all philosophy is a commentary to Kant. Kant's influence on many philosophical issues is immense, particularly on the subject of free will. Looking at the way he set up the problem can be of help to us. This does not purport to be a commentary on his work, nor an exposition, nor an historically founded interpretation of it.[3] Rather, in Kant's work we find all three areas addressed in fairly clear diction—the three areas that in my opinion constitute the main points of the philosophical problem as it is discussed in contemporary analytical philosophy. So we can *use* Kant's ideas and definitions similarly to the way in which Descartes' thoughts on consciousness are often used as a point of departure for discussing the mind-body problem, without going into his original ideas in full detail.

A thinker with a lifelong interest in natural science, Kant explored themes of natural philosophy in his early work, for example in his first paper, *Thoughts on the True Evaluation of Living Forces*, written in 1746. It is interesting to note that in the debate between the Leibnizian school and the Cartesian school over the correct definition of force, Kant took sides with the Leibnizians, who postulated that there are "living forces" for "the freedom of human reason" (Höffe 1983, p. 24). In an anonymously published work titled *General Natural History and Theory of the Heavens, Dealt with According to Newton's Basic Laws* (1755), Kant developed a qualitative theory of the genesis of the world. Known as the Kant-Laplace Theory, Kant's theory, together with the quantitative world genesis hypothesis of Laplace (1796), played a dominant role in astronomy for a long time.

Even in his later, more critical phase, the conflict between physics theory on the one hand and the freedom of human reason on the other remained a central topic for Kant. In *The Critique of Pure Reason*, Kant describes four antinomies that result when pure reason—theoretical, pure cognition—deals with issues for which it is not competent: the question of the world's origin, the divisibility of matter, the determinedness of being and the existence of God. According to Kant a statement is antinomous when the proposition and its contradiction can both be well founded with the instruments of pure reason, meaning that laws of reason conflict. In discussing the third antinomy Kant describes how pure reason entangles itself in unsolvable contradictions when it tries to comprehend the causal, natural law order of the world as something universal. His thesis in the third antinomy is: "Causality according to the laws of nature is not the only type of causality from which all the phenomena of the world can be derived. We must also assume a causality given through freedom in order to explain them." (Kant 1787/1983, B 472) Kant proves this via *reductio ad absurdum*, that is, by demonstrating a contradiction when assuming the contrary. The antithesis: "There is no freedom, everything in the world happens solely according to the laws of nature" (Kant 1787/1983, B 473) can, however, also be "proven" by a *reductio ad absurdum* of the opposite. Thus we have a second order contradiction. For now both the thesis and antithesis have been proven, yet both cannot be simultaneously true. Must we live with this antinomy? That would not be satisfying. And in fact Kant does find a way to solve the contradiction in a certain sense. Besides the causality of nature, we need to assume the "freedom of cosmological reason"; it marks the ability of a state to "originate in itself" (Kant 1787/1983, B 561). Kant calls this "absolute spontaneity" (B 474). "Causality through freedom" lies not in the empirical, but in the "intelligible character" of an agent (B 567). The contradiction between thesis and antithesis results only when we try to understand freedom as an empirical concept, which is objectionable. Thus Kant postulates two different worlds in which different laws hold: the intelligible world and the empirical world. These are evidently imagined to be so different from each other that their laws may contradict one another. Each of these worlds has its own type of causality. So in the end, Kant's solution must be understood as a dual-world theory.

But how can the inconsistency among both worlds be solved or accommodated? According to Kant, this is done by making the will *practical*. He defines the will as the ability of beings possessing reason "to determine their own actions consonant with ideas of certain laws" (1786/1983 BA 63). The antinomy can be solved in ethics, the realm of practical reason. Our freedom, Kant says, is not bare freedom, freedom *an sich*, it is *moral* freedom. Our actions are only free when they are due solely to insight in moral law,[4] so that consequently "a free will and a will under moral laws become one and the same" (BA 98). Using the idea of agency, Kant links theoretical reason (intelligibility) to practical reason (morality): Reason "must consider herself the originator of her own principles, independent of foreign influences, therefore she must consider practical reason . . . to be free" (BA 101).

In sum, we find three aspects of free will in Kant's work: First, determination by natural law and freedom appear to be mutually exclusive. Second, autonomous action means *intelligible* action, acting according to principles. Third, morality is linked to intelligibility via the idea of origination; in practical terms free will and morality are even identical. The close relation between the three components of my model and these three features in Kant's work will become conspicuous when I explain the three-component theory of the free will in the following section.

1.3   The Three Components of Free Will

In analytical philosophy all three mentioned aspects play roles in principal theories and arguments.[5] They obviously express central ideas that are not only part of philosophical theories, but also part of our everyday ideas—our intuitions. Joining Seebass (1993, p. 25), I hold that free will has three relevant features: freedom (being able to do otherwise), volition (as an intelligible, i.e., understandable action), and agency.[6] My provisionary definition of free will reads:

A person has free will (commands freedom of will) if three pivotal conditions are satisfied in a critical number of his acts and decisions. The person:
i. *could* have acted *otherwise* (he acts freely),
ii. acts for understandable reasons (intelligible form of volition), and
iii. is the originator of his actions.

On no account do I maintain that this component view is an analysis of "what we have always meant" or what we "really" mean when we speak of free will—especially not what *the philosophers* mean. I do claim, however, that these three features rest on central intuitions that can be found in nearly all theories about free will. Those various theories differ solely in the fact that they either deal only with part of the components, or they declare one of them to be particularly significant, or they support variously strong interpretations. In a way, the component view is ecumenical. It combines divergent views under one roof by expressing shared intuitions in a general and consensual manner, while preserving a broad interpretation.

It is obvious that expressions such as "could have done otherwise," "for understandable reasons," "willingly," or "origin" are anything but unequivocal. In the following paragraphs I will explain and discuss these terms in more detail. At this point a few general warnings are appropriate.

First: I do not distinguish strictly between the freedom of action and the freedom of will. Traditionally, philosophy has understood the freedom of action as the freedom to do what one wants to do, and freedom of will as the freedom to want what one wants. Volition is, however, in my opinion, a philosophical concept so overly ambiguous and controversial that I would rather not use it fundamentally in my study. Later on (3.1) I will in fact explain volition, but detailed involvement with that term is dispensable for our purposes.[7] Many of the analytical philosophy theories on free will that I selected for my study deal only with free action and free choice. In my work, free will is taken as a predicate attributable to a person in his actions and decision-making. As long as I do not explicitly state otherwise, in the ensuing exposition I am referring paradigmatically to choices, that is, situations in which a person is confronted with the choice between alternatives and makes a decision. This choice (or decision) can be considered an act, namely when the person must express his decision through behavior.

Second, my three component explication makes no reference to moral responsibility. I'd like to briefly justify this. It is fully correct that free will and moral responsibility are related, as I will later show in more detail when it comes to arguments. I am not including moral responsibility in my explication because I am dealing with free will as an issue of *natural philosophy*, not as an ethical issue. In other words, I am not trying to characterize free will as something that supports moral responsibility, in order to subsequently examine whether or not it exists. A naturalistic strategy takes the opposite course: Free will is explained as a characteristic of persons without reference to the concept of moral responsibility. It is either attributable to them or not. First we investigate which characteristics the persons have, that is, which interpretations of free will are applicable to real persons. Then we examine whether this interpretation is also the one that supports moral responsibility. Of course I will occasionally state my position on the problem of moral responsibility, but for the purposes of this work it remains secondary.

Third, a naturalistic strategy does *not* imply assuming that we can find empirical proof or refutation for free will. But we can test each suggested explication for free will and discover whether or not it conforms to our knowledge of the world. I am particularly interested in whether or not it aligns with our knowledge of the brain. So in chapter 3 I shall lay out a neurophilosophy of free will. As soon as we accept that the way the world is limits the possible answers to our questions about free will, we realize the advantage of the component solution. We can examine various interpretations on the individual components to see whether they are consistent with our knowledge of the brain. We can also heuristically use neurobiological knowledge by exploiting insights on the functional principles of brain organization to favor and test particular interpretations and components. The main task of neurophilosophy for free will is nevertheless rather conservative. It lies in discovering which interpretation provides the greatest possible empirical plausibility.

Whether or not we should still call whatever comes out in the end "free will" is a purely terminological matter, albeit a terminological issue of psychological bearing that we shouldn't underestimate. I believe we should guide this decision by considering how much of the strong libertarian component is lost and the implications that result from that. At this point I can only reveal that enough is actually lost that we should consider finding a new name for what remains. I suggest the term "natural autonomy." I understand natural autonomy (literally: giving oneself laws) to mean self rule without reference to supernatural powers. But I am getting ahead of myself a little.

Now that we have, I hope, gained a first impression of free will, I intend to more closely analyze the three components of it. I will describe some intuitions, give further explanations, address some arguments and finally show how the components are connected to certain philosophical issues. In each case one thing always remains in the foreground: For freedom (as being able to do otherwise) it is the problem of determinism; for intelligibility it is the phenomenon of intentionality and the problem of its naturalization; and for origination it is the challenge of justifying our ascription of moral responsibility and the personal attribution of actions.

2   Freedom and Doing Otherwise

2.1   Folk-Psychological Intuitions

We Can Do Otherwise.
—Movie title by Detlef Buck

Most people take for granted that they have a free will. The idea that it is within our power to do other than what we actually do plays a central part therein.

Imagine that one morning you go to the bakery to buy a roll. What a beautiful day! The sun is shining and you don't have to work because you are on vacation. No work has been left undone, nothing must be taken care of immediately, you have no obligations at the moment, no appointments in your daily planner, no debts at the bank. The world is wonderful, you're in a great mood. Suddenly along your way you meet a misanthropic looking person and she eyes you critically. You notice her student garb, deep rings below her eyes, sallow skin from smoking heavily, and a facial expression exiled to spheres of the abstract. "O.K.," you think to yourself, "a humanities student!" In the back of your mind you make a note that your worldview has been confirmed. But something is wrong. A recorder and a mike? What for? And now this person approaches you with her microphone—why? She's not going to interview you, is she? Yes, she is. She's from the philosophy department of the local university. They are conducting a course on free will. And now they want to know, what—pardon the expression—*normal* people with common sense think intuitively about it. And since at the university they are biased (or should we say spoiled? Well, whatever) due to their philosophical training, they are prejudiced and no longer trust their own intuitions. They thought they would go out onto the street, so as to make philosophy a little more empirical. That is why she is here now and picked out the first best person who didn't look like he would refuse, for this is her initial interview and she would like to begin with her inquiry. What she wants to know is: Do you have a free will?

Surprised and feeling a slight pity that someone can waste a nice day on such matters, you answer considerately: Yes, of course. All people naturally have free will. And before the tired student can state her second question you leave her standing there holding her microphone and you head for your favorite bakery. Engrossed in making the difficult decision between whole cereal rolls and chocolate-filled croissants you have already almost forgotten the incident.

Too bad, actually. The fact that most people, when asked, confirm that they command a free will is neither particularly exciting nor interesting. The second question would have brought us straight to the core of the problem: How do you know that you have a free will? Imagine that the same interview was given to Mr. Vorberg, who happens to take a little more time. He also affirms the first question. To the second question he replies: "How do I know? That's easy. I can give you an example. I can lift my arm now, but I can also not lift it, if I want to. The fact that I can do one or the other, depending on what I decide to do, clearly demonstrates that I have a free will." This response is intelligible and demonstrates a basic intuition about free will: It is up to me to do one thing or another and whatever I decide, it is always *my* decision. What does our student comment? "I'm sorry, but naturally you will or will not move your arm. It might even be the case, that you don't know yet, which of the two you will perform. But it is possible that your actions are determined by the way things are. Because everything that happens, happens necessarily; everything happens the way it must happen."

"Oh really?," Vorberg asks, "How will I behave?" The student ponders for a moment and finally replies: "You will not raise your arm!" Vorberg: "Thanks for telling me. Without you I wouldn't fathom what to do, Miss Know-it-all. But despite your thesis—whoops—I've raised my arm! Okay?"[8]

Unfortunately it is not. It gets quirky here. The student patiently explains that the fact that he lifted his arm actually proves that his behavior is determined, since her prediction contributed to his arm-raising. The reason he lifted his arm was to prove that he has a free will. In that case, Vorberg claims he can also do otherwise and next time he will not be tricked. Will she challenge him a second time? As you please; this time he will not lift his arm. You see, claims the student, exactly by explaining her method she has altered the conditions for his actions and contributed to his lack of arm raising. And even if her prediction had been incorrect, she continues earnestly, that would not be evidence against the determinedness of his actions. It is just a sign of her own incomplete and willy-nilly fallible knowledge. She's jesting, replies Mr. Vorberg angrily, and he won't allow it! Her arguments are not scientific, not even philosophical, they are pseudoscience. Apparently, for whatever happens, whether he lifts his arm or not, she can claim that this shows determinism to be correct. It is obviously an immunization strategy—that much he does know about the theory of science. And how does she know that everything is determined? From physics? He doesn't mind. Physicists can claim whatever they like, he knows about his free will from years of experience. When she's his age, she'll understand. Of course he has been reared in a certain way, perhaps even in a slightly old-fashioned manner; admittedly he has a specific genetic make-up that he cannot change (not yet anyway). He doesn't deny this, that would be silly. But in his case, as for every human being, there is something more to him—and that is his free will. And if she wants to use physics to support her arguments, she should take a look at a modern textbook on quantum physics. There she will find that even in physics no one seriously still holds a deterministic world view. He alone, as well as every other person, determines by himself his life and his actions. He has just decided, for example, to leave. End of the interview.

2.2 Freedom as Being Able to do Otherwise

I think that this little story well describes those intuitions we have about free will that relate to the first component. I call this component "freedom," with the adjunct "as being able to do otherwise." Why not simply "freedom?" Like "love," "freedom" belongs to those concepts that are highly valuable and yet so difficult to apprehend; we can discuss them for hours and—apparently—philosophize over them for thousands of years. The concept of freedom spans just too much. We have civil freedom, freedom of the press, freedom of conscience, freedom to speak, political freedom, and much more. These types of freedom are important beyond controversy. But none of them has to do with free will. For free will the question is not whether someone else permits us to do or want something. It is also not a question of whether we are free of coercion exercised by others.[9] The issue is whether our actions and decisions could turn out other than they actually do.

It seems self-evident that in certain situations we could act or decide otherwise. There may be exceptions. Sometimes we behave automatically; sometimes we are tired and just do something without reflecting on all the alternatives; sometimes we are not even conscious of our actions; sometimes we lack concentration or are ill—all these things prevent us from doing otherwise. But in a normal case, under normal circumstances, we are able to do otherwise. For Mr. Vorberg, our fictitious interviewee, the freedom to do otherwise does not mean that one time he decides to lift his arm and the other time to leave it at his side. It means, rather, that *in the first incident* it was possible for him to decide one way or the other. The fact that in the second incident he chooses to leave his arm down does not prove that in the first incident this alternative was actually available to him. The initial situation for each incident was different; the events are not identical. The question is whether Mr. Vorberg, Ms. Pinkert, or any person at all is actually *free* in a given situation, to act thus or otherwise.

It is not a question that can simply be answered empirically. For the *exact* same, identical situation always occurs only once and is never iterated. But we can still ask the question meaningfully. And it is irrelevant whether we are asking if it is an act, a decision, or a desire that "could have been otherwise." At some point there is always the question of being able to do otherwise. I want to briefly demonstrate this by returning to the difference between the freedom of action and the freedom of will.

Traditionally the freedom of action has been understood as the possibility to do what one wants to do. Mr. Vorberg was free in this sense. In the first incident he wanted to raise his arm and he did so. *If* he had not wanted to do that, *he could have done otherwise*, as the repetition of the experiment shows. This kind of relative freedom—also known as conditional analysis because of the aspect of *if–then* freedom it contains—is, of course, possible. It does not contradict the statement that a person at a very specific time and under the conditions holding at that time could only act in a certain way and not otherwise. Naturally the question immediately arises: Could he want something other than what he wants? The issue of being able to do otherwise goes up to the next level. Here, we can also formulate a conditional solution, a conditional solution at the second level. If he had desired to want otherwise, then he could have wanted otherwise. What does the next level look like? Certainly we can always define higher levels of relative freedom. But at each level we can ask: Do we have here the possibility of doing otherwise in a nonconditional sense? This is sometimes called the principle of alternative possibilities (in the following called alternativism) and it allows us to inquire whether we have *real* alternatives. The issue of whether or not we have real alternatives is relevant for acts and decisions. If we want to avoid an infinite regress we will have to settle this matter at some point.

But why shouldn't we at some—probably lower—level be able to do otherwise in a "genuine" sense of the word? Are there objections? Yes. If determinism is true, then there is no nonconditional ability to do otherwise, there are no real alternatives. The hypothesis of determinism states that for everything that happens there are conditions such that if these conditions hold, then only that thing can happen. Since determinism plays such a central role in the free will debate, we will take a very close look at it in the following pages.

2.3   Determinism

2.3.1   The Concept of Determinism   To get a first impression of this concept let us consult the *Duden* reference book for foreign terminology. In the fifth edition we find:

Determinism [Latin-New Latin], masc.: 1. Doctrine of the causal (pre-)determinedness of all that happens. 2. Doctrine of the determinedness of the will through internal or external causes (ethics) which negates the freedom of will; Opposite: cf. Indeterminism.

This lexical entry is quite informative. It condenses many of the elements of philosophical discourse on the topic. First, it shows how close causality and predeterminedness are linked to the idea of determinism.

Second, it states that determinism negates free will but is not its oppo-site. According to the final note its contradictory opposite is *in*deter-minism. Third, it mentions that free will belongs to ethics or is at least connected to it. And finally, it shows that there are (at least) two concepts of determinism. This substantial description offers more than some philosophers are willing to admit for a conceptual definition of determinism.[10]

The *challenge* of determinism was discussed in philosophy long before the term even existed. The terms "determinism" and "indeterminism" were initially adopted in the second half of the eighteenth century under the influence of natural science. Ch. W. Snell's book *Determinism* (1789) is considered one of the earliest treatments of the problem using this title.[11] Older efforts usually were more concerned with the question of fate (Latin: *fatum*) of a person. Is it determined by the gods? Can and should one revolt against this predeterminedness?[12] Or should a person comply with his fate, since there is nothing at all we can do about it (fatalism)? A famous Stoic metaphor compares man to a dog leashed to a cart. He is forced to run after the cart whether he wants to or not. In this case, the most sensible thing to do, is to prudently trot behind the cart in order not to injure oneself by fighting one's fate. Concrete inter-ests, particularly influence on political and social decisions, have always played a part in the question of determinism. If the future is fixed, it should theoretically be possible to predict events. Consider the prophe-cies of seers, the predictions of astronomers, the oracle at Delphi, and biblical prophecies. In Christian philosophy it was particularly the doc-trine of original sin that created a challenge to the question of free will. Adam was free to choose to take an apple or not. But for both Augus-tine and Luther, man no longer had a free choice between good and evil after the Fall. He does not have the power to make a free decision. Because of the original sin, he is destined to be a sinner despite all his efforts. Only God's grace can save him. Calvin's predestination doctrine postulated that only a select few would partake of this unmerited mercy. Luther's famous statement, "Here I stand and cannot do otherwise," thus not only expresses his personal steadfastness, but also his concept of determinism.[13] Yet, even without the doctrine of the fall of man, an omni-scient and omnipotent God is a problem for the idea of free will. If God knows what a human being will do, and if he has created this being with all its traits, then by God's creation the actions of that being are fixed at the moment it is created: No human being is really free. For many philosophers God's knowledge of what will happen is just as threatening for freedom as scientific determinism is (cf., Fischer 1989, 1994). So what is exactly determinism? Here are some philosophers' explications:[14]

• "Everything in the world happens solely according to the Laws of Nature" (Kant).
• The "metaphysical theory that everything is necessarily as it is and that there are no genuinely open possibilities beyond what actually happens" (Ayers).
• "When we call a result determined, we are implicitly relating it to an antecedent range of possibilities and saying that all but one of these is disallowed" (Anscombe).
• "Determinism, in a nutshell, is a philosophical position which denies the existence of real, that is, causal, alternatives in nature" (von Wright).
• "In the case of everything that exists, there are antecedent conditions, known or unknown, given which that thing could not be other than it is" (Taylor).
• "The thesis that there is at any instant exactly one physically possible future" (van Inwagen).
• "Causal determinism is roughly the claim that everything that occurs at any time is causally necessitated by prior states of the world and the laws of nature" (Watson).
• "The events in the world follow laws in such a way that one state of the system called "world" can be followed by one and only one other state of the same system" (Pothast).
• The "thesis or hypothesis that the real world—understood as the embodiment of spatial-temporal events—is entirely fixed, determined, in its being and its manner of being" (Seebass).
• The "supposition that everything has a cause and can be understood as part of a comprehensive causal network" (Gerent).

What do these conceptions of determinism have in common? For one, they share certain terminology. They all involve concepts of laws of nature, necessity, causality, and causes. A clear deterministic theory should therefore also address those notions. Unfortunately, all these concepts are themselves very problematic.[15] Then again, they express a standard idea. It can be symbolized by the idea of a world line. There is only one thread of events, only one actual way an imaginable course of the world could be. One explication, which is very general but does mirror the intention of determinism concepts as quoted above, is given by Paul Edwards under the entry *philosophic determinism*. "Determinism is the general thesis which states that for everything that ever happens there are conditions such that, given them, nothing else could happen."[16]

Now it is clear why the thesis of determinism is a threat for the concept of alternative actions. If there are conditions for everything that happens that allow for only one possible outcome, then we have no real alternatives. Determinism excludes "free will" in the sense of having "real" or "genuine" alternatives. Of course we can ask: Does determinism matter? Or is it just a threatening *idea*, a conceptual possibility? Is determinism true? To answer these questions let's take Mr. Vorberg's advice and go to the branch of science that has something to say about it: physics.

But first, even scientific determinism (at least philosophers agree on this) is a metaphysical position, because it is a position that can be neither proven nor disproven. But the fact that a position or theory has metaphysical character does not mean that choosing or declining it is arbitrary. Findings of the empirical sciences are indispensable for ontological questions about what is the case. Philosophical theories that contradict research results in practical science cannot be true—as long as the scientific theory is correct. Of course, it is possible that an accepted scientific insight is wrong. Two theories that contradict each other cannot both be right. Where there is contradiction, we must therefore make science and metaphysical theory compatible. This is why we are interested in the question of whether determinism is actually true.

However, with physics it is not as simple as Mr. Vorberg imagines. Science theorists who examine physical determinism emphasize that in order to really understand determinism we would need to construe a comprehensive philosophy of science, one that we at present do not have (Earman 1986). But should the metaphysical character of determinism and lack of an adequate philosophy of science prevent us from tackling the conceptual chaos about physical determinism? Not at all. It is a wellspring of philosophical misunderstanding and we can dissolve some myths of popular science and perhaps even discover suggestions for solutions and novel ideas for the challenge of free will.

2.3.2 Determinism and Predictability   The idea of determinism predominant in philosophy and everyday experience today is still characterized by classical physics. Newton reduced the abundance of phenomena, both macro and micro, to a few laws of nature. With some initial data and knowledge of the laws of nature as Newton formulated them, it became possible to calculate and predict the movements of bodies, whether these be distant planets or items we use everyday. The validity of those laws of nature, understood as eternal and immutable, was projected back into the past as well as forward into the future. On this perspective taken from physics, determinism makes our world into a block world in which everything is fixed and basically predictable. William James summarized this frightening world view as follows:

What does determinism profess? It professes that those parts of the universe already laid down absolutely appoint and decree what the other parts shall be. The future has no ambiguous possibilities hidden in its womb: the part we call the present is compatible with only one totality. Any other future complement than the one fixed from eternity is impossible. The whole is in each and every part, and welds it with the rest into an absolute unity, an iron block, in which there can be no equivocation or shadow of turning. (William James, quote taken from Earman 1986, p. 4f)

James did not distinguish between the fixedness of the past and the future. But from the standpoint of classical physics that would not be necessary anyway. In physics the past and the present differ only in terms of time variables. All developments are, in principle, reversible because natural laws are invariant regarding time. Our knowledge about constraints and initial conditions can be construed for bygone world development as well as predicted for the future progress of the world, at least in principle. This symmetry of time explains why determinism and predictability go hand-in-hand and are sometimes considered two sides of the same coin. Pierre Simon Laplace expressed this classical position using a demon metaphor:

All events, even those which, due to their insignificance do not follow the great laws of nature, are a result of it just as necessarily as the revolutions of the sun.

... Given for one instant an intelligence which could comprehend all the forces by which nature is animated and the respective situation of the beings who compose it—an intelligence sufficiently vast to submit these data to analysis—it would embrace in the same formula the movements of the greatest bodies of the universe and those of the lightest atom; nothing would be uncertain to it and the future, as the past, would be present to its eyes.[17]

The Laplacean demon exhibits at least one property traditionally attributed to gods—namely omniscience. He is not omnipotent, but he does possess the supernatural quality that practical, even theoretical limits of calculation are unknown to him. Laplace's demon has quite a few kin. James Clark Maxwell, for example, who discovered electromagnetic equations, dreamed up a demon capable of violating the second main axiom of thermodynamics. His thought experiment was, nonetheless, heuristically valuable because right up to modern times it served to increase precision in theories of predictability and calculability.[18] Another, secularized descendent of Laplace's demon ancestor is Popper's demon. We can imagine this one to be more like a super scientist than a mystical figure. Popper equated scientific determinism with a thesis of fundamental predictability. Scientific determinism in his words is:

that the state of any closed system at any given future instant of time can be predicted, even from within the system, with any specified degree of precision, by deducing the prediction from theories, in conjunction with initial conditions whose required degree of precision can always be calculated (in accordance with the principle of accountability) if the prediction task is given. (Popper 1982, quote taken from Earman 1986, p. 8)

The fact that of all people one of the founders of modern philosophy of science introduced this thesis with all his authority perhaps partially explains the failure in current discourse to sharply distinguish between determinism and predictability. This is unfortunate, because determinism *does not coincide* with predictability. Even in classical physics, we have unstable systems for which any tiny changes in the initial conditions lead to huge changes in the system's conduct. We can find reasons for why it is not always possible to precisely and sufficiently determine initial conditions. And there are good arguments for denying that it is always possible to make predictions about the future behavior of a system when it is considered in isolation. Also, we do not know whether the real time we need to calculate something is sufficient to make an exact prediction. True, these three arguments do not demonstrate that there could not be such a demon. But what they do show is that predictions of a system's behavior can be impossible, even though that system may be deterministic. One class of such systems is that of chaotic systems, to which we will return later on.

In this context we must introduce a renowned and important distinction erected in the theory of science (cf. Vollmer 1986, p. 178). For different types of questions it is useful to distinguish various levels of inquiry: The *ontological* level (What *is the case*?), the theory of knowledge, or *epistemological* level (What can we *know*?), and the *methodological* level (*How* did we arrive at this knowledge?). For example, we can ask whether Helmut Kohl drank a cup of coffee on January 24, 1967. At the ontological level we ask whether or not he actually did that. This fact is independent of our knowledge about it, our theories about it, and our effort to find out. At an epistemological level we can ask whether we can know anything about the facts and how reliable this knowledge might be. Is personal memory sufficient proof? What criteria do we have for the credibility of a memory? Does the report of an independent witness provide more proof? Why? How reliable are memories in general? Do we have more objective methods, like unmanipulated photographic documentation? At the methodological level pragmatic considerations become important. Which method do we use for ascertaining facts? Which method gets us to our goal the fastest? What is the best method regarding the means available to us?

The same is true for determinism. Whether or not *ontological* determinism is true depends on whether nature herself is fixed—in the past (historical determinism), the future (futuristic determinism), or both (total determinism). *Epistemological determinism* means the fundamental possibility that events of nature can be either retrospectively unequivocally explained (postdictive determinism), or that they can be predicted for the future (predictive determinism), or both (total predictive determinism).[19] The relation between ontological and epistemological determinism is not symmetrical. It is correct, that the ability to scientifically predict everything presupposes determinism. Yet from the validity of determinism we cannot automatically conclude that all events are predictable (cf. also figure 1.2). Therefore, we must clearly distinguish between ontology and epistemology. A verbal distinction is often made between ontological and epistemological determinism. Actually, it would clear up the matter if we only meant ontological indeterminism when using "indeterminism" and used "nonpredictability" when we meant epistemological indeterminism. In the following I will comply with this usage as far as possible and only speak of epistemological indeterminism when it is necessary to do so for historical reasons.

2.3.3   How Deterministic Is Physics?   We cannot tell whether determinism is true or not simply by examining theories in physics. But we can deploy those theories for investigating various conceptions of determinism. Is determinism—judged by any theoretical standpoint in physics—true? We need clear answers for three questions: (1) Is spacetime generally relativistic and do tachyons and singularities exist? (2) Is an undetermined version of quantum mechanics the final word in micro physics or will a deeper theory resecure determinism for the microworld? (3) Can mental phenomena be explained deterministically by a combination of neurophysiology and cybernetics? (Weatherford 1991, p. 191) Chapter 3 answers that question, but for the time being we will primarily address the first two issues. John Earman's definition of determinism is useful for that purpose. Earman published a comprehensive and comprehensible introduction to determinism in physics in 1986. He illustrates determinism using a concept of possible worlds as follows: "Letting W stand for the collection of all physically possible worlds, that is, possible worlds which satisfy the natural laws obtaining in the real world, we can define the Laplacian variety of determinism as follows. The world $W \in W$ is *Laplacian deterministic* just in case for any $W' \in W$, if W and W' agree at any time, then they agree for all times" (Earman 1986, p. 13).

Using this definition, which leans heavily on the notions of determinism previously mentioned, we can examine whether or not prevalent theories in physics are deterministic. We normally identify the deterministic concept of the world with Newton's physics. This equation, however, is surprisingly false. Why? Because Newton did not exclude the *possibility of arbitrarily fast signals*. An example will demonstrate this. In Newton's physics determinism is valid forward and backward due to the symmetry of time. Also, in Newton's physics a particle can be accelerated to any speed. Although it cannot attain an infinite velocity, no matter how great the value of a particle's finite rapidity may be within a certain inertial system, it is always possible to construe another inertial system within which the velocity value is as great as we want. If we consider particles with finite, albeit unlimited, momentum, we find that a particle can be accelerated until it asymptotically approaches an infinite velocity and disappears in infinite space, despite finite rapidity (Earman 1986, p. 34f). If we introduce time symmetry we can observe this process in reverse. We try to ascertain the state of the universe at time t_1 with the complete knowledge we have of the state of the universe at time t_3. At time t_2 there is no trace of the particle. At time t_1 it would suddenly emerge "from nowhere." Not only would this emergence be unexpected; it would also not be determined by the state of the universe at time t_3.

Specific relativity theory (SRT) does not have this problem. Newton's absolute concept of space is replaced by the so-called Minkowski space-time cone. In SRT energy-mass movements can be faster than light. The speed of light is the absolute (and finite) limit for the velocity of particles. That is why for any chosen space-time point there is a space-time cone that includes all the space-time points of the expanding universe that can exchange signals with the selected space-time point. This restriction allows our first formulation of a truly deterministic theory. Paradoxically, then, there was no "threat" to freedom by any determinism in physics until everyday notions and philosophical discussion conjured it up. However, even in SRT determinism does not *always* hold. One of the most important arguments contra mass-energy, which can move faster than the speed of light is the fact that an infinite amount of energy is needed to accelerate mass-energy faster than the speed of light. This problem can be avoided by postulating particles that do not need to be accelerated because they have already always been that fast! The existence of such relativistic super-fast particles—tachyons—cannot be debarred by SRT. They could develop causal effects, if Minkowski's space-time cone is designed permeable, which is theoretically possible. There is, albeit, no evidence of the existence of tachyons, but we can maintain that if they were to exist, then we would have no guarantee of determinism even in SRT.[20] So once again, present theories do not offer us determinism. The notion of determinism is, rather, a test for whether the theory in question is valid or needs to be amended. Indeterminism is at least possible.

The question of global determinism in general relativity theory (GRT) is complex. The way Earman discusses this issue (Earman 1986, pp. 170–198) demonstrates nicely what the idea of a test (employing the concept of determinism) is supposed to mean. If we want to know whether determinism is true we can inquire which constraints in GRT must be satisfied to make it true. For example, if within the class of cosmological GRT models we accept those that contain noncausality or paradoxes such as time-traveling, determinism is lost (Earman 1986, p. 175f). In contrast, certain suppositions can prevent determinism from being introduced in GRTs solely as a premise.[21] Earman also asks whether *local* determinism is possible within GRT. The answer is yes— as long as it can be shown that it holds for space-time sectors of any small size. In using certain other presuppositions, however, both local and global determinism are at risk. While for SRT the tachyons ruined the victory for determinism, in GRT the existence of singularities does the same. For our purpose it suffices to imagine a singularity as a black hole. A black hole pulls in with gravity everything surrounding it with an irresistible force. It destroys not only matter, but also space-time itself.[22] We do not know whether such singularities really exist. If they did, they would not automatically prove that determinism is false. But it would no longer be *guaranteed* that it is correct. The issue of determinism's validity in GRT is thus difficult, since the answer depends on whether or not we accept certain assumptions. Determinism serves a regulative purpose for physicists: It motivates them to test physics' theories and improve them, in order to formulate them in terms of determinism.

Quantum theory is the most interesting form of physical indeterminism, and the one most often discussed in connection with free will. Here lurks the first real threat to determinism. In quantum mechanics it appears that we have absolute contingency. Quantum events are absolutely contingent if they are not determined by a previous state of the world. Using Earman's terminology for determinism, two worlds W and W' are imaginable, that are identical at time t_5, but no longer identical at t_6. A favorite example for such an absolutely contingent event is the deterioration of a radioactive nucleus. But we have to take a closer look if we want to understand what indeterminism in quantum theory really is.

Quantum theory seems to involve many contra-intuitive, unintelligible, and mysterious consequences such as: An electron is simultaneously a particle and a wave (wave-particle dualism); registering a particle in one place can alter the state of another particle at any distance without information transfer in the normal sense (Einstein-Podolsky-Rosen paradox); Schrödinger's cat can be in a state in which it is, in a way, neither dead nor alive; there are infinitely many parallel universes, existing next to each other (Everett's plural world interpretation), and so on. In contrast, Heisenberg's famous uncertainty principle (position and momentum of a particle cannot be simultaneously measured accurately) appears almost harmless. (A brief description of such "perplexities" is given in Davies and Brown 1988). At this point, however, we want to know: How and where does quantum theory include indeterminism? I have taken the following description from Penrose (1991, 1995).

Quantum theory arose in the 1920s and is founded on the Schrödinger equation. This equation corresponds to Newton's second axiom in classical mechanics and describes how a system develops under the influence of outside forces with given initial conditions. We often hear that we can only specify the location of an electron with a certain degree of probability and that this is the source of quantum physical indeterminism. But this idea is misleading. Contrary to the widely held misconception there are no undetermined quantum events. The processes at the quantum level itself are highly determined.

How can this be? Observe the quantum mechanics description of the state of an electron. In quantum theory the electron is described by the totality of its states at position A and position B. (For simplicity let's assume only two positions.) The description of those states is weighted by certain factors (w and z). These do not, as is sometimes claimed in popular explanations, indicate the *probability* of where the electron is:

w and *z* are *complex* numbers, so such an interpretation makes no sense at all. The ratios of the quantum weightings *w* and *z* are *not* ratios of probabilities. They cannot be since probabilities always have to be *real* numbers. It is *not* Cardano's *probability* theory that operates at the quantum level, despite the common opinion that the quantum world is a probabilistic world. Instead, it is his mysterious theory of *complex numbers* that underlies a mathematically precise and *probability-free* description of the quantum level of activity. We cannot say, in familiar everyday terms, what it "means" for an electron to be in a state of superposition of two places at once, with complex-number weighting factors *w* and *z*. We must, for the moment, simply accept that this is indeed the kind of description that we have to adopt for quantum-level systems. Such superpositions constitute an important part of the actual construction of our microworld, as has now been revealed to us by Nature. It is just a *fact* that we appear to find that the quantum-level world *actually* behaves in this unfamiliar and mysterious way. The descriptions are perfectly clear cut—and they provide us with a micro-world that evolves according to a description that is indeed mathematically precise and, moreover, *completely deterministic*! (Penrose 1994: 258f)

But when can we correctly speak of probable events (and count on them)? Whenever we progress from the micro-physical quantum level to the level of macro-physical events which can be described using traditional physical theories:

The element of probability, which we commonly associate with quantum mechanics, comes about when you magnify the quantum event up to a classical level for observation and measurement. That is to say, the element of randomness occurs in the transition between the upper and lower boxes of the diagram [see figure 1.1], and is indicated there by the letter *R*. It is described as the "collapse of the wave function" or "reduction of the state-vector." Whenever quantum events are magnified to a macroscopic scale we must, on conventional theory, use this procedure, and one has merely a probabilisitc description. (Penrose 1994, p. 246)

The transition *R*, according to Penrose, is the true mystery of quantum mechanics. Mathematically this is evident in the fact that we work with complex numbers at level *U* and not until level *R* (by generating absolute squares and quantum amplitudes) can we speak of probabilities. Opinions differ on how to interpret *R*. The so-called Copenhagen interpretation, which essentially originated with Niels Bohr, claims that it is the subjective consciousness involved in the measurement process that mysteriously causes a reduction of the state vector. Einstein, on the other hand, was convinced that quantum theory must be incomplete just

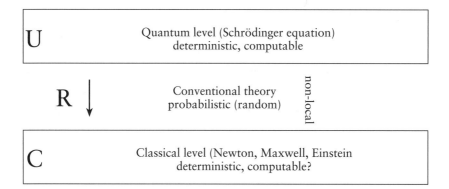

Figure 1.1
The reduction of the state vector. The figure illustrates a physical system's transition from quantum description (U: unitary development) to "classical" description (C) via reduction of the state vector. From Penrose (1994: p. 246).

because of its lack of determinism. His famous statement "God does not throw dice," meant to express that there must be "hidden variables" in physical reality which deterministically explain "absolute chance."[23] Penrose rejects both interpretations and is convinced that a theory can be produced that objectively explains the reduction. His suggestion for this theory is the theory of quantum gravitation. We need not deal with this theory in detail at the moment, since it has been only vaguely worked out and only exists as a program. But we will return to it.

At this point, keep in mind that there is no generally accepted interpretation of quantum theory—even the experts are in dispute. It does not help much to appeal to quantum theory's founding father Niels Bohr, nor to the genius Einstein, nor to the acclaimed physicist Penrose to defend the "true" or "really correct" interpretation of it. Appeal to authorities happens often enough, but it is not an argument. Scientifically, the serious possibility of indeterminism is at least given and it seems to leave room for "being able to do otherwise." Quite a few theorists have attempted to localize free will just there (cf. section 2.1 in chapter 2). Before turning to the second component, let us discuss the point in time when an undetermined event happens and how that is relevant for a theory about free will.

2.4   At Which Point in Time Does Indeterminism Occur?

If being able to do otherwise means doing otherwise under identical Laws of Nature and under identical constraints and initial conditions, then determinism does exclude free will. This seems to imply that a voluntary act, choice, or decision must contain an indeterministic element, which is effective *at the time* of the act, choice, or decision.

Some authors think that indeterminism must not necessarily be effective at the time of the act, but prior to it, inasmuch as it contributed to the decision in a relevant way. An automobilist who causes a fatal accident due to speeding and disregard for sufficient safety distance is not free to prevent the accident at the very moment it happens. But prior to the collision he was free to drive slower and more considerately. An action may be completely determined by the character of the agent and the circumstances; but his character may have been shaped during antecedent incidents of being able to do otherwise. In this way a current determined act can be voluntary. Double calls such theories of freedom *delay libertarianism* or valerian theories. Traditional (non-valerian) libertarian theories, in contrast, postulate the undetermined element at the moment of decision. The distinction "valerian vs. non-valerian" was introduced by Dennett (1981: 297). It refers to a quote of the poet Paul Valery, who said "Invention is the intelligent selection from among randomly generated candidates."[24] The notion of selection will become important later on.

In Plato's writings we find a valerian theory, for example (Plato, 1990, Book 4, Politeia, 10, 617–621), presented as a myth. A reborn soldier tells how he acquired his present self. Each soul is presented a selection of lives before it is reborn. These lives are prototype characters called *daimons*. One has the choice among such illustrious items as the *daimon* of a tyrant, a wealthy man, a beautiful woman, a lion, or a swan. Each of these characters has predetermined characteristics, certain mixtures of physical strength and intelligence, and other vital conditions, such as degrees of health and illness, wealth or poverty. Each soul selects a *daimon* for its future existence. They are free in this choice. But once the decision has been made it is tied to the spiral of necessity. The *daimon* of the future person is fixed. Future acts are only voluntary inasmuch as they are due to the original free choice. Plato is valerian! Of course, here the problem has only been shifted. Shifted not in the decision hierarchy—as in the case of the conditional solution discussed earlier (cf. section 2.2)—but in time. What does it mean to *freely* select a *daimon*? Once again, the question arises: Did the soul really have an alternative at that time or was it not possible to make any other selection than the one which it did make? Careful observation discloses that the soul's very act of selecting was itself determined. For the choice of a particular daimon is determined by the knowledge of the available characters (the circumstances) and the way the soul lived in previous incarnations. We can always raise the question of being able to do otherwise in an indeterministic sense.[25] If it doesn't turn up at a lower level in the hierarchy of wishes, it will show up at a higher level. If it doesn't manifest itself at the time of action, it was there prior to the act.

An indeterministic possibility of alternative action may be a necessary prerequisite for free will, but it is certainly not sufficient. If indeterminism is true, perhaps even an amoeba can behave other than it does, but we do not attribute free will to it. Which special characteristics distinguish being able to do otherwise within the context of free will? We will discuss this question in the next section.

3   Intelligible Volition

3.1   Volition and Intentionality

I planned each charted course, each careful step, along the byway.
—Frank Sinatra

At first it seems so easy to approach the question of free will; we just need to contemplate what the will is and then examine whether or not it is free. So, what is the will? Surprisingly enough, the concept of the will plays no part at all in many discussions about free will. My guess is that the main reason for this lies in the fact that the concept of the will is either dispensable or replaceable in practically all important arguments for or against free will. As Jürgen Mittelstrass noted in an essay called "*Der arme Wille*" ("The Poor Will," 1987), in philosophy there is no conceptually uniform usage of the term "will." This can be seen by the fact—among others—that despite its profuse history, the term no longer even appears in leading philosophical dictionaries! Wolfgang Gerent (1993, p. 238ff) researched the usage of the term "voluntarily" and discovered fifteen different uses. Instead of reviewing the myriad of historical examples available for the concept of the will, I will explain the concept of will in the way it will be used in this book.[26]

Kane (1985, 1996, pp. 21–31) distinguishes three forms of the will, which are easiest to introduce by considering the various meanings of the expression "I can do what I want to do." In this phrase "what I want to do" can mean:

(i) what I *want*, *desire* or *prefer* to do,
(ii) what I *choose*, *decide*, or *intend* to do, or
(iii) what I *try*, *endeavor*, or make an *effort* to do.

The first form of wanting is *simple wishing*. It refers to what one would like to do or what one has a tendency to do. It is sometimes also called *appetetive will*. The second form of will is the *rational will*. The rational will has to do with practical reasoning. It includes skills such as deliberating, thinking practically, choosing and deciding, making practical judgments, developing intents and purposes, critically examining reasons for actions, and so on. The third kind of will has been named the *striving will* by O'Shaughnessy (1980). It refers to an effort to do something. This kind of will is important for the concept of the weak will: The will's effort is not strong enough to achieve what is desired.

According to Kane (1996, p. 27) all three forms play a role in the problem of free will: In practical reasoning, says Kane, we can consider our desires (motives and reasons) as the input in decision processes. The decision itself is the result (output) of practical contemplation. Effort, or voluntary striving, is somewhere in between. Is there anything that unites all three forms of the will? Yes, namely being oriented or having a propensity for something objective or a goal (Gr.: *telos*), which is desired (will type 1), chosen (will type 2), or attempted (will type 3), respectively. "In other words, the idea of will is essentially teleological, and different senses of *will* and *willing* represent different ways in which agents may be directed toward or tend towards *ends* or *purposes*" (Kane

1996, p. 27). Seebass thinks similarly: "Human striving displays . . . a character of intentional-teleological, motivationally effective *wishing* and *wanting*" (Seebass 1993, p. 225).

In an initial approximation voluntariness can be considered equal to "being actively directed toward a goal." For in our actions we are not passively aimed like a gun, we are not passively straightened like a table-cloth. Being directed towards a goal, rather, guides our actions. Voluntariness shares that aspect of being aimed with two other closely related concepts: those of *intention* and *intentionality*. To do something *intentionally* is often used to mean the same as "to do something voluntarily." "Intentionality" is a philosophical term that originated in medieval literature, where it meant reference to mental objects or operations. At the end of the nineteenth Century it was taken up by the psychologist and philosopher Franz Brentano, who used it to denote the peculiarity of mental states in comparison with physical states (intentionality as a *mark of the mental*). Since then it has played a significant role in continental phenomenology as well as in analytic *philosophy of mind*.[27] To have intentionality means that a mental state is directed toward something. What it is aimed at, is its semantic content.

We see, then, that voluntariness, intention, and intentionality are interconnected. Today the primary topic of discussion is intentionality, while the matter of what comprises the will, is considered secondary. In the following, I concentrate on the phenomenon of directedness, that is, the phenomenon of intentionality. In chapter 3 I will lay out the foundation for a neurophilosophical theory of voluntariness, in which I develop a theory about how a neural, that is, a physical state can exhibit intentionality. That also provides a concept of intention. The type of will emphasized is—borrowing a little from Kane—the rational will: choosing and deciding.

3.2 Intelligibility and Reasons

In order to command free will we must be able to do otherwise. But usually we want more. We don't want blind, random, reflex-guided or animalistic choices we prefer "the power to decide our courses of action, and to decide them wisely, in the light of our expectations and desires" (Dennett 1984, p. 169).

Possessing this power is logically dependent on being able to do otherwise. In philosophy, "reason" traditionally was considered a sufficient condition, even a guarantee for free will. "Reason is the root, the fountain, the origin of true liberty, which judgeth and representeth to the will, whether this or that be convenient, whether this or that be more convenient" (Hobbes, *Works*, Vol. V, p. 40).[28]

The concept of "reason" is notoriously multifaceted. From the Ancient Greeks (*lógos, nous*) right up to Hegel (world spirit), reason has been viewed as a cosmological metaphysical principle. Medieval philosophers were more likely to equate reason (*ratio*) with conceptually analytic and discursive thinking. Kant finally severed pure (nonperceptual) reason from reason understood in terms of psychology. If we attempt to clarify the somewhat vague notion of reason by distinguishing it from related notions such as voluntariness, contemplation, rationality, reflection, or intention, we find it very difficult to draw exact boundaries. Kant, for example, considered reason and the will to be junctional: "Only a being with reason has the power or a will to act according as laws prescribe, i.e. to act according to principles. Since we need reason to derive our actions from laws, the will is nothing other than practical reason" (Kant 1786/1983, BAA 36).

As I mentioned before, in philosophy itself the notion of the will has become unpopular. In action theory, for example, you won't find anything like "reasonable volition." The issue, however, is occasionally discussed under the heading "reasons vs. causes." It is said that actions are characterized by the fact that they are determined by reasons (acting *for* reasons, cf. Audi 1986). This prerogative is usually viewed as a specifically human skill, an ability, it is said, that cannot be explained naturalistically. In the philosophy of mind it is said that intentional states (desires, opinions, intentions) cause an action (*intentional causation*). All these mentioned and quoted conceptions consider a *special reference to something that is to be realized* as the common essential characteristic for voluntary actions; it causes the agent to do what he does. We need a *terminus technicus* that not only portrays what is meant, but also is not so overly colloquial that it arouses misleading associations. I have selected the term "intelligibility" (capable of being understood, inducible to insight) for this purpose. In section 1.3, I initially characterized intelligibility as "acting for understandable reasons." We now need a fuller account. In order to make an intelligible decision a person must at least partially know the reasons for her actions. She should also know that there are alternatives and that she has a choice. When making a decision she should take the consequences of her decision into consideration in some way (anticipation). This results in the following definition:

A person acts (wants, decides, chooses) intelligibly, if she at least partially mentally represents alternatives and their possible consequences, apprehends their meanings, and using this knowledge actively realizes one of the alternatives for reasons which are—in principle—inducible to insight.

"Intelligibility" is an appropriate term in several respects. First of all, in the debate about free will itself, it plays a role cloaked as the "intelligibility argument." Second, using it I can avoid the consciousness terminology, which is sometimes introduced at this point of the discussion, but which I feel is too murky, ambiguous, and tainted to serve as a *terminus technicus*.[29] Third, this term conveys an active as well as a passive aspect. The process is active, inasmuch as the reasons must be understandable to the subject herself for an act executed in this way is to be intelligible. It is passive inasmuch as intelligible action must be—at least theoretically—understandable (i.e., the reasoning can be followed) to other rational beings. This introduces a normative aspect into the concept of intelligibility. Fourth and finally, in Kant's tradition "intelligibility" is understood as something that is not accessible empirically. It is something that belongs to another world, to which man must believe himself to belong, by using reason. Some nondualistic philosophers also characterize reason as something that cannot be naturalized (cf. Putnam 1982). However, I do not consider such antinaturalistic connotation to be an insurmountable difficulty for an empirically founded theory of intelligibility. On the contrary, we are faced with the challenge of finding a naturalistic, neurophilosophical alternative.

It is notoriously trivial that people are able to act *for* reasons. We go to the cinema because we want to see the movie *Free Willy*. After giving it a lot of thought, we phone a friend because we hope that he can give us advice for making a decision. Although we urgently desire to read the news, we do not go to the newsstand and purchase a paper because we know that once there, we cannot resist also buying a bag of potato chips.

But the idea that actions are determined by reasons (psychological determinism) is evidently not compatible with an indeterministic interpretation of being able to do otherwise.

Imagine the German citizen Hans Michel, who does not belong to any political party, and his behavior shortly before an election for parliament. Guided by his prejudices he tends to vote for one of two moderate parties, all the rest he finds revolting. He is more or less politically disinterested, a typical undecided voter. But this time he has resolved to make a well-founded choice. He peruses the parties' programs, collects information about the current political scene from daily newspapers in his local library, and asks himself which party is the better choice. He carefully weighs arguments pro and con for the SPD (German Social Democratic Party) and the CDU (Christian Democratic Union)—the two popular people's parties in Germany—and after thorough contemplation arrives at a well-founded decision. Since the vote is secret, we do not know what he chooses. But since he almost always acts in accordance with his convictions, we can be pretty sure that he selected one of the two major and large people's parties. Yet we can still say for this choice, if the choice was made of his own free will—as in a libertarian world— then his reasons cannot necessarily have determined his choice. Because he could also have voted other than the way he actually did. In nonvalerian libertarian theory this could be guaranteed by an indeterministic process, which let his decision drift in one or the other direction at the moment of voting. But if the indeterministic aspect was truly the *decisive* factor, then it was neither his carefully weighed arguments, nor his political preferences, nor his enduring pet sympathy nor disgust for any particular politician, nor his hopes for a better future that were decisive for his vote. An undetermined choice is therefore not intelligible (not understandable, not open to insight); it is arbitrary, random, irrational, unexplainable. So runs the *intelligibility argument* happily employed by compatibilists and determinists. I will return to it later (cf. 6.2 in this chapter and 2.5.2 in chapter 3).

At this point I would like to note the following: The argument relies on thinking of reasons as entirely ordinary causes (this is a causal view of action).[30] Reasons cause actions. An *anticausal concept of action* denies that reasons *are* special causes. Neither the intentionality of behavior, nor intentional explanations—so this thesis claims—require a causal condition. Explanation by reasons does not give us causes, it only places an action within a system of rules and practices and thus makes it comprehensible.[31] The idea is that if we do not take or mistake reasons for causes, we would not be in the predicament of having to postulate reasons as determinant causes. There are well-known objections to this view;[32] but most important: It makes reasons causally ineffective. For the intentional causes which are attributed as reasons play no role in behavior.

In summary, our idea of free will not only contains the notion of being able to do otherwise, but also a belief that our voluntary (goal-oriented) actions and decisions occur for understandable reasons. I call this characteristic of free will *intelligibility*. In order to evaluate the intelligibility argument we need a theory about how reasons are causally effective for our actions. And this itself presupposes a theory of intentionality.

4 Agency and Its Consequences

4.1 Agency and Moral Responsibility

It looks like we have covered almost all essential constituents of free will. We have intelligible action, which could also have been different. What more can we demand of voluntary acts? Agency. Agency is the idea that our actions and decisions are *ours*. We are their author, their source, their origin. Libertarians think that this is only possible when this provenance is not embedded in the causal order of the rest of the world. Thus for Kant free will means that a person himself can initiate a causal chain, and that he can set up his highest principles himself. Chisholm speaks similarly when he calls man an unmoved mover. But even determinists and compatibilists use terms that involve this element of agency (Seebass 1992): *origination* (Honderich 1990a), *self-determination* (Watson 1987), *self-mastery* (Lindley 1986), and genuine *self-determination* (Gerent 1993). The metaphor of beginning a new causal chain best illustrates the intuition of agency. In the German edition of a book by Honderich (1995), Joachim Schulte translates origination pertinently using the term *initial cause (Erstauslöser)*. Even if the notion of agency is included in the idea of open alternatives (being able to do otherwise), the two are, nevertheless, logically independent. If a person were able to begin a causal chain by himself, we could view him as an initial cause. But this does not necessarily imply that this person could have begun a causal chain other than the one he actually initiated!

I find the severance of alternativism from agency particularly important, because agency is more significant for the issue of moral responsibility than is generally recognized. (Compatibilists seem most ready to accept this.) The following thought experiment illustrates the matter.

Imagine that we could construct a robot that utilizes the indeterministic nature of quantum theory *and* simultaneously has the power to make intelligible decisions. Call him Martin. Does Martin command a free will? If the freedom of will consisted solely of these two components, we would have to say yes. But intuitions on this issue certainly vary; many people would totally deny it. What reasons support the opinion that Martin does not command a genuinely free will? The answer coheres to agency and the notion of moral responsibility. Is Martin morally responsible for his movements? No, for the robot's "character" was not contrived by the robot itself; it was produced by us. The robot itself is not responsible for its own design. But is this a good argument? Neither did we create ourselves, and yet we are responsible. Aren't we? The situation is quite ambiguous. If our souls were created by God and free will is a trait of the souls that were given to us, we would still be able to make decisions freely, but would we—in the end—still be responsible for those decisions? If we attribute the three classic powers to God—omnipotence, omniscience, and infinite goodness—the issue gets even more complicated. For then He can foresee what will happen and it would be in His power to cause or prevent certain events.[33]

Perhaps Martin, despite his origins, is responsible after all, since he does satisfy the first two components according to our premises. Let us imagine that after he has become accustomed to us and proves to be a valuable member of our society we return Martin to the laboratory. Out of pure curiosity in experimental philosophy we slightly alter his wiring. This tampering does not change his exploitation of the indeterministic nature of quantum theory nor his ability for contemplation. But let us say it makes him a criminal robot. Would we still think he bears responsibility? This decision is even more difficult, for it was not his fault that we tinkered with his wiring. The percentage of readers who would now not hold him responsible has presumably increased.

At this point our intuitions appear to be inconsistent. We could object and claim that this intuitive dilemma is due to a trick! Either the alterations we made were so insignificant that through his own strength the robot will soon revert to a good guy. In that case the manipulation was merely a disturbance. Or, the changes were so massive *that he cannot do otherwise*, and he is doomed to be a criminal little machine. If this is the case, then naturally he is no longer responsible. But then the alterations have been so extreme that he no longer commands a free will. According to the definition, something must be different about the abilities that were described in the first two components, despite the assumed claim that tampering with the robot's wiring did not influence those abilities. Obviously, we can no longer give him credit nor blame him for being good or bad. He is no longer the originator of his machine acts.

Is this objection plausible? We don't really need the robot example to discuss this. Aren't there also people who have undergone changes that have made them criminal? These need not be laboratory manipulations; they could be traumatizing actions, methods of upbringing, or other influences people experience while maturing. True, we normally assume that a person with intact mental capacities is the originator of his actions and thus morally fully responsible, independently of what has occurred in his past and independently of how he has become what he now is. But this assumption is not without controversy.

Martha Klein (1990), for example, defends an interesting thesis for explaining why—despite determinism—we still consider some persons—due to their pasts—to be less responsible than others. Her *payment in advance* thesis states that socially deprived persons should not be held responsible to the same extent as persons who grew up in happier circumstances, because the disadvantaged group has already suffered for its deeds in advance.

For many philosophers, however, free will and responsibility are so interwoven that they consider free will a topic for moral philosophy, rather than one for theoretical philosophy. It is perhaps for this reason that discussions about free will easily slip into what I call *the Palmström argument*: "It just cannot be true, that we do not have a free will. Thus, we have a free will." Naturally, this is not a conclusive argument (cf. 6.5). Nevertheless, it is an effective strategy to devise a nihilistic scenario in order to motivate others to believe in free will. But is it really true that without free will ethics is impossible? This seems to be implied by the general conviction that we can only demand moral behavior from one another when that is actually achievable. In Kant's words: "For if moral law commands us to be better people: it follows inevitably that we must also be capable of it" (Kant 1794/1983).

Stated in a well-known and salient phrase: Ought implies can! (Moral responsibility presupposes free will.) Reciprocally, it appears to follow that if people cannot satisfy moral demands—due to their lack of free will—it is unjust to make those demands.[34] In short, there is no morality without free will. Now this is a rather disturbing thought. Fearing dire consequences, many people find it absurd to claim that there is no moral responsibility. How troubling or bizarre is this notion really? Contrary to the nihilistic scenario of some libertarians, the nonexistence of free will by no means implies that the principle of responsibility breaks down entirely or must be abandoned. Even if there should not exist free will in the strong sense, we should not ignore that fact. We should be realistic concerning human capabilities, instead of assuming that our fellow men command a power that they do not, and instead of expecting from them something that they cannot achieve. Our answer to the question of whether free will exists has consequences for many of our socially anchored notions. To illustrate this I shall use an example from German penal law.[35]

4.2   Punishment, Guilt, and Attribution

Why do we punish people? Our penal law appears to have answered this question in line with a libertarian standpoint. The following was established in a frequently quoted fundamental ruling by the German Federal Court of Justice:

Punishment presumes guilt. Guilt is the object of reproach. By judging the guilt unworthy, we reprimand the agent that he did not behave according to the law, we rebuke him for deciding to act unlawfully, although he could have behaved lawfully, he could have decided to do what is right. The deeper reason for admonishing guilt is that man is free, responsible, and self-determined and thus capable of choosing what is lawful and rejecting what is unlawful.[36]

For what do we rebuke the "guilty" person? We blame him that he decided to do what is unlawful, although he could have chosen to do what is right. He had alternatives. But that is not all. The decision to do a morally reproachable alternative, the decision to violate the law, was his own. This is the component of agency on which personal accountability is founded. We can consider this concept of guilt a combination of the first and third components.

What if this sort of guilt concept turns out to be an illusion? We would have to change our penal law. But it would not necessarily collapse. Many active determinists have argued for a deterministic penal law.[37] For them responsibility is identical to the susceptibility to influence future behavior. Punishment is seen as a means to influence behavior in the future—more precisely, a means of prevention. Particular prevention is the attempt to hinder an individual culprit from committing a new crime; general prevention is the strategy of deterring all potential culprits from committing crimes by threatening to punish. Punishment is no longer considered a retaliation for guilt, but rather a kind of therapy. People who offend social norms should be prevented from doing so again. Naturally, penal law of this kind has its challenges. One problem is what to do with criminals who knowingly exploit this attitude. Repetitive criminals for whom preventive measures exhibit little prospect of success are another problem. Finally, a third issue is how to deal with the very common desire for retaliation.[38]

Interestingly enough, the actual practice of our legal system is not founded on a strong version of free will in the sense dictated by the Federal Court of Justice. In practice it is not philosophers of law who must decide on whether to attribute responsibility or not; it is done by judges and psychiatrists. Glancing into a widely used textbook for forensic psychiatry (court psychiatry) we find that in spite of all the philosophical debate obviously a kind of "pure retaliation-oriented penal law finds no support today" (Schreiber 1994; p. 5). Can we reconcile this with the concept of justice quoted above? What is guilt?

Penal guilt means subjective accountability for unlawful behavior. It cannot be understood as misuse of free choice in an indeterministic sense, but rather—based on experience—understood pragmatically as falling short of the standard for behavior that can be expected of a citizen under normal circumstances; it is the misuse of an ability which we attribute to each other for daily purposes in our individual and social life. A concept of guilt like this remains below the unsolvable alternative of determinism and indeterminism. . . . It does not assume a free will, which is always inaccessible for individual assessments in penal procedures, it presumes solely a normal ascertainment of behavior via social norms (Schreiber 1994, p. 10).

This advances a *normative* notion. A person is guilty when he falls short of a commonly *expected* standard of behavior. Two essential criteria for evaluating this are the capacity for insight and an ability to control (Venzlaff 1994, p. 107). The capacity for insight corresponds to the component called intelligibility; the ability to control is the topic of many compatibilistic expositions on the free will.[39] The quoted forensic view dispenses with a strong concept of guilt. However, it does maintain an element of personal accountability: We must "remember that individual behavior cannot be attributed solely to a social system, but also to an individual." We "need behavioral control via social norms. To achieve this . . . sanctions are necessary. These sanctions can only be executed when we have subjective accountability combined with the behavior of the individual and his related responsibility" (Schreiber 1994, p. 7).

Here we no longer have the claim that an agent could have acted otherwise. The claim here is only that an individual has fallen short of a standard and his behavior is attributed to him personally because this makes sanctions effective. Attributing responsibility is a social strategy for getting people to behave according to standards. The lesson to be learned here is that penal justice without reference to a strong version of free will is not only feasible, it is at least theoretically already partially accepted. Thus the contention that there is no moral responsibility in a Libertarian sense of the word is not absurd. It is correct, however, that the concept of responsibility undergoes a change if it shall be maintained. This is also true for other concepts related to agency.

4.3   Agency: Implications of Determinism

It is often overlooked that the issue of moral responsibility is only a part of what we mean by personal accountability. Matters of approval and disapproval, of offense and benevolence, of pride and shame, and much more, also accompany the term. Strawson (1962) analyzes accountable reactions as the totality of personal and moral sentiments. He divides the theorists into two camps: the optimists, who believe that the lack of pressure itself justifies accountable reactions, and the pessimists, who hold that they are only possible under conditions of contra-causal freedom. Strawson tries to mediate by leading both parties toward an acknowledgment. The optimist should admit that his theory is faulty, the pessimist should forego the conditions of contra-causal freedom. According to Strawson, accountable reactions are part of human dignity and are, to some degree, a transcendental condition for interpersonal relations. They belong to a system of attitudes and reactions that is neither readily debatable nor disposable.

Personal accountability is intertwined with the notion of agency. According to Pothast, accountable reactions are distinguished by seven characteristics: They contain a personal element that is tainted by affect and includes approval or disapproval and an evaluation of the agent. The acceptance or rejection of that person based on that evaluation leads to manifest behavior and is accompanied by the feeling that the evaluation attributed to the person is justified (Pothast 1980, pp. 370–79). This would include, for example, disdain for a traitor, pride about an achievement, recognition for enduring sacrifice, and much more. We cannot only have accountable reactions to others, but also toward ourselves.

The consequences of determinism for personal and moral sentiments have been most impressively and comprehensively demonstrated by the determinist Ted Honderich (1990a, 1995, cf. Weatherford 1991). Admittedly, Honderich does not distinguish three components of free will; but in his study he does explicitly deal with the notion of agency as *origination*, which is not compatible with determinism. He mentions seven areas that are significant for the truth of determinism: Life hopes, nonmoral personal sentiments, the concept of knowledge, moral responsibility, the moral quality of persons, moral praise and reproof, as well as social institutions, practices, traditions, particularly punishment, and finally upbringing and politics.[40] While philosophers are primarily occupied with the question of moral responsibility, it is life's hopes that are directly relevant for each of us. So I would like to take a closer look at them instead of the other areas.

Among our life's hopes we find the notion that we can achieve something within our lifetime. Normally, we are convinced that *it is up to us* to really achieve it. We are the real originators and planners of our lives only if we do not let them be determined solely by heredity, chance, assistance, or other lucky circumstances, but when we build their essential elements out of *our own strength*. Once we have reached our goals *by ourselves*, we are proud. We attribute success to ourselves personally, and lack of success counts as personal failure. We can only be justifiably proud or ashamed of ourselves if what happened was within our power, when our actions originate in ourselves and are not caused by circumstances cannot control—because, for example, they happened before we were born. We must be the initiators of our own actions so that we can justifiably attribute them to ourselves. But if determinism is true, if there is only one path the development of the world can take and everything necessarily results from previous events, then our actions are mere consequences of events that took place before we were born, and we are not responsible for those. At least this is the argument of the strict determinist. Assuming that determinism is true: What can we still hope for our lives?

A life hope consists first of all of the content, *what* it is that we desire, and second, of the ideas and hopes about *how* we achieve it. Honderich distinguishes two kinds of life hopes. The first consists of viewing the future as open. Depending on one's decisions, the future will be one way or another. What happens is up to oneself. We have the power; the future is undecided, a garden of many paths (Borges). This is the notion, the kind of hope that we must deny if determinism is true. Most people react to this with dismay. But is it a reason to give up all life hope? No. One may continue to hope that one achieves one's goals; not through pure chance, but in a certain way. With determinism one cannot continue to claim that one is the true, real, genuine originator of one's actions. But one can continue to hope that one achieves one's goals not through blind luck, but *according to one's efforts and skills*. One can hope to arrive at one's goals in the way one desires and hope that one's own life story has a causal course that meets up to one's own wishes and ideas. Life hopes of this second kind are by all means compatible with determinism. When we understand this, perhaps we no longer react with *dismay* to the idea that determinism could be true, but with *intransigence*. We need not despair. Even without free will, life hopes of the second kind can be fulfilled. But something is lost. The proud claim, "It's more, it's more than this, I did it my way," is a farce.[41]

We can develop the attitudes of dismay and intransigence in all seven areas of life that Honderich mentions. When we realize that even our personal feelings such as affection, loyalty, recognition, love and rejection, indignation, contempt, and hate are consequences of world circumstances, we will initially react shocked. We have to drop the metaphor of agency as origination if we are to develop an appropriate attitude. Even in a deterministic universe nothing can stop us from enjoying certain things or suffering for certain reasons, even when we are convinced that these feelings do not rest on the fact that someone is his own cause or the cause of his actions. But the same is true here: Something is lost, something must be lost.

Based on this approach Honderich makes a suggestion for how we can achieve a psychologically adequate attitude toward the truth of determinism. The solution consists of developing a secondary reaction of a kind of affirmative answer to determinism as a reaction to the primary feeling of dismay and intransigence. This solution is motivated by the fact that in everyday life, psychologically we cannot help reacting with dismay to the possibility of determinism, because in daily life we apparently presuppose free will. However, Honderich does not claim that this affirmative attitude is freedom. He also does not claim that it is possible to develop this attitude at all times, for this itself would presuppose freedom to do so. He only shows that it would be an appropriate attitude not to entirely discard our views about the abovementioned areas, but to *revise* them if we want to remain consistent while assuming determinism. In chapter 3 I intend to show how neurophilosophy can contribute to an explanation of personal ascription that underlies our intuitive moral reactions. I intend to justify it in a certain sense and particularly to revise our rationalistic opinions about the role our feelings play in moral behavior.

5 Definitions, Constraints, Context

Whoever ventures into the thicket of philosophical opinions about free will for the first time quickly notices that there are two fundamentally different strategies used to approach the issue. The first is to give a clear, unambiguous, and understandable definition of free will right from the start and then to prove or refute that there is free will. The second strategy consists of coping without definitions and simply appealing to the reader's or audience's intuitions, either because everybody knows what we are talking about, or because the author is convinced that it is the task of philosophy to discover the "real" concept of free will. My strategy is mixed. I began with a working definition. It was very general and I have appealed to intuitions and preconceptions several times. I will now enrich this definition with interpretations of various degrees for the concepts that appear in it (table 1.1).

I will explain this strategy using the paradigm of being able to do otherwise. In a strong interpretation "freedom" means being able to do otherwise under identical circumstances (natural laws, constraints, and initial conditions). This implies indeterminism. But we could also chose a conditional interpretation, which construes being able to do otherwise as meaning that one would have done something differently, if one had wanted to. Or we could, alternatively, select a hierarchical approach (conditional analysis of an higher order) and interpret being able to do otherwise as meaning that we could want differently, if we wanted to. Or we could opt for a very weak interpretation and think of being able to do otherwise as the fact that one is not hindered by extraneous pressures from choosing one of the alternatives. And there are more intermediate interpretations. Not surprisingly, advocates of free will value the "strong" interpretations, while its opponents prefer the weaker versions.

The situation is different for the intermediate positions. For example, Frankfurt (1988), who defends conditional analysis of an higher order, claims to argue *for* free will, while those who favor a strong version say

Table 1.1
Three Components of Free Will

Freedom	Being able to do otherwise
Maximal interpretation	In *identical* circumstances
Moderate interpretation	In accordance with higher order volitions
Minimal interpretation	Free of external coercion
Associated issues	Compatibility with both determinism and indeterminism, external vs. internal coercion, genuine choice, control
Intelligibility	Acting for understandable reasons
Maximal interpretation	Aided by supernatural reason
Moderate interpretation	Involving reflection and intention
Minimal interpretation	The strongest motive is the reason for action
Associated issues	Intentional causation, weakness of will, rationality, the role of consciousness
Origination	Origination within oneself
Maximal interpretation	Initial causation by a transcendent(al) self
Moderate interpretation	In accordance with one's self
Minimal interpretation	Originator equals executor
Associated issues	Notion of causality, concept of the self or person, personal ascription

The three components of free will are characterized briefly, with their variously strong interpretations. Also mentioned are issues associated with each of the three components.

that his interpretation has nothing to do with free will, particularly because he suggests a weak interpretation of being able to do otherwise, namely a version that is compatible with determinism. The *compatibility debate* revolves around just this question: Is free will compatible with determinism? I suggest that it depends on how we define free will! We can view the compatibility debate as a contest for the correct concept of free will.

If it were only a matter of the strength of the concept of being able to do otherwise, things would still be difficult, but at least graspable. But for the other components there are interpretations of varying degrees as well. The demand for intelligibility can mean that free choices are only free when made by pure reason, which is not of this world. A weaker, yet still sophisticated interpretation would demand that the choice be made "rationally and consciously." Perhaps "intelligible" only means "with reflection and intention." Or—just to mention a very weak version—perhaps it means to act for *any* reason *at all*, namely the most potent motive? Then every act would be intelligible, inasmuch as it doesn't happen entirely unmotivated. It is not irrelevant to ascertain to which interpretation one is referring. Interpretations of various strength can also be demarcated for the concept of "agency." The notion of initial causation by a transcendental or transcendent self is certainly one of the most drastic interpretations. It is often said that to be the originator of an action means to act in accordance with one's own standards and traits of character. Or, the originator is considered merely the executor of an act.

While we started with the distinction of two camps (the advocates and opponents of free will), the situation becomes increasingly complicated. For certainly all kinds of combinations of variously strong standpoints are imaginable. Not all of the possible positions are actually claimed by anyone, but nevertheless, decidedly more than two are. How should we name these positions? The most plausible solution is to say that someone who pleads for all three components in their strictest versions is an advocate of free will (a libertarian). By distinguishing stronger and weaker interpretations and versions I have opened the door for accepting a very weak version of free will. This is not a particularly welcome result, because it lets everything appear to be a matter of interpretation. However—and this should calm us down—it is certainly not the fault of the component theory I have chosen that those who claim weaker or moderate versions turn out to be free will supporters. The reason is more likely to be that more people want to advocate than oppose free will and therefore tend to find even weak versions sufficient. Motives color terminology. It is actually extremely difficult to draw a generally acknowledged demarcation, unless only the strongest version of free will remains valid. The advantage of my method is that first we can find out which interpretation is satisfied and then we can still decide whether we want to call whatever is left free will. We need sophisticated terminology, but it should not be so complex as to be futile. I opt for terms very close to standard usage, as shown in table 1.2.

Some explanation is due here. Libertarianism is explicated not only by the element of being able to do otherwise, but also by a combination of

Table 1.2
Standpoints on Free Will

Libertarianism: The thesis that we have a free will: At least some people sometimes act freely in the sense that all three components are simultaneously fulfilled in a strong version.

Anti-libertarianism: The thesis that libertarianism is not true.

Determinism: The thesis that for everything that happens (actions, decisions, choices included) there are conditions such that these cause everything to happen the way it does and not otherwise.

Indeterminism: The thesis that determinism is not true.

Compatibilism: The thesis that there is a sufficiently strong version free will that is compatible with determinism.

Incompatibilism: The thesis that every sufficiently strict sense of free will is *not* compatible with determinism.

---

several other constituents of the three components. "Determinism" is often chosen as the opposite of libertarianism (e.g., in the German dictionary definition). But I do not agree with this usage. For then we would have to distinguish two kinds of determinism: physicalist determinism (in natural philosophy), which has something to say about physical reality, and determinism in the issue of free will. We have already been confronted with similarly muddled concepts in our attempt to distinguish indeterminism from nonpredictability. Using the same word for different matters creates unnecessary confusion and leads to apparent, purely linguistic paradoxes. If in nature there were indeterministic processes, which, in the form of constraints, influence our actions and decisions yet are not directly involved in our determined actions and decisions, then we could simultaneously advocate—in terms of natural philosophy— both indeterminism and determinism in the matter of free will. It follows that we would have indeterministic determinists! Such games block our view of the real issues. Therefore; in the following I reserve the terms determinism and indeterminism for the question in natural philosophy and use the terms libertarianism and anti-libertarianism for the issue of free will. Figure 1.2 shows this relationship once again.

Indeterminism does not mean that *all* events are undetermined, only that *some* events are not determined. Analogously, the libertarian is not

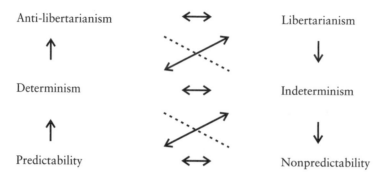

Figure 1.2
Libertarianism, indeterminism, and inpredictability. Legend: → means "implies";
---- means "is compatible with"; ↔ means "mutually exclusive."

obliged to claim that *everyone always* has free will. The weakest description of a libertarian position would be that it claims that one person acted freely once. This would be logically correct, but of course we mean more by free will. We mean that most people normally can act freely, and this conviction was watered down to *some* people *sometimes* can act freely—just to be safe.[42]

The term "compatibilism" is not always used clearly in philosophical literature.[43] Normally it denotes a compatibility of free will and determinism. Often however, it *additionally* implies the compatibility of determinism and moral responsibility. This is probably why William James calls the compatibilistic standpoint *soft determinism*; in contrast, he calls a determinism that denies both free will *and* moral responsibility *hard determinism*. Both libertarians and "hard determinists" are incompatibilists, for both hold the opinion that free will and determinism are incompatible. *As a fact*, however, most libertarians call themselves incompatibilists. By the way, in the debate on compatibility the fact that anti-libertarianism is often called determinism takes its toll. For it is often overlooked that within the logical topography of the standpoints (see table 1.3) one position is excluded, namely the one that claims that free will is also not compatible with indeterminism. Following James, we could call it "hard incompatibilism," or following Double, call it a "no-free-will-either-way theory."[44]

We are now ready to look at the arguments for and against the existence of free will. In the ensuing section I understand this to be the

Table 1.3
Free Will and Determinism

	Determinism	Indeterminism
Free will	Soft determinism (compatibilism)	Libertarianism (incompatibilism)
No free will	Hard determinism (incompatibilism)	?

question of whether or not a strong form of free will—libertarianism—is true. We must not necessarily mean the strongest possible interpretation. While explaining and evaluating the arguments I will note—whenever needed—whether the argument refers to a particular interpretation of a component.

6   The Debate

Do humans possess free will? Asking it this way implies an alleged kind of free will, and the answer can be positive or negative. If we adopt even the weakest version of free will, the question becomes: Which kind of free will do humans have? Or we could ask: What is it that humans possess, that makes philosophers say they have free will? We will find an inquiry along these lines in chapter 3. Presently I shall turn to the most important and frequent arguments for and against free will, to describe, discuss, and evaluate them. To my knowledge, a compilation of this nature does not yet exist. I want to take into consideration arguments that are brought forth in nonscientific discussions as well as those brought up in relevant philosophical literature. The reason for this list is to classify types of arguments so that we recognize them in related forms. This classification should not, however, divert our attention from the fact that types of arguments can cross-cut each other or be connected in terms of contents.

6.1   Pseudo Arguments
Without a doubt, most people are convinced that they have free will. It is intuitively self-evident; it is rather conspicuous, why one should doubt

it. For some reason it seems, at least in our culture and going by our phenomenal model of the self, that the libertarian attitude is natural, while one does not become an anti-libertarian until one has done a bit of thinking. Ask a friend, whether he or she believes to have free will. Most people react like Mr. Vorberg (cf. section 1.2.1). But the fact that in many cases I can often act other than someone has predicted (*defiance argument*)[45] says nothing about whether I could act differently in any particular unique situation. The experience of being able to act differently in similar situations is certainly a main source of our intuition that we possess free will.

How can we tell whether *intuitive arguments* like this are evidence for free will? In general it is true that every intuition can be correct, but in itself it is not an argument. This becomes particularly apparent when different people have different intuitions. What criteria decide which intuitions are right? The one that is most common? Then we would have to admit to free will. But why should we rely on the fact that most people have the right intuition? History teaches us that intuitions mutate, and experience shows that intuitions depend on cultural and individual knowledge. Even if everyone had the same intuition, they could all be mistaken. Even though for thousands of years most people found it intuitively natural that the sun sinks into the sea in the evening, it did not make that description of events true.[46] Particularly in the case of strong cultural prejudices—and free will doubtless belongs to them—it is often difficult to separate learned and acquired preconceptions from phenomenal intuitions.

Not only in daily life do intuitions play an important role. In the philosophy of mind they are customary in the form of thought experiments. Thought experiments are done by imagining situations (which are often not possible) and placing oneself into them in order to evaluate something. Dennett calls them "intuition pumps."[47] They are vivid, easy to access by thought, and can also be understood by laymen. Imagine that a cosmic child had designed us as playthings for his own fun; imagine that even under hypnosis we could hold the opinion that we do certain things entirely voluntarily, even though we have orders to do things post-hypnosis; imagine that neurosurgeons have manipulated our brains and make us do things that we do not want to do. Such ideas make us shiver.

"We're not like that," cries the libertarian; it is so evident. We are different—namely free. "Of course we are just like that!" says the determinist appealing to our intuitions; the difference lies solely in the fact that not a cosmic child, but God (or Mother Nature) created us; or that it is not a hypnotist who determines our actions, but our genes and our upbringing; or that it is not the ruthless neurosurgeon that commands our brain, but the brazen laws of neurophysiology.[48]

Who is right? Our intuitions cannot answer the question. They serve other, basically heuristic purposes. They help us to understand what we think; they lead us to explicit theories; and they challenge us to find explanations, particularly when they are inconsistent with our convictions. But taken by themselves they are seldom real arguments.[49]

Appeals to tradition or authority are also pseudo-arguments. First, an appeal to authority is not concerned with the content of the concept of free will, it has little to do with the problem at hand. Second, it is easy to see that every position can be backed, as soon as we find some authority who does so. We can accept this stalemate, shrug our shoulders, and concede that there simply are different opinions and one's penchant depends on one's devotion to a particular authority. A Calvinist would then be a determinist, many a Koran teacher would be libertarian.[50] But an argument demands more than that we believe in insight of an authority. It demands, at least, reasons for believing that authority. For example, if someone claims the truth of determinism because Einstein was determinist, he is asking to us to *trust* Einstein. Even if he thinks Einstein should know what he's talking about, since he was an ingenious physicist, this would still be a feint argument. No matter how highly gifted he might have been, Einstein certainly had reasons and arguments for his views that had nothing to do with his own personal authority. The arguments that are independent of his person are the ones we are interested in from a philosophical standpoint. A claim based on authority is either replaceable by real arguments or merely a matter of belief. This is also true for the *argument for unknown explanation*. This states that it is logically not impossible that we could still discover hitherto unknown powers (such as skills in parapsychology) or other empirical evidence that shows free will to be a fact. Certainly; it is logically not impossible that we may discover an unknown natural power. It is also logically not impossible that as of tomorrow the laws of nature will no longer be valid. If this should happen, we might even be able to demonstrate it empirically. But we have no serious evidence for the existence of such unknown powers.

6.2 Determinism's Threat

As we have seen, determinism threatens the concept of freedom as being able to do otherwise. If the world is deterministic, then there is no free will. This *argument for factual determinedness* sounds correct. But is it? Variations on it refer to different kinds of determinism. Many people feel that their free will is threatened by *genetic* determinism. But the general problem of determinism is chiefly entirely independent of the issue of genetic determinism. Even if genes predetermined only about 1 percent of our behavior, which would imply that genetic determinism is false, then *general* determinism could still be true, because our behavior is also influenced by our upbringing, our surroundings, learning experiences, and other environmental factors. And these could be entirely deterministic. If, on the other hand, our genes determined our behavior in 99 percent of all cases, freedom could still lie in that remaining 1 percent. Some philosophers think that the determinism of neurophysiology is the real threat for free will (Thorp 1980). This is not wholly incorrect, as neurophilosophy does assume that mental properties are manifested in the brain (see chapter 2). But not without reason have I described determinism so generally that it should hold true for all imaginable processes that are involved in creating our will (namely in all possible worlds)—in the brain or wherever.

If general determinism is true, that is, if one of the necessary conditions for free will is not met, then there is no free will. This claim of the incompatibilist is currently known as the *consequence argument*.[51] If determinism is true, then our actions are results of natural laws and events in the distant past. But we are responsible neither for what happened before we were born, nor for the state of natural laws. We are also not responsible for naturally necessary consequences, including our present actions. Therefore, there is no free will. In other words; only if we could influence the past or change natural laws would we really be free in a determinist's world.

The interesting thing about putting it this way is that it expresses the problem using terms that refer to natural laws and a notion of necessity customary in physics. But at bottom the element of agency plays a central role in the principle of transitivity that is decisive for the claim. If a past action is not really up to us (agency), then we are also not really responsible for its consequences. Van Inwagen (1986) calls this modal principle the β-rule; Fischer (1994) calls it the transfer principle, more precisely the "principle of transferring powerlessness." Formally they look the same:

$$N(p), N(p \rightarrow q) \vdash N(q)$$

p and q are any propositions, which express the matter. N is a modal operator. For van Inwagen it means "and no one ever had or has a choice whether . . . " (van Inwagen 1986, p. 93), for Fischer it means "*power necessary.*"[52] A proposition is "power necessary" relative to a person when this person has no choice whether the proposition is true (Fischer 1994, p. 8). Basically both arguments end with the same results. In Fischer's terminology the transfer principle means roughly (for illustration I will now speak of matters and not propositions about matters): If someone is powerless with respect to a matter, and powerless with respect to the fact that this matter leads to the next, then he is also powerless with respect to that second matter. For example: Suppose a comet hits my house (expressed as proposition p). I am powerless in the face of this event (N(p)). If a comet hits my house, it will also destroy my house (p → q). I am also powerless with respect to this connection (N(p → q)). Thus I am also powerless with respect to the destruction of my house (N(q)).

You might now suspect how the argument for incompatibility is construed. We can ask ourselves, namely, whether or not I was free with respect to certain events q, that is, whether I was not powerless. In determinism this is only possible when I was not powerless with respect to antecedent conditions of q, that is with respect to p, or not powerless with respect to natural laws. But I am powerless with respect to both p and natural laws. For I can change neither the past nor the laws of nature.[53]

I find this argument basically valid. Whoever disagrees must attack the transitivity principle in some way.[54] The consequence argument refers not only to being able to do otherwise. This is clear in the phrases "our responsibility," "no real choice," and "powerless." Here, being able to do otherwise is connected to agency. The implicit idea is that we cannot be held responsible for something for whose origin we are not responsible. One way to criticize the consequence argument is thus to find fault with the notion of initial causation hidden within it. Dennett's objection to the consequence argument is that it is similar to the so-called *Sorites paradox*: One does not make an accumulation of seeds become a pile simply by adding one more seed. We can add one seed, we can add another and another, but according to the first premise we can never make a pile out of them. Of course, we know that this is wrong. If we add one seed at a time over a period of time, we slowly create a pile. But it is hard to tell just when that point is reached. It is exactly the same with decisions, Dennett says. Even if their particular origins are not our responsibility, because they lie in the past, that does not mean that the sum, or consequences are not our responsibility—in a sense that we must specify more precisely. It is easy to see that a theory of the self is important here. I call this retort the *Sorites argument*. Yet independent of the theory of the self, it is right, that if determinism were true it would annihilate any undetermined ability to do otherwise. Every discussion on free will returns to this problem sooner or later. Leder (1995) says it is a bounce-back argument: Every time we believe we have knocked it down and let go of it, it bounces back to its feet.

If we accept the consequence argument and are still convinced that there is free will, then it absolutely follows that determinism is false. But what could an undetermined free will look like? Or asked fundamentally: Is undetermined free will at all possible? The *intelligibility argument* denies this.[55] Stated briefly it says that a real choice is intelligible and follows from understandable reasons. An undetermined choice, however, is *per definitionem* not determined by reasons. Thus an undetermined choice is not intelligible; it is arbitrary, random, irrational, not an act—or at least not a real choice. Therefore, (intelligible) free will is not compatible with indeterminism. Rather, it demands determinism by reasons. Van Inwagen (1986, p. 126–152) discusses these arguments in detail, particularly the one that claims that an undetermined choice is no real choice. He concludes that this claim could by all means be true. But then, according to van Inwagen, the consequence argument would also have to be true; for both rest centrally on the β-rule. Just as the incompatibilist says—using Fischer's wording—that in an indeterminist's world powerlessness is transferred from the past to the present, so also the fact is transferred that undetermined factors make a choice become an unreal choice. If we follow this line of argument, we have shown with one stroke that free will—in a strong sense—is compatible with neither determinism nor indeterminism.[56] But since van Inwagen is a libertarian and believes in free will, he finds himself forced(!)—even though he maintains that the critical premise β is valid—to find the intelligibility argument false. For what reasons? His only reason is that he prefers the puzzling issue (an undetermined act should be intelligible) over the inconceivable issue (giving up certain other premises). He considers a theory called *agent causation* to be a plausible solution. But as I will show (in section 3.1 of chapter 3), this theory itself is questionable. This gives us one reason more for validating the intelligibility argument.

At this point we can also introduce another variation of the Sorites argument: Perhaps a purely determined choice is not a real choice and a purely undetermined choice is not a real choice either. But from this it does not necessarily follow that a mixed determined and undetermined choice is not a real choice. Whether or not we accept the Sorites argument depends on the point at which we are willing to accept any choice as being a real choice.

Describing the concept of free will by using three logically independent components helps us to better understand the debate among incompatibilists and compatibilists. Their arguments deal with the compatibility of different components. The consequencialist claims that only undetermined acts can be associated with agency, which means that the third component implies the first. Advocates of the intelligibility argument claim in contrast that, if strongly interpreted, the first and second component cannot be satisfied simultaneously. If, for free will to exist, we demand strong interpretations of all three components, then it follows from acknowledging both arguments: This type of free will does not exist because it would be incompatible with both determinism and indeterminism! The reason that incompatibilism sometimes seems convincing, and compatibilism seems convincing at other times is that, in a certain sense, they are both right. They simply appeal to different intuitions, which means that the concepts of free will underlying their arguments differ.[57]

6.3   The Dualist Strategy: Doubling the Problems

Any theory for explaining free acts is a two-world theory if it postulates things, powers, or properties, which do not adhere to the laws of physics. A dualistic argument goes something like this. The physical world is causally determined. Physical causality excludes free will. But we do command a free will. Therefore, free will exists in another world to which we also belong; it exists in a nonphysical substance—the soul, for example—or in the "realm of the intelligible." These two kinds of dualism can be distinguished by calling one substance dualism and the other rationality dualism.[58] Rationaliy dualism is a variation on property dualism found also in other contexts.

At first glance, dualism appears to be an elegant solution. But it is also true here: You don't get something for nothing. Problematic consequences are attached to that apparent elegance. First of all, the determinism issue and thus also the question of whether the first component is satisfied, will not disappear; it has simply been placed in another world. And that world itself could be deterministic. Perhaps the problem of determinism is more easily solved in that other world. How? The second world is usually thought of as a realm not accessible to science or human understanding. And why not? Why should everything be accessible to science? Couldn't we just accept the fact that the problem of determinism in that other world cannot be solved or adequately grasped? We can. But do we have a reason for that? If the challenge of free will is our only motivation for doing so, then our reason is ad hoc. Which other reason could we find? Reference to an authority? Aside of the fact that many people reject that method and prefer to adhere to Kant's maxim of using one's own power of reasoning, even if we did eliminate reason, grave problems would remain. One is the problem that Eccles's interactionary dualism could not solve: How do both of those worlds mutually effect each other? How can the second world influence the first and how are the two worlds coordinated? Every reciprocal effect would violate the law of the conservation of energy and is thus a scientific anomaly. But even if we could accept this in spite of all doubts, we are faced with another problematic consequence. The first world can, by all means, be partially determined. Neurophysiological, psychological, and genetic determinism have not been annulled. The more events in the first, natural world we can explain with special determinisms (adding indeterministic processes), the more the second world becomes obsolete. (This is also known as *Ockham's razor*; superfluous ontological assumptions get shaved off.)[59] If we can explain the evolution of new kinds with a theory of natural selection, we do not need to postulate continuous intervention in the universe. If we can explain the "sacred illness" (as it used to be called) of epilepsy as a disorder in the excitability of neurons, explanation via a theory of demoniacal possession becomes superfluous. If we can explain life in terms of a self-organizing biological process, the so-called *vis vitalis*—"life power"—becomes obsolete. In my terms this means that factual determinedness really only gains significance in the context of a two-world theory. For the second world can no longer be effective in terms of free will where the first world is determined. This means that every deterministic element of the first world reduces the chances of the second world contributing effectively to the way the first one functions. A dualist thus has only two alternatives: Either he limits himself to supplying explanations for only a very small portion of our so-called free decisions, or he is on the retreat. The more monist explanations we can offer, the fewer dualist explanations we require. The dualist resembles opponents to artificial intelligence who claim that man-made systems could never accomplish this or that. Slowly, but surely, he loses credibility, and the more artificial systems succeed at "intelligent" performance, which he considers to be typically human.

For the reasons mentioned above, I will not further pursue the substance dualist's solution. Rationality dualism does play an important role, however, because not only is it still stubbornly professed in various forms, it is also fairly influential. It is closely connected to the self-contradictory argument. The following section discusses it in that context.

6.4 Stumbling Over Our Own Feet: Self-Refutation?

There is a kind of argument that we can call genuinely philosophical, because it endeavors to demonstrate that determinism is an untenable philosophical theory due to the logic of the concepts involved.

Self-refuting arguments are as old as Epicureanism.[60] According to Epicurus, anyone who claims that everything happens with necessity cannot criticize someone who denies it, because he would thus be admitting that his own criticism was predetermined and is thus not genuine criticism (Honderich 1990b, p. 360). The general form of the argument goes: A determinist who pleads the case for determinism is in a dilemma. Fighting for the cause of determinism either occurs on the assumption that it is not right, or one is contradicting oneself. In short; determinism is either wrong or self-refuting! The common denominator shared by various forms of this argument is the move from premises about epistemological or normative concepts to the conclusion that ontological determinism is false or self-refuting. Such deductive reasoning on self-refutation is also often directed toward positive arguments for free will. It aims to demonstrate that free will is necessary for exactly those epistemological or normative concepts (predictability, truth, knowledge, debate, rationality, reason, morals). A rational being cannot help but think of himself as free (Kant 1786/1983); a causally determined choice is not a genuine choice (Rickert 1921); free choice is a necessary condition for fulfilling standards of rationality (Boyle, Grisez, and Tollefsen 1976).

Are these arguments convincing? At a glance we recognize that a few of them are not. The claim, for example, that a statement cannot be *true* simply because it is the result of a causally predetermined process, is not tenable. If truth is the correspondence of a proposition to a fact (correspondence theory of truth), even a wholly determined statement can be true. We must also examine the arguments for self-refutation to see whether they beg the question; whether they presuppose whatever it is that they claim to prove. Pothast (1980, p. 258–276) has shown *petitio principii* can be found in the analytical form of Boyle, Grisez, and Tollefsen's argument (1976).

More common, however, is the objection that a belief, statement, or argument must originate in reason and may not be traceable back to causal connections. When we agree with an opinion, statement, or argument, we do so because we think that it is correct. At first it seems implausible that such insight or understanding is due to a causal chain of events determined by something long past. If we do not have a genuine way for achieving true knowledge through insight and understanding, then it would seem as if beliefs, statements, and arguments lose their special status. Basically there are two fundamentally different views of this argument. One is to locate reason outside of the picture of the world as a causally determined system. I have already stated grounds for rejecting this dualistic notion. But even within the monist's camp there are philosophers who deny that it is possible to naturalize reason or rationality (like Putnam 1982, 1992b). Rationality is more a normative ideal that we simply must assume if we are going to debate at all and which resists naturalization, in spite of the threat of circularity. How can we reply? It is true that in the determinist's idea of the world our endeavors for knowledge and understanding develop a character different from the kind we intuitively take for granted (Honderich 1995, p. 115f). For our faith in our own knowledge rests on the fact that we are free, or at least were free to do certain things. My faith in the correctness of any particular claim rests on the fact that I am free to ask myself certain questions, to think up possible evidence for or against the claim, and so on. If determinism is true, however, then I am no longer in a position to undertake real investigation and research; therefore, I can have no real faith in truths provided by determinism.

It is difficult to ignore this argument entirely. It is correct that in a determinist's world there is no room for unlimited freedom of thought and research and the idea that we can, in principle, gain access to any particular kind of knowledge we would like. But perhaps the problem is that we have a philosophically exaggerated notion of reason. Perhaps reason is not really unlimited, perhaps even our epistemological skills have limits. In fact, to a crucial extent, they do actually depend on our past. Without the appropriate education, the right history of learning, the historical development of language, the invention and tradition of thinking aids—particularly systems of symbolic representation—we would not be in the position to think and argue as we do today. We would be able to refute the claim of non-naturalization of rationality if we could show how reasonable actions of rational beings can be determined by past events, without this implying a loss of rationality. In other words: How can we gain faith in our own knowledge even though our thinking is predetermined? The self-refutation argument can thus be seen as a challenge to design a naturalistic theory of reason or rationality, or to the point: a naturalistic theory of intelligibility. Section 3 in chapter 3 sketches such a theory.

6.5   Arguments from Moral Philosophy

Arguments from moral philosophy couple free will with moral responsibility. The difference between them depends on the factor each takes to be basic: some start with the existence of free will, some with moral responsibility. Meta-ethical issues, like the question of whether or not there are objective values or objective moral properties, also play an important part. Because moral issues tend to have emotional connotations, I will discuss these arguments rather dryly by examining their logical structure.

In section 4 I said that the claim "ought implies can" is a generally accepted notion (moral responsibility R implies free will W) and that we can conclude that without free will there would be no moral responsibility. Closer analysis shows that the conclusion depends decisively on how we interpret the expression "R implies W." In order to reach the conclusion "without free will, no responsibility," the phrase must read: "W is a *necessary* condition for R." Then the relation can be expressed as implication: Moral responsibility R implies free will W. Because Kant held the freedom of will to be a necessary prerequisite for responsibility, in the following I will call this interpretation *Kantian implication*. It is used by hardcore determinists when arguing that there is no moral responsibility. Since there is no freedom of will within determinism (incompatibilism), there is also no moral responsibility. In logical notation:

$$R \rightarrow W, \neg W, \vdash \neg R$$

All incompatibilists agree with this valid modus tollens conclusion. Of course it is not an argument for or against free will. The premise is, that free will is nonexistent. Using Kantian implication, however, we can plead for freedom of will by accepting as given the existence of moral responsibility.

$$R \rightarrow W, R \vdash W$$

This *claim of truly existent moral responsibility* reminds us of the Palmström argument, which went: "It just cannot be true that we have no free will. Thus we have a free will." Why is the Palmström argument poor philosophy? Whether a person has free will or not is a fact that can be described. In contrast, "It just cannot be true!" is deontological statement—a statement about what should or should not be the case. We cannot deduct descriptive statements from deontological statements. Doing that is making a logical mistake, committing a "deontological fallacy."[61] Van Inwagen's position does, at first, look false: "If incompatibilism is true, then either determinism or the free-will thesis is false. To deny the free-will thesis is to deny the existence of moral responsibility, which would be absurd. . . . Therefore, we should reject determinism" (Van Inwagen 1986, p. 223).

If we read "it is absurd to deny the existence of moral responsibility" as meaning "it just may not be," then we do in fact have a deontological fallacy here. But van Inwagen's argument can be rescued by introducing another premise. Instead of saying "it is absurd to deny the existence of moral responsibility," van Inwagen should posit that "there *is* moral responsibility." The argument is then valid (a modus ponens), it is an argument about real existing moral responsibility.

Thus we have two very similar arguments that both use the Kantian implication as a premise. In terms of formal logic both are valid. So something must be wrong with the premises. Richard Double (1991) investigates the second premise of both by analyzing the concepts of free will and responsibility and concludes that "free will and moral responsibility, if they exist, are moral properties" (Double 1991, p. 138).

In his opinion, free will and moral responsibility depend on *objective* moral properties. The decisive—meta-ethical—question is, thus, are there objective moral properties? Double himself claims that there are not. In other words, he spurns moral realism. What we have, he claims, are simply diverse incompatible subjective intuitions about what we should do.[62] In this case he does have an argument against the freedom of will, the *argument of nonobjective morals*. If free will and moral responsibility depend on the existence of objective moral properties (OMP), then we have neither freedom of will, nor moral responsibility. In logical notation:

R → OMP, W → OMP, ¬OMP ⊢ ¬R, ¬W

Double's arguments make the problem of free will a meta-ethical issue. This corresponds to the strategy of various philosophers who view the problem of free will as a challenge to moral philosophy instead of to theoretical philosophy. I, in contrast, consider free will to be a natural property of persons who either possess it or do not possess it. So it must be possible to unlock the question of the existence of free will from the issue of moral responsibility. Instead of attacking the second premise, as Double does, we can question the first premise. The Kantian implication $(R \rightarrow W)$ is only a logically correct expression for "if you should do something you must be able to do it" if free will is a *necessary* condition for moral responsibility. If we consider it solely a *sufficient* condition for moral responsibility, the implication is reversed $(W \rightarrow R)$. Then it does not follow purely logically from the nonexistence of the free will that there is no moral responsibility. For moral responsibility nothing at all follows from the nonexistence of the free will. In formal notation:

Instead of $R \rightarrow W$, $\neg W \vdash \neg R$

we have $W \rightarrow R$, $\neg W \vdash ?$

These logical dependencies challenge us to design a concept of responsibility compatible with the nonexistence of a strong form of free will. The stance we take toward free will is evidently aligned by our standpoint in moral philosophy.

In this context there is another interesting argument showing, in my opinion, that deterministic theory of moral responsibility has more to do with consequential ethics than with ethics of principles. It is the *argument of moral luck*.[63] This argument begins with a fact of everyday psychology, namely that we make persons responsible for their actions, even when these persons *do not* fulfill the condition of being able to do otherwise. Consider two drunk drivers who each cause accidents during a state of unaccountability. One of them seriously injures a child, perhaps even kills her, the other is lucky enough—despite equal alcohol consumption—to only knock over a lamppost. The idea at play here is that the first driver deserves greater reproach and is at greater moral fault. Or, in another case, a person in a totalitarian state who becomes a concentration camp guard or torturer is morally condemned, while another person with the same sadistic inclinations is lucky to live in a country in which there are no such career opportunities for sadists. Unearned luck even plays a part in positive prejudices: After all, we admire people with impeccable manners, diplomacy, and moral integrity, even though we are well aware that their morally valuable traits are perhaps due—*among other things*—to privileges of decent or upbringing (Patzig 1994, pp. 204f). Justification for moral judgments evidently lies not in the fact that any moral deficit of one person is *actually* greater than that of another, but rather in the fact that the consequences of one person's actions are worse than those of another.

This argument does not mention free will.[64] But it does once again demonstrate just how our concepts of free will mingle with moral theory. In chapter 3 I will use a modified concept of agency to illustrate how not only consequences, but also the extent to which an action is considered an expression of an agent's personality, are relevant for ascribing moral responsibility.

6.6   A Moderate Standpoint: Compatibilist Arguments

Compatibilists hold the view that free will and determinism are compatible and they usually also support the thesis that people in a deterministic world are also morally responsible.[65] This necessarily leads to a modification of the libertarian concept of freedom. Even if determinism were true, so that there is no free will in the strong sense, the question remains as to why we distinguish voluntary acts from involuntary acts—and how to tell the difference. The question is not whether there are voluntary acts—there are—the question is, which feature is characteristic of such an act? This *argument of the paradigm case* is at the bottom of every analysis that attempts to formulate a weaker concept of freedom. One paradigmatic case is the phenomenon of the weak will.[66] Everyone knows that people sometimes do not go through with what they have planned, they regret it afterward and feel that their will was just not strong enough to do what they wanted. Basically this is the point of departure for every conversation about free will. No one denies that before we become philosophers we characterize various actions and decisions as "voluntary." Only because we do fairly intersubjectively distinguish among certain cases of behavior does the question arise of what is at the bottom of this distinction. Controversial is, which kind of "freedom" justifies the distinguishing characteristic. If, for example, we take the first component as a basis and if determinism is true, then we evidently call some actions voluntary, even though they are not really that. Freedom built solely on the second component would be compatible with general determinism, but it is threatened by teachings of psychoanalysis.

Proceeding in this way creates three difficulties. First, we have to know what kind of paradigmatic case we are using. It should be relatively easy to get agreement on that. Second is the issue of whether a concept of freedom is really the common characteristic of those cases or whether they are not more likely characterized by varying features that are thrown together and then christened "free will." Third is the matter of whether a weak sense of freedom as used in these cases actually earns the name of free will at all, once we study all the implications.

One version of weak freedom is *freedom as the absence of coercion.* A person is free when he or she is not prevented by external (and/or internal) forces from doing what he or she wants to do. Classical examples for freedom as the absence of coercion can be found in Hobbes, Locke, and Hume (see Steinvorth 1987). Moritz Schlick (1930/1978) also views freedom as the absence of external and internal force. He holds free will to be a pseudo-problem. He emphasizes that confusing laws of nature with human laws leads to the notion that humans are not free. Understanding freedom as the absence of coercion is unproblematic, as long as it refers to external forces;[67] we can also possess this type of freedom in a deterministic world. It is no accident that this solution has been chosen by most authors in political philosophy—the notion corresponds widely with our conception of political, individual freedom. This type of freedom *is* important, desirable, and unfortunately still not available for many people today. But it has little to do with free will. It is a different topic. In our terminology it can, at most, be understood as an extremely weak version of the first component. Being able to act otherwise would read as: A person can act otherwise when he or she is not prevented from doing so by external or internal force.

Another version that modifies and reinterprets the first component is *conditional freedom.* It emerged through analytic philosophy of language, G. E. Moore being its originator.[68] He shows how the ability to do otherwise is possible in a deterministic world by reinterpreting (weakening) the word *can*. "A person could have acted otherwise" does not mean that he would have acted exactly the same in identical circumstances. It means he would have acted otherwise, if he had wanted to (Moore 1912/1970).

Finally, to mention a third mode of the concept of freedom, there is so-called *epistemic indeterminism*.[69] This name is unfortunate, because determinism and predictability are by no means identical. The point of these positions is *nonpredictability*.[70] (For historical reasons I will use the expression here.) According to this view we are free when we cannot predict our actions for fundamental reasons. The reasons vary from author to author. Henri Bergson argues that it is subjectively and objectively impossible to predict how conscious beings will decide. That would presuppose that phenomena of consciousness are calculable (which they are not). Bergson pointedly summarizes his view with the phrase that we cannot predict decisions, we can only make them. Holm Tetens formulates an "uncertainty principle" in neurobiology, which says that the attempt to predict the behavior of a person using knowledge of his neural states is not feasible because of the hypersensitivity of the brain and the resulting influence on measurements (Tetens 1991, p. 12).[71] Other epistemic indeterminists have a weaker claim. They do not argue that decisions and actions are *fundamentally* unpredictable, but rather that they are unpredictable for the subject making the decision or acting (Planck 1936/1978). Donald McKay (1967/1978) argues with reference to Popper's (1950) ideas on indeterminism as nonpredictability for a "principle of logical relativity." Agents are free in as much as prophecies or predictions about their future behavior would not bind them for logical reasons. This would be true even if the agent were designed as mechanically as clockwork.

A frequent objection to compatibilistic solutions, which postulate hierarchies of actions, choices, and states of desire, is the *regress argument*.[72] This argument rebukes compatibilistic views for not solving, but merely shifting the problem of free will. If I define free will as the freedom to be able to do what I want to do, then we can inquire: Do I have the freedom to want differently? In general, the argument says that theories that define free will as being determined by other processes end up in an infinite regress or do not address the crucial issue. Compatibilist authors do see this problem.[73] This is why they are concerned to find a criterion for avoiding such a regress. We will deal with this when discussing agency.

Another way to organize moderate arguments is by the components they take into consideration. The most frequent modifications relate to the first component. The ability to do otherwise is enfeebled. Frankfurt's conditional analysis of higher order, however, does make reference to the second and above all the third component, as we shall see in our neurophilosophical analysis of agency in chapter 3. Finally, epistemic indeterminism relates to the first or second components. When evaluating the arguments in section 6.7 I will claim that it will always be necessary to deprive the components of some strength in some form or another, because in their strongest interpretations the three components are not compatible. In contrast to the traditional view, however, the issue of determinism alone is not decisive; some components must or can be weakened in an indeterministic world. The two essential questions of every compatibilistic theory of free will are, then, which modification is needed where and to which extent and, which consequences result from a thus weakened free will. Ultimately, as discussion on the intelligibility argument and the Sorites argument in section 6.2 has shown, when we evaluate a compatibilistic theory, we should consider the component able to do otherwise, but we must also inquire as to what makes a choice intelligible and when we can rightly say that a person is the originator of his actions.

From a philosophical point of view it would be nice to be able to show that all the arguments mentioned thus far fully exhaust the debate that none further are to be found. If this is not doable, it would be desirable to at least be able to show that they are ordered systematically and there is hope that that system has some gaps for new lines of thought. Unfortunately, I cannot prove that my list is complete, nor do I see a well-formed system. Table 1.4 gives only a survey of important and frequent claims. References for individual arguments can be found in sections 6.1 through 6.6.

Table 1.4
The Most Frequent and Important Arguments Supporting a Freedom of Will

---

Pseudo-Arguments

Intuition argument: We have a strong intuition in favoring free will. An intuition this strong cannot be a delusion. Thus, we must have free will.

Defiance argument (revision is possible): We can always do the opposite of what we are supposedly determined to do, even if only to prove that we have free will. Thus, we have free will.

Authority argument: Some authority claims or teaches that we have free will, so we do.

Palmström argument: It just cannot be true that we do not have free will, thus we do.

The argument of unknown explanation: Science cannot explain how free will is possible in our world. But it is real. Therefore, there must be unknown factors which could explain it.

Dualistic Argument

Two World Theory (causality argument): We know that we can act freely. The physical world is causally determined. Physical causality excludes free will. Therefore, we belong to another, noncausally determined world (of the mind, or reason).

Incompatibilist Arguments

Argument of factual determinedness: The world is in fact determined. We are part of the world. Since we are determined, we have no free will.

Consequence argument (transfer principle): Free will requires at least that we are responsible for our actions. If determinism is true, our acts are consequences of laws of nature and events in the distant past. We are responsible neither for the laws of nature nor for events of the distant past, thus (β-rule, transfer principle) we are also not responsible for the consequences of these things, namely our actions. Determinism thus excludes free will.

Self-refutation argument (Epicurean argument, reasons versus causes, mentalism argument): The claim that determinism presupposes something which it denies (effectiveness of reasons, possibility of knowledge, mental causality, etc.). Therefore determinism is either self-refuting or false.

Regress argument: Theories that define free will as determination by other processes merely shift the actual problem to another level. These theories either enter an infinite regress or they do not really address the crucial issue.

Table 1.4
Continued

Compatibilist Arguments

Intelligibility argument (MIND argument, psychological determinism): A real, intelligible choice results from reasons. An indeterministic choice, however, is not determined by reasons. An indeterministic choice is therefore not intelligible, it is arbitrary, random, irrational, not an act at all or at least not a real choice. Therefore, intelligibility is not compatible with indeterminism. On the contrary, it demands determinism by reasons.

Argument of the Paradigm Case (weakness of will): We call certain acts and choices free. The question is not whether there are such acts—there are—the question is, What is the distinctive mark of such acts?

Sorites argument: From the fact that we had no choice about the origins of our actions it does not follow that we have no choice now. For the fact that a system has a certain property it is not necessary that this property is attributable to its parts or an earlier version of it.

Freedom as absence of coercion: Acting freely *means no more* than being able to do what one wants without being hindered therein.

Conditional analysis: That a person could have X-ed otherwise means no more than that she would have X-ed otherwise if she had Y-ed otherwise. Most common variant: X = act, Y = want.

Freedom as insight in necessity: To act freely means to act with the knowledge of the determining factors.

Freedom as unpredictability (epistemic indeterminism, Newcomb's paradox): We are free when we cannot predict our own actions. Since it is in principle impossible to do so, we are free.

Arguments from Moral Philosophy

Argument of real, existent moral responsibility: Moral responsibility implies free will. Since we do really have moral responsibility, we also have a free will.

Argument of non-objective morals: Free will implies the existence of objective moral properties. There are no objective moral properties. Thus we do not have a free will.

Argument of moral luck: Moral responsibility does not depend on being able to do otherwise in an indeterministic sense, because we also make different moral judgments about people even when their actions depend on good or bad luck.

Thrift Argument

Ockham's Razor: Assuming free will explains certain mental phenomena and experiences. The better we can explain these without the notion of free will, the more superfluous it is to assume one.

6.7 Summary and Evaluation

Having traversed various arguments I would like to take a summarizing and evaluative position on the ontological question; Does free will exist? Without a doubt, many people have strong intuitions *in favor of* its existence. There is also no doubt that there are acts that we intersubjectively call free. These two facts say little by themselves, because they are compatible with every possible standpoint on the issue of existence. If we want to take a stance toward the question of whether or not free will exists, we must say which concept of free will we mean. For starters I will use the strongest possible concept of free will, as it is normally defended by libertarians: A person has a free will, when under identical conditions—that means identical laws of nature, constraints, and initial conditions—she could also have made her choices differently, and that the person makes these choices for intelligible reasons and is their sole originator (initial cause).

We do *not* have a free will like this, one that satisfies all three components in their strongest interpretation. This is true whether determinism is true (consequence argument) or not (intelligibility argument). Thus a free will that simultaneously fulfills the first two components in their strongest interpretation is impossible. A theory of two worlds suggests itself as a way to rescue the free will from one kind of determinism, namely physical determinism. Defendants of dualism, however, are in an uncomfortable position. Whatever is factually determined undermines the effectiveness of the "other" type of freedom. And then there is also the question of determinedness in the second world. Invoking reason to refute determinism (self-refutation arguments) only works when reason is thought of as something that lies outside of our natural world. It only works as a dualistic argument. But then we get all the problems of dualism. The only alternative is to consider reason or intelligibility as belonging to the physical world. If anyone is convinced of the existence of free will solely because its nonexistence would have drastic consequences (Palmström argument), he may use this as motivation for continuing research on the matter, but, being based solely on the fear of consequences, it is not an argument—for purely logical reasons. Whether moral responsibility can be seen as evidence for free will depends on whether there is anything at all like moral responsibility or objective moral responsibility. This meta-ethical problem can be avoided by understanding free will not as a necessary, but rather solely as a sufficient condition for moral responsibility. Then there is the question of what the nonexistence of a strong form of free will implies. As the argument on moral luck shows, our moral judgments are at least sometimes not dependent on being able to do otherwise in an indeterministic sense.

Compatibilist theories of free will weaken individual components of it. The traditional solution, namely to emphasize the diluted version of being able to do otherwise in the form of conditional analysis (I could do otherwise, if I wanted to), is not convincing. More significant is how the concept of agency and the component of intelligibility are to be understood. Even if we cannot control the origins of our acts, that does not mean that during the course of our lives we cannot control and determine our acts and choices ourselves (Sorites argument). Self-determination without dualism and initial causation demand the dilution of one or more components. Neurophilosophy of free will aims to discover which dilutions can be justified, without losing sight of the intuitions that lie at the bottom of all three components.

I shall not tackle this task until chapter 3. First I shall wander a bit through the contemporary theoretical scene to see whether the three-component model and the arguments we have found adequately describe current philosophical debate. The component theory of free will and the way I have organized the arguments used in the debate helps us keep track of and understand all the theories about free will. It will become obvious that most of the theories do not incorporate all three components and that critics of each position employ exactly the neglected component as leverage.

7   The Component Model and Rival Theories

7.1   Dualistic Libertarianism

I include substance dualism, as well as the theory of agent causation and rationality dualism among the dualistic theories.[74] Classical *substance dualism* postulates an additional substance, which does not obey laws of nature; a substance that is, however, mutually causally effective with the physical world and which is the realm in which we find free will (Foster 1991; Eccles 1990; Swinburne 1997). These theories are confronted with all three consequential difficulties of dualism mentioned earlier. For classical theists the component of agency and the connected issue of moral responsibility emerge as the theodicy problem. Even if we had souls and they were not subordinate to the laws of physics, the issue still arises of whether our actions originate in us and we are morally responsible, or whether the creator of our souls is responsible for them. Philosophical theists see the major difficulty in the omniscience of an omnipotent God, which would be just as threatening to free will as determinism (Fischer 1989, 1994). In order to rescue free will, some thinkers go as far as to weaken omniscience (Swinburne 1995).

The other two variants are more subtly dualistic in that they postulate a second kind of causality. On one hand we have the theory of *agent causation*. It claims that human behavior is caused by the substance of the agent, which in turn is not caused by any other events.[75] The talk is of an "unmoved mover"; in paraphrase we could say an "uncaused cause." The main problem for the theory of agent causation is that according to it, reasons cannot be causes for free actions. For the agent is the *only* and exclusive reason (or cause) of his actions (see Kane 1989: 226–230). In this respect it is a variation on the intelligibility argument.

Third, there is rationality dualism, as Kant defends, for example. He postulates a realm of reason that is different from the realm of natural causation. Rationality dualism must work around the issue of mental causation and stops at a dilemma. If reasons are abstract, they cannot be causally effective. If they are to be considered causally effective, rationality dualism is in danger of turning into substance dualism. One escape route would be to think of reasons as something that is not outside of nature. That might be the way to a promising solution. But then it turns into monistic naturalism and is no longer rationality dualism.

7.2 Monistic Libertarianism

Not all libertarian theories need be dualistic. Libertarians, we all agree, rely on indeterminism. And our world does actually seem to be partially indeterministic. What would seem more natural, then, than to formulate a respectable theory of the free will using physical indeterminism. One suggestion would be, if causal determinism is inconsistent with free will, our voluntary actions must be uncaused or undetermined.[76] Another variation does not claim that voluntary actions must be uncaused, but rather that they are caused by probabilistic or undetermined laws.[77] Now we *can* ask whether there is such a thing as probabilistic causality.[78] The most important objection to both variants is, once again, the intelligibility argument. Can undetermined or probabilistically caused actions be intelligible? It seems inconsistent to assume that they can be. How can being undetermined and being intelligible be made compatible?

One way would be to drastically limit the cases in which free choices can be made. This strategy is called *restrictivism* (Fischer and Ravizza 1992: 239). According to this view we are only free when, after considering all reasons, it is still not clear what we should do, that is, when those reasons *do not* vividly determine which choice should be made. Van Inwagen (1989), for instance, defends a restrictive position.

Theories working with *teleological intelligibility* (Wiggins 1973; Kane 1985, 1996) try to preserve the rationality of free, undetermined choice by attempting to show the extent to which an undetermined choice must not necessarily be arbitrary. They concede that being undetermined alone is not sufficient for voluntary actions. But it is possible that our biographies nondeterministically, yet intelligibly, fit into our actions, intentions, and goals. Thus Kane (1985, 1988, 1989) defends a thesis of *dual rationality*. He claims a choice is only free (undetermined and intelligible) when it is rationally founded or can be rationally founded in *both* directions. He considers the *effort of the will* as the indeterministic element. But then there is the question as to which extent this indeterministic element originates in ourselves. The element of agency, which essentially justifies personal accountability, is neglected. In order to establish agency, the indeterministic element would have to be part of the agent himself. Based on our present knowledge, that would mean that it must be part of his brain. Therefore, many libertarians postulate undetermined quantum processes in the brain. In chapter 3 I will deal with these theories in detail.

7.3 Compatibilism
Compatibilistic theories diminish at least one of the three components. Classical compatibilists (Moore, Hume) restrict themselves to a conditional analysis of *being able to do otherwise*. Contemporary compati-

bilists also seriously deal with our intuitions about being able to do otherwise, but they shift the concept of open possibilities from the ontological to an epistemic level. It is important that we envision possibilities, although we do not yet know whether we can make them become real. And it is important that we know of possibilities, for which we know how we could make them become real, and which play a part in our deliberations (Dennett 1984; Nathan 1992).

In contrast, other theories concentrate on the second and third components. They try plausibly to explain what intelligible action is or when intelligible action of such and such a kind can be understood as the action of a person, when a person can justly be considered the agent of her intelligible actions. This last point draws these considerations strongly toward the ethical implications mentioned previously, which are connected to the idea of agency. These theories can be divided into three groups:

i. *Hierarchical compatibilism* emphasizes the fact that the volitional structure of human beings is hierarchical. For a diminished concept of freedom (that implies moral responsibility) it is decisive to which extent a person *identifies* herself with her will, which means to which extent she acts with conviction. We have identification, when, at a higher level, a person wants to have the desires that she actually has.[79] *Capacity theories* on the other hand can be distinguished from *identification theories*. Capacity theories emphasize the skills or capacities a person must possess in order to be able to make intelligible choices.[80] The most potent and most natural criticism of hierarchical compatibilism says that a person is not free to have particular higher level desires and capacities or to command certain skills. As in the regress argument, we are thrown back to the question of being able to do otherwise. Even though they think that this first component is unimportant, the defenders of hierarchical compatibility nevertheless make an effort to find criteria for putting an end to infinite regress.

ii. *Responsiveness theories* try to reconcile intelligibility and agency by emphasizing responsiveness to rational reasons. They assume that a person acts freely when the *mechanism* that leads to a decision is responsive to reasons in a particular, weak sense. What is not meant is a form of rationality dualism, since these reasons can be natural causes. These theories are different from theories of agent causation in that they do not deal with an agent as a substance; instead they concentrate on a mechanism working within him. If a scenario can be set up in which the same *type* of mechanism is at work and in which the agent has reasons for acting differently, he will act differently for just these reasons (Fischer 1994, chapter 8). Obviously, here we no longer have the question of whether one would act otherwise in an identical situation, but whether one would act otherwise in a comparable situation. The difficulty remains of just how we come to have such mechanisms (regress argument) and to which extent the possession of such mechanisms means being the author of one's acts. The history of a person is particularly important for this last question.[81]

iii. *Valuational compatibilists* postulate that an action is voluntary when it takes place in accordance with valuations. "Valuations" presuppose both an evaluation, which in its classical meaning (Plato, Stoicism, Spinoza, and Kant) is necessarily rational, as well as a relation to values. Values and valuations can be objective or subjective.[82] In these terms we can say that Kant defends an objective valuation theory: Only acts which are morally right—that is, acts guided by the categorical imperative—are free.[83] This leads to a contra-intuitive consequence that wrong actions are always involuntary. Susan Wolf (1980, 1990), who propagates a combined subjective-objective valuation theory, tries to stay clear of this consequence by postulating "asymmetrical freedom." In her view actions of a person are *free*, if "and only if she is able to form her actions on the basis of her values *and* is able to form her values on the basis of what is True and Good" (Wolf 1990, p. 75). The relation between freedom and moral responsibility is asymmetrical because the condition of being able to do otherwise is used differently for each of them. Someone whose actions are good and right is free *and* responsible, because he thereby manifests a kind of normative competence characteristic of free actions. This is also valid when his good and right actions are determined. Someone who acts wrongly, in contrast, is only morally responsible if he could have done otherwise.[84] In chapter 3 I will formulate a variant of valuational compatibilism as a conceptual consequence to agency that does not found moral responsibility in Kant's or Wolf's meaning, but which does explain and justify personal accountability.[85]

This short survey of contemporary theories is certainly incomplete. But it does illustrate how the component view and this collection of arguments enable us to comprehend and evaluate those positions. The structure of all arguments remains essentially the same. This is true for the perennial challenges in philosophy. Often only the phrasing or the context of arguments is novel. It is quite difficult to find or invent new questions on free will. What can we do? How can we move forward—

where is knowledge to be gained? Loyal to my understanding of philosophy as I explained it in the introduction, I plan to test old arguments and theories against new facts. There are plenty of them. The brain sciences are on their way to researching and clearing up neurobiological foundations of mental events one by one. True, we do not have a total picture yet. We still do not have a theory that explains how our mind functions, but the puzzle is being put together piece by piece. We have already mentioned that most people have the "natural" conviction that they possess free will. This conviction is due to certain experiences and enriched by our cultural values of freedom and self-determination. The least that neurophilosophy can try to do is to attempt to explain the experience of being able to do otherwise, intelligibility and agency—by using the means and insights of neuroscience itself. If we simultaneously keep our eye on the ongoing philosophical debate, we can explain some of these experiences *naturally*, without retrieving the concept of libertarian free will, which is incompatible with causal determinism. This would give us an argument for demonstrating that the assumption of a strong version of free will is superfluous, even though we have not, strictly speaking, *refuted* it. That is not the goal of a neurophilosophy of free will anyway. Our goal is to find out how we must alter the traditional libertarian concept of free will so that it is compatible with our knowledge about the brain. That is the task of chapter 3, where I will discuss each component in detail. But first, chapter 2 explains what "neurophilosophy" is and what it means for the philosophy of mind.

2

Neurophilosophy: Empirical Challenges to Philosophical Theories

Synopsis

This chapter introduces the nascent discipline called neurophilosophy. Section 1 portrays its origins in the twentieth century along with some historic harbingers. A synopsis of mind-body theories follows. Working through these is mandatory for any kind of neurophilosophy. I then turn to the challenge of reductionism (2.1) and explain and critically analyze two influential advocates of neurophilosophy: Maturana's (2.2) neurobiological radical constructivism (2.2) and the Churchlands' eliminative materialism (2.3). Connectionism and some of its troubles follow as a fundament for a neurophilosophical theory of the mental. Finally, section 3 sketches a program for minimal neurophilosophy. Besides general and systematic reflections (3.1), I explore the notion of supervenience and the concept of emergence and relate them to the challenge of mental causation (3.2). Some notes on the naturalism of neurophilosophy close the chapter.

1 The History of Neurophilosophy

1.1 The Beginnings

Patricia Churchland's book *Neurophilosophy* appeared in 1986. It introduces modern neurosciences, discusses some central issues in analytical philosophy of mind and attempts to combine both sides of the discourse. Churchland (1986, p. 3) challenges us to team the top-down research approach of philosophy with the bottom-up methods of neuroscience in order to gain a common theory of the brain. The drive for neurophilosophy is obvious. Just as in other coalesced disciplines, like neuropsychology, the motivation in neurophilosophy is to bring two sciences closer together, let them be reciprocally influential and mutually fruitful in hopes of developing one integrative, common discipline or at least a joint research program. This preliminary characterization will suffice for the greater part of chapter 2; toward the end I will introduce my own concept of neurophilosophy, which emphasizes the philosophical corner.

In all fairness we must note that despite Patricia Churchland's coining the term, another publication—quoted with rather scanty respect in scientific circles—actually marks the birth of contemporary neurophilosophy: Karl Popper and John Eccles' *The Self and Its Brain* (1977). That book received huge scientific and public resonance and forced philosophers for the first time to come to terms with brain research. Eccles propagates interactionistic dualism, that is, the idea that a "self-conscious" mind has an effect on the brain. This notion enabled traditional dualists to accept the newest findings in brain research. It also compelled those who opposed this kind of dualism to retort in depth to neuroscientific research in order to be noticed at all against the backdrop of Eccles' scholarly competence as a Nobel Prize-winning neurobiologist. The result was fortunate: Fifteen years ago hardly a philosopher knew that the left half of the brain dominates language capacities, or anything about split-brain patients, what an EEG is, or what a homunculus in the brain might be. Nowadays these are basic lessons for all students in the philosophy of mind. Concepts like *readiness potential, blindsight, binding*, and *PET* are not foreign to them; they have at least heard of them, although they might not understand them properly.

Of course, Popper and Eccles and Patricia Churchland's books do not exhaust neurophilosophy. The twentieth century has known at least five well-established varieties: identity theory, interactionistic dualism, eliminative materialism, radical constructivism, and neurophilosophy as an integrative science.

Identity theory claims that mental states are identical with neural states. It is primarily a decidedly physicalistic position. The hypothesis of identity was more programmatic than actually being based on specific details about the brain. Identity theory prepared the way for ensuing theories, although it made philosophers *nolens volens* aware of neurophilosophical theses at all. Also, identity theory discourse was the cradle in which many currently significant issues were first rocked. I will portray some of them in chapter 3. Interactionistic dualism no longer has a good reputation, but for many reasons it is still present in the debate. Two reasons are: First, against the setting of interactionistic dualism it is easier to define other theories. Second, supporters of interactionistic dualism are once again cropping up, encouraged by philosophers defending property dualism. Radical constructivism and eliminative materialism have had great impact on contemporary theories. This is mainly due to the fact that radical constructivis is theoretically and practically narrowly connected to newer empirical-scientific work, namely the theory of self-organization. Similarly, eliminative materialism is not only related to the neurosciences, but is also interwoven with connectionism. Both varieties will be dealt with in section 3 of this chapter. At this point I would like to simply consider the concept of neurophilosophy as an integrative science.

There are many empirical, scientific joint disciplines exhibiting the attribute "neuro." Besides classic and established disciplines such as neurology, neurobiology, neurogenetics, neurochemistry, neurophysiology, neuroanatomy, and neuropsychology, recent years have brought forth fusions such as neuroimaging (Posner and Raichle 1996; Walter 1997b) and also witnessed the development of truly *interdisciplinary* approaches: (a revived) neuropsychiatry (Cummings 1985; Northoff 1997a), cognitive neuroscience (Gazzaniga 1995), psychoneuroimmunology (Schedlowski and Thewes 1996), and neurolinguistics (Kutas and van Petten 1994; Sproat 1995), some of which even have their own university departments, such as neuroinformatics (Rojas 1993). Considering that neurosciences make up the largest research program worldwide, it was only a matter of time before a discipline like neurophilosophy became established. It even already branches off into neuroepistemology (Oeser and Seitelberger 1988; Vogeley 1995), neurosemantics (Kurthen 1992), neuroethics (P.S. Churchland 1991) and most recently, neurophenomenolgy (Varela 1997).[1]

Now, it is one thing to invent a name for a discipline and something entirely different to actually do research along those lines. Even though philosophy is no longer the "principle science," perhaps it could at least take over the part of the superior science within the concert of disciplines. Klaus Mainzer defines neurophilosophy as a "necessary and critical position with epistemological and ethical, practical intentions within a research program of coordinated disciplines" (Mainzer 1994, p. 151).

Northoff (1997a, p. 30) speaks of a "critical position in the interdisciplinary context of various sciences which deal with brain function." If we were to take this seriously, we would have to add several other disciplines to neurophilosophy, besides neuroscience and philosophy alone: Calculation theory, computer science theory, robot theory, cybernetics, artificial intelligence, evolution theory, cognitive psychology, biological psychiatry, neuropsychology, connectionism, nonstable thermodynamics, chaos theory, artificial life, complex systems theory, mobotics, neuro-technology, and so on (says Mainzer 1994). Although it is true that these disciplines are important for neurophilosophy, the more interdisciplinary we conceive it, the more diffuse our integrative approach becomes. Above all, what happens to the specifically philosophical aspect of it all? In the confusion of disciplines philosophy either dwindles, loses significance, or is indignantly rejected as a meddling with genuinely scientific issues. In my opinion, what makes it neurophilosophy is the combination of philosophy and neurosciences. We can take for granted that it incorporates findings from other disciplines. In particular, computer science, cognitive science, and evolution theory have impacts on neurophilosophy. In part 3 of this chapter I will put forth a concept of neurophilosophy, which—in spite of the interdisciplinary character—limits itself to the essential. I call it *minimal* neurophilosophy. But we are not that far yet. In order to pave the way I must first explain some fundamentals of neurophilosophy. That includes a little early history, a brief introduction to the mind-body problem, and a short depiction of both neurocentered kinds of radical contructivism and eliminative materialism. Subsequently, the advantages of minimal neurophilosophy will become evident.

1.2   Historical Precursors

The idea of materialism is ancient, but that is not the focus of this brief historical outline. Here we are only interested in the extent to which the brain was considered the organ of the soul in the history of our culture.[2] The first historical evidence that humans might have suspected some connection between the brain and the soul is given by trepanations, that is the sawing of bone pieces out of the skull, a ritual proven to have been practiced 10,000 years ago. We can speculate whether that was meant to enable the soul to escape. But we must be careful not to project our own ideas into ancient times. The first written mention of the brain is found in the so-called "Papyrus Smith," a medical work from Egypt, dated 1700 B.C., although it might go back to the third millennium B.C. It reveals that Egyptians saw a relationship between the brain and some functions, albeit motor functions. We can conclude that the brain as the seat of the soul was not overly precious to them from the fact that embalmed Pharaohs were laid to rest without their brains. The sixth century B.C. gives us the first Greek neurophilosophical standpoint, formulated by Alkmaion of Kroton: "It is the brain which allows perceptions such as hearing, seeing and smelling; these create memory and imagination, and from memory and imagination—when they have settled down and found peace—knowledge is created" (Alkmaion of Kroton, quoted in translation from Oeser and Seitelberger 1988, p. 3).

It is probably no accident that Alkmaion was the first person known to dissect humans. He discovered the optical nerve, which he described as a channel leading from the eye pits to the brain, which he thought held pneuma (breath or air). The notion of the air-like character of the soul goes back at least to Homer. A hundred years after Alkmaion, Hippocrates guessed that the "sacred illness," namely epilepsy, was a brain disease. He further claimed that the brain was the messenger to consciousness and related to it what happens. But the medium of thinking, he thought not to be that "crumbly, white" brain stuff, but the air, which first enters the brain through respiration and then spreads throughout the body.

In terms of locating the soul, ancient Greek philosophers had two different notions: Plato's brain-centered thesis and Aristotle's heart-centered thesis. In the dialogue *Timaios* Plato (427–347 B.C.) discerned three constituents of the soul—the desirous, the courageous, and the knowing part. In his dialogue *Phaedo* he tells how Socrates in his youth ruminated on Alkmaion's idea that the brain creates mental processes (Plato 1987: 96b). Although he also seriously considered that possibility, he rejected such physiological speculations as being of little use, because they could not explain the *purposefulness* of human rationality.[3] Aristotle denied that the soul could be located in the brain, on the grounds of his empirical experience, gathered on the battleground. His observation was entirely correct, that an exposed brain does not react to mechanical stimulation and is cooler than the rest of the body. Confirmed by the furrowed look of cerebral convolutions with their similarity to cooling systems, he concluded that the function of the brain is to lower blood temperature.[4] And it also brings sleep. But the real seat of the soul, the place for feelings, passion, and understanding, was the heart. This idea is understandable from an everyday psychological point of view: We do experience many feelings around the heart. But for Aristotle the argument for the heart as the soul's site was particularly that this is where all the blood vessels from the periphery meet. The notion of a central organ where all the senses meet—according to Sherington, the founder of the theory of synapses—was heuristically an extremely prolific idea, even though Aristotle chose the wrong organ.

However, Aristotle's scheme had already been revised in ancient times. As early as 300 A.D. Greeks Herophilus and Erasistratos began systematically dissecting the human brain. Descriptive cerebral anatomy reached a peak not again ascended until the seventeenth century, because medieval religious traditions prohibited dissections. Herophilus and Erasistratos discerned nerves for sensation and nerves for movement. They also discovered brain ventricles and called them chambers. These three cavities lie in a row in the brain and contain brain fluid in living humans; when dissecting cadavers one finds air in them. In contrast to Hippocrates, Erasistratos claimed that first air enters the lung veins via the respiratory system, then it travels to the heart and then—in the form of an animal spirit—it reaches the brain ventricles. This was the first theory to locate mental capacities in the brain ventricles, a theory essentially polished to its final shape by Galen (131–200 A.D.), the ubiquitous commanding medieval medical authority. Although Galen himself did no medical dissecting, he did advise: "Don't look to the gods to discover the omnipotent soul through their insight, it is better to ask an anatomist" (Galen, translated quote taken from Oeser and Seitelberger 1988, p. 6).

Galen discerned a *pneuma psychikon* (animal spirit), which was made out of the *pneuma zootikon* (vital spirit) of the air we breathe and then stored (*pneuma*, Gr.: air, breath). He combined ventricle theory with

Aristotle's theory of knowledge and psychology. Mental capacities were thus located as follows. Understanding (*vis cogitativa*) and memory (*vis memorativa*) are in the second and third chamber, the first chamber holds the *sensus communis*, which—according to Aristotle—unites all the senses, as well as the imagination (*vis imaginativa*). In the fourth century A.D. Nemesius, Bishop of Emesa, reformulated the ventricle theory so that it was consistent with medieval Christian doctrine (see Doty 1965, p. 27). Medieval theologians as well as Arabian commentators on Aristotle absorbed it without question. Except for minimal supplements,[5] for the next 1,400 years succeeding Galen essentially little new knowledge surfaced, there were few novel conjectures or hypotheses about the relation of mind to brain.

Not until 1543, when Andreas Vesalius founded modern anatomy, did new questions arise and knowledge widen. Dissection was acceptable once again and Vesalius put an end to the Galen's ventricle teachings. His anatomic findings demonstrated that there was nothing but water in the ventricles. He shunned neurophilosophical speculation, however, and left—along with his immediate students—the question of the soul to the philosophers. He was the first to draw attention to the significance of cerebral convolutions, but he also noticed that anatomically these were pretty much the same in humans and donkeys.

The next decisive and directive step was taken by René Descartes (1596–1650), who can be considered the philosophical father of interactionistic dualism.[6] His renowned theory of interactionistic dualism is found in his posthumously published work *De homine* (1662). As a rationalist he felt that increasing scientific knowledge demanded an explanation about how the brain and mental skills of man are related. While earlier thinkers considered the soul to be independent, yet tightly entwined with the body (or brain), Descartes separated them radically. On one side, he said, we have *res extensa*, extended substance, to which also the brain belongs; on the other side we have *res cogitans*, the thinking substance. It would be erroneous to think that Descartes was anti-scientific because of his dualism. For it was his radical distinction between mind and matter that initially gave thrust to the idea of thinking of the body and the brain in terms of machines *without* degrading the divine privilege of reason. (Feelings and sensation, however, retained a purely mechanical nature, in his opinion.) Descartes, who was a cofounder of analytical geometry and the laws of mechanics, thought that the interaction among the two substances obeyed mechanical principles. He guessed that their reciprocal effects were located in the pineal gland (now known as the pineal body), for this was the only structure in the brain known to him of which there was only one. It thus had a special status. According to Descartes, the animal spirits pass through the pineal gland and the various ducts of the body to animate it and perform their work. He was concerned with the problem of interaction because the law of impulse conservation was already valid for the mechanics of his time. He tried to solve this difficulty by postulating that the mind alters the direction that the animal spirits take, but not their impulse.

We can say that Descartes's theory maintained popularity well into the twentieth century, even though it was criticized by many materialistic philosophers like Thomas Hobbes or the Frenchman LaMettrie, who wrote the book *L'homme machine* in 1747. But not all dualists shared his interactionism. Leibniz, universal scholar and philosopher, defended parallelism. He also considered it absolutely inconceivable that the brain could produce mind if it were a mechanical machine. He demonstrated this with a thought experiment that was a forerunner of one of our thoroughly discussed contemporary thought experiments, namely John Searle's Chinese room:

Furthermore, we must necessarily concede that perception and what depends on it is inexplicable in mechanical terms, i.e., with the aid of figures and movements. Suppose we had a machine designed to produce thoughts, feelings and perceptions. We would certainly be able to imagine this machine proportionately so enlarged, that we could walk right into it, as we do into a mill. Assuming this, when we inspect the interior we will find nothing but single pieces bumping against one another—and never find anything that would explain perception. Therefore, we must search for perception in the simple substance and not in compounds or in machinery! (Leibniz 1747/1979, § 14)

Kant discouraged any reputation for neurophilosophy for quite a while. His transcendental philosophy divided empirical knowledge and philosophical insight into two disjunct spheres. Philosophy is a matter for reason only, and can never be comprehended empirically. In concluding remarks to a book titled *On the Organ of the Soul* (1796) written by German brain anatomist Soemmerring (1755–1839), Kant writes that anything like neurophilosophy is unlikely. Soemmerring had picked up and repropagated Galen's ventricle theory, which science had long abandoned. It drew attention, but also ridicule. Using kind words, Kant found two arguments for constraint. First, he reasoned, ventricle theory cannot explain mind, because mind is organized and brain water is unorganized (Kant 1796/1983, A 83/84). And, he continues, even if we wanted to understand mind as "dynamically" organized matter, matter can never explain consciousness, because the capacity to know oneself would end in contradiction. The soul can have no specific location, because in order to recognize itself, it would have to be outside of itself, which is not possible (Kant 1796/1983, A 86). Ulrich Müller (1996) notes that Kant conjured up a grave schism by insisting that in the "squabble among faculties" medicine and philosophy have separate realms of competence. Ever since Kant philosophers have obeyed this division of labor, to the disadvantage of neurophilosophy.

At least Müller's description is right. A long time elapsed after Kant before any philosopher of importance had anything to say about the brain, while in science profound findings kept tumbling in, compelling many neuroscientists to consider the philosophical implications of their research. In 1796, the year in which Soemmerring's book appeared, a new epoch began that continues right up to today. In private lectures in Vienna Franz Joseph Gall (1758–1828) sketched the basic lines of a new subject called "organology" or "skull theory," later termed *phrenology* by Gall's student Spurzheim. Contemporary German neuroanatomist Karl Zilles considers phrenology to have been the decisive turning point: In phrenology, "the metaphysical question of locating the organ of the soul is replaced by a concept of individual areas representing sensory, motor, and associative functions in the brain cortex" (Zilles 1994, p. 191).

Gall explicitly refrained from dealing with metaphysical issues. Instead of *one* organ for the soul, he postulated twenty-seven organs in the cerebral cortex, each of which enabled special mental functions. Today, this principle is still influential in neuropsychology. But Gall's other theses, for instance, that prominent features of cerebral parts correlate positively with distinctive marks of mental functions, and that we can conclude mental functions by taction—feeling the shape of skull indentations or bumps—have been dropped, of course. We also no longer think that particular attributes like friendship, ambition, or generosity have their own sites in the brain. Gall was a talented speaker and cherished popular physician, but not an empirical scientist. His most significant concept, however, was empirically confirmed just three years before his death. In 1825 Jean Baptiste Bouillard declared a frontal area of the cortex to be the speech center (Zilles 1994, p. 194). Traditionally, however, the discovery of the motor speech center is attributed to French surgeon and anthropologist Paul Broca. In 1861, after the death of a patient with a certain speech defect, namely motor aphasia, he found damage in the left front part of the patient's brain, which he associated with that defect. This marks the beginning of modern neuropsychology, which correlates cerebral damage with specific losses of function. It was founded by Fritsch and Hitzig, Oskar and Cecilie Vogt, and Korbinian Brodmann. Neuropsychology first blossomed in the late nineteenth century in Germany. Many syndromes were discovered and described that people still talk about today: neglect (nonperception of certain space or body parts), all the apraxias (lack of ability to execute certain acts; see particularly Freund 1987), blind sight (ability to process visual information despite a lack of conscious visual perception), and many others (see Kolb and Wishaw 1996).

Sigmund Freud began his career as a neuroanatomist. Even today his comprehensive monograph on aphasias (speech defects due to brain damage) is still familiar in neuropsychological circles (Freud 1891). His 1895 manuscript, *A Project for a Scientific Psychology*, is less well-known.[7] In it Freud attempted to reduce the psychic apparatus to laws of psychophysics and connect normal and abnormal psychology. In this draft Freud stated ideas that come surprisingly close to cybernetics and particularly connectionism (cf. Pribam 1965). We could label Freud an early neurophilosopher. The evaluation of Freud's draft in terms of his own work, however, remains controversial. While classic Freudians view the fact that he abandoned the project as evidence that he considered it to be headed in the wrong direction, others view the draft as proof of his basically reductionistic standpoint, which he did not further pursue, merely because the times and scientific state of the art were not ripe for it. In *Beyond the Principle of Lust* Freud wrote: "The deficiencies of our description [of psychic events] would probably dissolve, if we could replace psychological terms with physiological or chemical terms" (Freud 1920/1940, p. 65).

Besides the correlation discovered between brain damage and functions, the discovery of the electrochemical nature of neuronal information transmission was important. The discovery of animal electricity by Luigi Galvani in 1786 deemed it unnecessary to postulate animal spirits or nerve fluids. Studies in the physics of nerves developed, becoming neurophysiology. When the German psychiatrist Hans Berger discovered the EEG in 1924, he hoped to have found a correlate to psychic energy. At this time the dispute between the Spanish neuroanatomists Golgi and Cajal about whether nerves are a connected continuum or whether they consist of individual neurons had long been decided in favor of the latter. And Sherrington's discovery of synapses, at which electrical impulses are transformed into chemical signals, ultimately amalgamated the anatomy, physiology, and chemistry of the nervous system into one large science.

Presently, we cannot delve in detail into the exciting history of neuroscience (cf. Breidbach 1997). We are interested in how these discoveries led to philosophical questions and answers. One important consequence was the dismemberment of mental abilities. Instead of seeking the seat of the soul, research soon emphasized the location of individual functions. This acutely illustrates a difficulty that Kant pointed out. Faced with the abundance of sensations, how do we arrive at a unity of consciousness? This issue, called the *binding problem*, has mutated to an empirically approachable question in contemporary neurophysiology. Heinz Schmitz (1996), a philosopher from Düsseldorf, gives the philosophical ruminations of the founders of neurophysiology the label "physiological Neo-Kantianism," that is, the attempt to find a solution for fundamental problems of knowledge, such as Kant suggested, with the assistance of science, or at least in light of scientific findings. He affirms that the intellectual forefather of the physiological Neo-Kantians (Johannes Müller, Hermann von Helmholtz, Ernst Heinrich Weber, and Ernst Kapp) was none other than empiricist David Hume. In particular, Müller's law of specific sense energy was central for Neo-Kantian contemplations on the theory of knowledge. This law involves the commonplace observation that the "sense energy" generated in the perceptual organ depends on the kind of stimulation present. A drastic example illustrates this. Normally, optical impressions are generated by light stimulation. But striking the eye causes us to see stars in the same way that electrical stimulation elicits specific visual sensations. On the other hand, when the same electrical stimulation irritates different organs, the result is differing sensations: visual in the eye, acoustic in the ear. " 'It makes absolutely no difference what kind of stimulation meets the sense organ, the effect is a matter of the energy of the sense organ' (Müller 1826, 45). The law of specific sense energies therefore says that 'we do not perceive external things, we perceive changes in our sense substances brought forth by the things' (Dubois-Reymond 1912, p. 151)" (Translated quote from Schmitz 1996, p. 48).

Observe the parallel to Kant's thesis that it is the thing itself that affects us, but that we know nothing about the thing itself, only something about the way our mind functions. Physiological Neo-Kantians in turn wanted to understand how perceptions generate ideas, how subjective reality and objective externals are related, how a coherent stream of consciousness develops from isolated stimuli, what Kantian a priorities look like in physiological terms, which role causality plays within the nervous system, how spatial perception works, why we have insight into some things and not into others, which regularities of thought follow from laws of physiology, and so on (see Schmitz 1996). New discoveries, in this case the law of specific sense energy, almost inevitably steer us in the direction of philosophical puzzlement.

Unfortunately, there was no academic contact between philosophy and neuroscience, just as Kant propagated. Philosophy developed in complete isolation from neuroscience and clung to pure reason. Schmitz (1966, p. 42) claims that Hegel introduced the chasm between the speculating mind, comprehending thinking and positive natural science into continental philosophy. He quotes from the *Phenomenology of Mind*:

Hence the important thing for the student of science is to make himself undergo the strenuous toil of conceptual reflection, of thinking in the form of the notion. This demands concentrated attention on the notion as such, on simple and ultimate determinations like being-in-itself, being-for-itself, self-identity, and so on;

for these are elemental, pure, self-determined functions of a kind we might call souls, were it not that their conceptual nature denotes something higher than that term contains. (Hegel 1807/1980, p. 41; English version taken from J. B. Baillie's translation, 1967, p. 116)

At the end of the nineteenth century, neurophilosophical conclusions drawn by scientists ebbed after neuropsychology had passed its zenith. Several factors explain this. One is the rise of behaviorism, which limited itself radically to the study of observable behavior and barred the investigation of inner mental processes as being unscientific. Then, in 1949, *The Concept of Mind* by the English philosopher Gilbert Ryle appeared. Ryle criticized the traditional dualistic notion of the mind as a "ghost in a machine." The concept of mind, says Ryle, is not based on innocent intuitions, but is the product of neglecting to analyze or incorrectly analyzing mentalistic vernacular. Ryle's book simultaneously brought relief and disaster. Falling on the fruitful ground of behaviorism, it silenced dualistic speculation in philosophy. On the other hand it elicited the dominance of conceptual analysis in the philosophy of mind that is effective up to this day. Not until identity theory moved in was the brain once again a focus of philosophical interest. In the following section let us systematically explore the mind-body problem as the question of the relation between mind and brain.

2   Facets of Neurophilosophy

2.1   A Brief Introduction to the Mind-Body Problem

Today the mind-body problem is usually understood as a mind-brain problem[8] and can be stated as the question: How are brain and mind related? More generally, how are mental and physical phenomena related? Naturally, within our context, I cannot describe the entire complex of this issue in a historical or systematic way that would come anywhere near being complete.[9] Still, for the project of neurophilosophy it is extremely important to at least be familiar with the mind-body problem and know just what is the topic of the philosophy of the mental. For this purpose I will briefly portray and explain the most common positions.

2.1.1 Substances The so-called "substance quarrel" is the classic mind-body problem. It begins with the question of whether the soul (or mind, or consciousness) is a special, second kind of substance or whether it is merely a different form of one single substance (cf. Vollmer 1986, pp. 66–99). The assumption that body and soul—today we speak more of matter–energy and mind—make up two different substances, will be called (substance) dualism in the following; the opposite assumption is monism. Depending on which assumption one shares, one gets different questions. The dualist inquires: *Are there* reciprocal effects among the substances? The answer is usually positive. Though parallelism is one exception. The next question is: *In which directions* are these effects transitive? Generally reciprocal effects are assumed. Substance dualists view the mind as immaterial and not locatable—in contrast to a matter–energy substance. Therefore, we have the next question: *Where* do the mutual effects take place? But the real puzzle for dualists is finally: *How* do these reciprocal effects happen? For if the mind can effect the material–energy world it must have causal influence and be able to change it.

The monist on the other hand must ask himself: *What is* the one and only existing substance? He can envision it as mind (spiritualism), or matter–energy (materialism) or another unknown and unnamed substance (neutral monism). But because our inquiry assumes that there are at least two different kinds of phenomena, the monist must still face the question: *How* is it that one substance displays both aspects? Identity theory, in particular, which identifies mental states with brain states, must address this question: *What are* the structural and functional peculiarities of those neural states and processes, considered to be mental experiences, in comparison to those that are not mental experiences?

Table 2.1 contains a survey of the prominent historical positions on the substance issue. According to the clock allegory in dualism—introduced by Geulincx and used by Leibniz—mind and matter are like two clocks that show the same time. Their synchronization can occur through various kinds of mutual effects, shown in table 2.1 by the direction of the arrows. This scheme, of course, cannot show all the possible positions in detail. We cannot rally ancient and medieval thinkers into the

Table 2.1
The Mind-Body Problem

Substance Dualism Clock Allegory	Substance Monism

Parallelism
Brain and mind are independent
of each other, but synchronized.
How are they synchronized?

Neutral monism (double aspect theory)
Mind and matter are merely different
aspects of a single (unknown) substance.
(Heraclitus, Spinoza, Schelling, Ostwald,
Russell, Feigl)

(a) Autonomism
Synchronization is random.
(No advocates)

Spiritualism
Everything is spirit. There is no matter.
(Berkeley, Fichte, Hegel, Schopenhauer,
Mach, Whitehead)

(b) Occasionalism
Synchronization is continually
kept up and controlled by God.
(Geulincx, Malebranche)

Strict materialism
Everything is matter. There is no
spirit. (Hobbes, LaMettrie, Holbach,
Vogt, Moleschott)

(b) Prestabilized Harmony
Fixed by God for all time at the
time of creation. (Leibniz)

Philosophical behaviorism
Mental entities are behavioral
dispositions. (Skinner, Ryle, Wittgenstein,
Malcolm, Quine)

Eliminative materialism
There are no mental entities. Mental
expressions will be replaced by
neurophysiological terms. (Feyerabend,
Rorty, Stich, Churchland)

Dualistic epiphenomenalism
Brain controls mind without
feedback.

Monistic epiphenomenalism
Mind is merely an epiphenomenon, (a
reflection, a shadow, a secretion) of
neural processes without causal feedback
(Epicurus, Lucretius, Nietzsche,
T. H. Huxley, Broad, Ayer)

Table 2.1
Continued

Substance Dualism Clock Allegory	Substance Monism
Animism Spirit animates all matter. (Plato, Plotinus, Augustine)	**Functionalism** Mental states are functional states. *Hylemorphism* (Aristotle, Thomas Aquinas, New-Thomism) *Machine functionalism* (Putnam, Fodor) *Teleofunctionalism* (Papineau, Millikan)
Interactionism Brain and mind are actively mutually effective. (Descartes, Penfield, Popper, Eccles, von Ditfurth)	**Identity theory** Mental entities are identical with complex neuronal states and/or processes. *Type Identity Theory* (Place, Smart, Bunge, Vollmer) *Token Identity Theory* (Davidson, Kim) *Causal role IT* (Lewis)
	Nonreductive materialism Mental entities are always realized physically, but not reducible to physical entities. *Anomalous Monism* (Davidson) *Property Dualism* (Honderich, Chalmers) *New Emergence Theory* (Stephan)

Various proposals and advocates of substance monism and dualism (taken from Vollmer 1986, p. 78, and modified). The clock allegory symbolizes the sort of causal mutual effects posited between mental and physical substance.

scheme without doing them injustice because they were not familiar with the question of substance dualism in its contemporary form. Some positions will be nailed to neither dualism nor monism. For example, for epiphenomenalism the substance issue is insignificant. Important is the fact that causal effectiveness works only in *one* direction (from matter to mind). And functionalism can be defended by dualists as well as by nonreductive materialists. But on the whole a survey such as this proves valuable for getting an initial grasp of the subject.

2.1.2 Contemporary Families of Theories Nowadays few philosophers defend *interactionistic substance dualism.*[10] Nevertheless, I intend to discuss it in a little more detail for two reasons. First, as I suggested earlier, it is a variety of neurophilosophy that gained widespread attention. Second, in many expositions it is still very much alive and kicking, partially because our traditional way of thinking has been heavily influenced by Descartes. In the worst case, it provides us with a straw man to beat upon without injuring ourselves; in the best case it works like an opponent's proposal. It pokes at exactly those sore spots for which it is most difficult to find satisfactory answers. Why is it hard to find supporters for this position in the philosophy of mind; why is it considered anachronistic? The answer is simple. This theory is a scientific anomaly. On one hand, Eccles proposes that the self-conscious mind is not subject to normal laws of nature; on the other hand he explains that the self-confident mind is in a position to effect and be affected by a part of the physical world, that is, the brain. He thus clings to the concept of mental causation. A change in the physical condition of the brain, however, requires energy. A kind of mental causation that introduces energy into the physical world, which was not previously there, violates the law of conservation of energy. Furthermore, information on physical influences on the brain, such as reactions to drugs or consciousness-altering drugs, must be conveyed to the mental substance. According to notions to date, this would not be possible without energy transfer. The interactionism dualist has two options. First, he must claim that information transfer occurs without energy transfer. Only a wonder can handle that. This is logically possible, but quite useless: Wonders can prove anything. Second, the dualist can suggest that the violation of the law of the conservation of energy is so minimal that it is practically not measurable. In fact, this is Eccles' strategy—summoning quantum physics (Eccles 1990). But a violation of the law of the conservation of energy remains just that, no matter how minimal. The scientific anomaly does not disappear, it just escapes testing.

Can the thesis of dualism be tested in any way at all? The way brain research is dealt with in the media we are made to believe that it should be possible (because we can observe some brain processes directly on living brains) to decide whether dualism is true or false by collecting empirical data. Those hopes are misleading. Scientific proof of a mental substance is impossible, because the mental substance suggested by dualism is *by definition* not accessible scientifically. All that remains is negative proof, such as evidence that certain phenomena cannot be explained by monistic theory. However, it is not enough to simply claim—or prove—that something cannot be explained in monistic terms. Perhaps it is merely *not yet* explainable. We need an argument stating why a particular phenomenon cannot, in principle, *be* explained in terms of monism. Favorite candidates for this avenue are subjective states of consciousness, although they can only be tested indirectly. Can dualism be refuted? Unfortunately, no. Even *if* everything were explainable in monistic terms—something that will probably never be the case—that would still not refute dualism! Whatever can be explained by one substance can naturally be explained by two (or more) substances. Of course there are prudent reasons for thrift and getting by without the second substance (Ockham's razor, cf. section 6.3 of chapter one). Perhaps it is this insight that makes interactionistic dualism so unprofitable for science.

One method of retaining dualism without maintaining substance dualism is to assume strict *parallelism*. This position has found some contemporary advocates. Modern parallelists either leave the above-mentioned critical aspects of interaction open (Linke and Kurthen 1988) or they postulate a necessarily nature-given linkage between mental and neurophysiological properties: common occurrence without interaction (Honderich 1990a, 1990b, 1995). This clears away the problem of interaction, but it remains uneconomical. A parallelist can avoid the query of whether someday it will be possible to explain all phenomena with monism. He simply proposes that for reasons of research heuristics we should assume two different worlds, because our access to the world of the mental is itself mental. In fact, it actually appears that many research projects are implicitly based on parallelism. This is evidenced by the widespread usage of the phrase *"correlates of mental states."*

The search for correlates would be in vain, of course, if we should discover that there are no mental states. This position is *eliminative materialism*. Mental entities are relics, theoretical entities, and as useless as phlogiston is for explaining combustion or as ineffective as demons are for explaining mental illness. According to Wilfried Sellars, we should think of our everyday locution of mental states—also known as *folk psychology*—as a kind of *theory*, and a poor one at that. In spite of its benefits, in many situations it has very little explanatory value. It has been stagnating for over two thousand years. It has become increasingly incompatible with much of our knowledge about ourselves and must urgently be replaced by a better theory. Scientific theories could explain many mental phenomena better than folk psychology, as the theory of oxidation better explains combustion and scientific psychiatry better explains mental illness than do phlogiston and demons. The feeling that this position is contra-intuitive is merely a consequence of our language habits. Sooner or later we will be accustomed to a different vernacular, or we could retain the old jargon for the sake of convenience. Although early eliminative materialists like Feyerabend (1963) formulated this more as a program or to be provocative, some contemporary eliminative materialists—exemplified by the Churchlands (P. S. Churchland 1986; P. M. Churchland 1989, 1995)—try to complete this program. They strive to show how talk of mental states could eventually be replaced with terms of other theoretical entities. For example, certain mental states commonly are described as being *beliefs* and *desires* (a.k.a. *propositional attitudes*). We assume that thinking consists of combining these beliefs and desires in adherence to psychological laws. But eliminative materialists say that findings in the neurosciences and particularly in connectionism prove this assumption to be wrong. Cognitive activity does not consist of reasoning using rules within a system of propositional, sentence-like mental states. Scientific psychology founded on this assumption is prone to fail; brain science in search of physical correlates for beliefs and desires will find them nowhere. The basal units of human cognition are activation vectors of neuron populations; mental processes are transformations of one activation vector into another. While P. M.

Churchland advocates eliminative materialism in its contemporarily purest form, P. S. Churchland belongs more to the reductionist camp, because she does not hold that there are no mental states at all, but only that these are not what we think they are in terms of everyday psychology. Since the reductionist method reconstructs mental states as cerebral states and thereby strongly alters their character, we could—as she herself suggests—more correctly label her position: *revisionistic*.

Eliminative materialism in its most radical form can best be understood as a reaction to spats within the family of identity theories. The zoo of identity theories is made up of various animals. Cynthia MacDonald (1989) discerns three main species of theory: type identity, causal role identity, and token identity. The distinction type–*token* refers to the difference between a *class* of events (type) and one specific *element* of such a class (a *token*). Type identity theory claims that all occurrences of a particular type of mental states are identical with a certain type of neural events. An often cited example is; "Pain is nothing but the firing of C-fibers."[11] However, this kind of identity claim soon aroused opposition, because it does not fulfill certain logical conditions of identity. In this argument, attributing properties to mental or physical states is important. If pain or thoughts are really identical with neurophysiological states, they would have properties that they do not have. According to Leibniz's law of identity—*principium identitatis indiscernibilium*—(the principle of indiscernibility), two things are only identical to each other when they share all properties.[12] The activation of C-fibers is spatially extended; the phenomenal content of pain, thought, and other mental states is not. Therefore, they cannot be identical.

We can reply to this argument in several ways. Either we claim that mental states *are* located in space-time and we are just not accustomed to speaking of them in that way, or we conclude from the indirect proof of nonidentity that there just are no mental states (eliminative materialism). Or we advocate some form of parallelism or double aspect theory, which leaves the question unanswered about which kind of fundamental substance it is, which evidently can have two kinds of properties. Another, metaphysically relatively neutral, option would be to consider the identity theory as a research program and thus as a thesis that will prove wrong or right. Philosophers tend to imagine that questions about identity must be discussed and decided independently of empirical findings.[13] But we can always ask whether it is particularly meaningful to apply Leibniz's law of identity to the mind-body challenge at all (see Bechtel 1988a, p. 98f).

Causal role identity theory classifies types of mental states by the kind of causal relationship they have to other mental and body states. Mental states fulfill a particular causal role and are thus identical to neural states that take over the same causal role (Lewis 1994, p. 418). We cannot automatically equate the concept of pain with certain neural states, because perhaps Martians or abnormal people have entirely different internal states that fulfill the same causal role (Lewis 1989). Lewis thus considers a species-specific kind of identity theory to be true. Pain is defined—among other things—by certain behavioral dispositions, which can be described as causal roles. Causal role identity theorists are also often called functionalists.

Functionalism is the thesis that solely a functional role defines a mental state, no matter what kind of substrate or substance it is made of. One significant argument of functionalism is that of *multiple realization*. One and the same functional state can be realized in different ways, therefore it is wrong to equate a functional state with one specific kind of realization, such as a neural realization. Functional arguments like this are true not only for mental states. A bottle opener, a chair, or money are all things defined *solely* by their function in a particular setting. True, every bottle opener, every chair, every piece of money, and every mental state is in a particular physical state, but its concrete materialization is unimportant. Each of these objects could be made of something else, and yet, if the function remains the same, it would still fulfill the same functional role and thus still be what it is (a chair, money, and so on). So it would be wrong to identify a mental type with a neurophysiological type. From a purely functional standpoint (sometimes called *algorithmic functionalism*) a theory of mental states that describes types must be independent of a substrate, that is, not specific to the brain. (We will meet another variety, teleofunctionalism, in chapter 3.) It is no surprise that many (albeit not all) functionalists think highly of artificial intelligence. Still, most functionalists are materialistic monists. They retain the basic intuition that there is only one substance. We can also call them token identity theorists.

Token identity theorists opine that each *token* of a mental event is identical with one neural *token*. But they do not demand that *types* of mental events are identical with *types* of neural events. If a person A is in a certain mental state, this individual mental occurrence (*token*) is identical to a certain neural occurrence. At other times or in other people the same type of mental state could also manifest itself in a different physical state. One version of this thesis is Donald Davidson's *anomalous monism*. Davidson calls his monism anomalous because in his view there are no strict laws governing the connection between mental and physical states, although mental and physical events are token-identical. Strongly summarized, we can outline his argumentation for token identity as follows (Davidson 1970, pp. 292–316). The theory is based on three premises. First, there is causal interaction between mental and physical events. Second, causality requires that there are general laws to which these events are subject. Third, there are no strict determining laws to which mental events are subject and to which we can make reference when predicting and explaining mental events (the anomaly of the mental). Davidson holds all three principles to be true.[14]

This conceded, we can construct the following argument for physicalism. Since mental and physical events causally interact, they must instantiate a law. They cannot be an example for psychophysical laws, however, because there are no psychophysical laws. Therefore, they must instantiate physical laws. In order for mental events to exemplify physical laws, however, they must have a physical description. To have a physical description, in turn, means to be a physical event. Therefore, all mental events are physical events (in terms of token identity theory).

Many monistic positions share Davidson's thesis that although they are token identical, mental events cannot be reduced to physical events. Nowadays a number of thinkers use the label *nonreductive materialism* for their work, without illumining what it is actually supposed to mean. Many functionalists also designate themselves as nonreductionists. For if we want to reduce mental (qua) functional states to physical states, we can only reduce them to a disjunction of infinitely many manifestations, which would be inefficient. Among the nonreductive monists we also find emergence theorists (Sperry 1980; Stephan 1999); their theses will be discussed later. Most recently, property dualism has joined the scene. This thesis assumes one single substance but (at least) two different classes of properties that cannot be traced back to each other (Honderich 1995; Chalmers 1996a, 1996b).

Two further important theories need mentioning, namely abstractionism (instrumentalism) and pragmatism. These theories question exactly what all the others presuppose: specifically that mental entities are either real or not. They reject this dichotomy by retaining a special kind of realism. According to *abstractionism* mental entities are abstract things or instruments deployed by the subject seeking knowledge (Dennett 1987, 1991). These *abstracta* are useful for ordering experience, recognizing patterns, and predicting behavior, although in a certain meaning of the word they are not real, do not really exist. They are not simply inventions, however, they are justified by the indirect reference they make to entities that do exist. Pragmatic or internal realism holds an intermediate position among the standpoints (Putnam 1982b; Dummett 1982; Goodman 1978). This kind of "Realism with a Human Face" (Putnam) exhibits an antirealistic tendency in that it criticizes positions that try to ascertain the reality of mental (and other) entities beyond the limits of human practices, human language usage, and human reason. Advocates of this position (such as Baker 1993; Brüntrup 1994) plead for pragmatic criteria in discussing mental entities. This plea is based on the conviction that our theories cannot surpass our conceptual systems; there is no standpoint over and above ours (no divine standpoint) and thus our explanations are always relative to our human being. Theories about the world are always also theories about our epistemological skills and limits.

In summary we can say that the trend of the last forty years looks like this. After World War II discussion was first dominated by ontological and metaphysical questions (substance quarrel, identity proposals); it then turned to rather methodical questions of scientific theory (reductionism). Most recently, epistemological, pragmatic issues dominate (concept of explanation, knowledge as practice, embodied cognition). Almost all theorists agree to ontological monism or physicalism. Seldom does a philosopher postulate a spiritual substance for explaining the function of the mind. But there are also several nonreductive materialists and property dualists who support the view that certain classes of properties cannot be traced back to or explained by others. Brüntrup calls this "dualistic ideology with monistic ontology" (Brüntrup 1996, pp. 64f). In other words, today the question of ontological reduction has been replaced by the issue of explanatory reduction. Just what this means we shall see later when discussing mental causation. Doing justice to its unbroken importance, I now turn to the problem of reductionism as seen from the perspective of scientific theory.

2.1.3   The Trouble with Reductionism   In general, reductionism sets up claims of the type that statements of one kind can be traced back—or reduced—to statements of another.[15] The most interesting cases are those that set up daring claims, such as these: Psychic occurrences can be traced back to material occurrences; moral language can be reduced to imperatives; or ethics and the theory of knowledge can be replaced by sociology, psychology, and behavioral biology. The term "reductionism" is often disparaged in these contexts, characterized pejoratively or at least viewed as dangerous. The concept has been discoursed abundantly since the late 1950s. The center of dispute is the reductionistic claim that the behavior of complex systems can be explained by understanding the cooperation of their parts.

The classic concept of reductionism (Nagel 1961) can be traced back to the notion of the unity of the sciences and the deductive-nomologic scheme of explanation developed by Hempel-Oppenheim (the HO scheme). It says that a scientific explanation is a valid conclusion with which we can explain a fact by beginning with constraints and initial conditions and adding natural laws. Strong reduction can then be thought of as deducting the statements of one theory from statements of another. Weak reduction means deducing concepts of one theory from those of another (Hempel 1974, chapter 7). Candidates for reduction can be statements, concepts, laws, or entire disciplines. One frequent example is the successful reduction of thermodynamics to classical mechanics. Thus it is possible, starting with the principles of statistical mechanics, to deduct the Boyle-Charles law of classic thermodynamics, which describes the ratio of temperature and pressure in gases. Critical expressions in the Boyle-Charles law, for example temperature and pressure, are *identified* with terms referring to kinetic properties of ideal molecules. This leads to identity statements such as, "Temperature is the mean kinetic energy of molecules." Assisted by bridge laws and certain constraints (choice of gas and container, etc.), the Boyle-Charles law can then be logically deduced from the laws of statistic mechanics. Three points of this "Nagel reduction" are decisive for the discourse on reduction in neurophilosophy. First, explanation and reduction share the same logical form. Second, discovering identities is important. When such identity is discovered, we speak of *ontological* reduction, in contrast to epistemological and methodological reductions. From the perspective of classical scientific theory a reduction is a scientific explanation for a question of the type "What is x?." Third, reductions rely on bridge laws.[16]

The motivation for this kind of project came from logical positivism and roots in the reduction of formal theories to other formal theories in mathematics and logic. Among the empirical sciences it was most successful in physics, where it was possible to reconstruct the replacement of older through newer theories as a kind of reduction. Seen this way, Galileo's earthly and Kepler's heavenly physics were reduced to Newton's mechanics. Newton's mechanics and theory of gravity were reduced to Einstein's theory of relativity. Geometric optics were reduced to wave optics, and wave optics to electrodynamics. Other sciences also record successful reductions. Organic chemistry can be reduced to inorganic chemistry, chemistry reduced to the atomic physics, and Mendel's genetics reduced to molecular genetics.

Scientific theorists have worked on making the relation of reduction more precise. Careful scientific historical analyses have shown that successive theories are often incommensurable. It also became evident that deduction in the strictest sense of the word is not really possible in mathematics and physics without introducing additional assumptions, which themselves do not result solely from the theories to be reduced. Hooker (1981) suggested a modified theory of reduction. In his approach a successful reduction includes a *correction* of the reduced theory. Strictly speaking, the older theory T_1 is not deduced from T_2, it is a new, corrected theory T_1^*. Strictly speaking, Galileo's law of gravity cannot be logically deduced from Newton's mechanics. We need what is called approximate reduction.

Viewed in terms of scientific theory the mind–body problem is a matter of whether psychological theories can be reduced to neuroscientific theories. Many nonreductive materialists claim that strict reduction is impossible, but this is not surprising. The reduction model was developed for complete formal theories, not for theories still in progress. It is less an issue of proving successful reduction than of asking whether it is meaningful to attempt such a reduction, or whether there are arguments showing that it is in principle senseless, unprofitable, or counterproductive.

One antireductionist motive is fear of eliminating the superior theory. For as soon as reduction is successful, the higher theory becomes at least obsolete, or merely a simplified model of the in-depth theory. Fodor (1974) attacked reductionism in the debate on the unity of science. He tried first to show that it is not possible to construct traditional bridge laws between psychology and neuroscience. He refers to the functionalistic argument about multiple instantiation. At best, bridge laws could connect psychological laws and concepts with an infinite number of disjunctions among various realizations; this would be impractical, pointless, and not really a nomological reduction. Technically speaking, bridge laws are not transitive; they are not biconditional. Reducing psychology to neurophysiology would involve making many generalizations no longer appropriate that are now acceptable in psychology. Also, the concept of rational explanation inherent in psychology would be lost because regularities among neural events have nothing to do with rationality, but at the most with causality. Fodor concludes that psychology is independent of neuroscience (psychology is autonomous) and should also progress with independent methods of research (methodological solipsism).

Now, it is correct that postulating bridge laws between psychology and neuroscience is problematic. Most psychological laws merely take on the form of generalizations that are usually or—on a statistic average—right. However, the independence of psychology itself is also problematic, because many psychological laws can be best explained or even corrected with knowledge of their neurophysiological underpinnings. Advocates of reductionism thus propose the coevolution of psychological and neuroscientific theories. This idea was prompted by Schaffner (1967), who—inspired by examples in biology—suggested that we understand reduction as a two-level process. Applied to our issue this means that the attempt to reduce psychological theories to neuroscientific theories leads to difficulties. These problems force us to modify and further develop both the theory to be reduced and the theory to which the first is to be reduced, in order to produce a reductive relationship at a second level. Patricia Churchland correctly points out that if Fodor's argument were right, even examples of successful reduction would have to be considered failures. Even laws of thermodynamics can have multiple realizations, because temperature is something different in gases, plasma, or solids. Reductions are *relative to domains*.[17] If we accept successful reductions in the rest of science, we also have to accept the reduction of psychology to neuroscience: "if human brains and electronic brains both enjoy a certain type of cognitive organization, we may get two distinct, domain-relative reductions" (Churchland 1986, p. 357).

A further argument in support of coevolving reduction is that closed autonomy hinders reciprocal fertile effects among different disciplines. Bechtel (1993), for example, demonstrates how trying to derive biological processes from chemical ones using biological examples (fermenting alcohol to sugar, cell respiration) advanced both sciences. One example of the pitfalls of uncoupling psychology from neuroscience is Gall's phrenology. His basic approach of locating mental functions in the brain—a conclusion he derived from the shape of the skull—did turn out to be valuable, as state of the art neuropsychology confirms. But one reason Gall's project did not survive was his refusal to acknowledge Flouren's lesion studies. In an experiment on animals Flouren damaged brain sections for which Gall had postulated certain functions. By demanding autonomy for his science and rejecting corrections provided by neuroscience, Gall hindered the coevolution of both theories (Bechtel 1988b, pp. 80ff). The study of biological systems reveals that in biology reduction is always an attempt to understand the relation of a whole to its parts. It is not enough to observe components in isolation; we must also know to which extent components are tied in with the structure of the entire system if we want to claim to have achieved a reduction.

For Patricia Churchland (Churchland and Sejnowski 1992, pp. 11ff) two ideas are crucial to the relationship between psychology and neuroscience: (1) the idea of hierarchically ordering nature into various levels and (2) the idea of coevolution. Different functions occur at different levels. One microreductionistic strategy consists of finding explanations at a certain level within a system by using theories from a lower level. Churchland considers the existence of different levels to be a fact and coevolutionary research a methodological desideratum. She believes that research at one level can lead to corrections, constraints, or even inspiration for other levels. Neuroscience needs psychology because psychology discovers what systems do and neuroscience, in turn, tries to explain that by microreduction. One example of successful reduction of important psychological phenomena to neuroscience is the explanation for conditioning given by processes at the neural level (cf. Bickle 1995).

The biologist Ayala (1974) discerns three varieties of reductionism: Ontological reductionism, which says something about the world; epistemological reductionism, which clears up logical and semantic relations between theories; and methodological reductionism, which claims we should search for reductionistic explanations. Vollmer borrows this distinction and proposes the following thesis. Whoever is interested in the progress of knowledge at all must support methodological reductionism; reductionism must be his program. Only by attempting reduction do we propel science forward, and the antireductionist himself can only use failed reductions for proving that reduction is impossible in certain domains. Scientifically, there is no alternative to methodological reductionism. As to the question of the truth (of ontological reductionism), no standpoint has been taken.

Within this triangle nonreductive materialism can be understood as follows. It adheres to ontological reductionism, but with the claim that certain mental phenomena cannot be *explained* through reduction. That is, it postulates *explanatory* antireductionism. This leads some to postulate property dualism, others refer to the pragmatic character of scientific explanations and recommend that we refrain from ontological statements entirely (Putnam 1992; Baker 1993). The result of the debate: Because psychological as well as neuroscientific theories are still works in progress, the best strategy is methodological, coevolutionary reductionism. We do not know how far this will take us, we shall see as we attempt reduction. We can ignore the argument of multiple instantiation by limiting research to domain-specific reductions. Another result is the insight that the concepts of reduction, laws, and explanation are intertwined. But let us now return to neurophilosophical theories.

2.2   Radical Constructivism: Is The World Inside Our Heads?

The term "constructivism" meanwhile has been used for so many different areas in and outside of philosophy that the word is hardly more than an empty phrase.[18] If by "constructivism" we mean the simple thesis that during the process of knowledge the subject himself makes an active and *constructive* contribution, that is, if the subject himself does not merely represent the objects of knowledge passively and without participation, or again, if the structure of our apparatus for gaining knowledge is somehow constitutive in knowledge, then there is hardly anyone who is not a constructivist. Therefore, we must supplement and define "constructivism" in a way that contrasts it to other constructivisms.

Radical constructivism had this supplementary description from the start. It had at least three sources. On one hand, it developed from philosophical-epistemological considerations at home in nascent cybernetics (cf. Von Glasersfeld 1987; Von Foerster 1985). Second, it has roots in anthropological psychotherapeutic approaches mainly associated with the name Gregory Bateson and the *Mental Research Institute* in Palo Alto, California. Third, and most important in our context, there is the decidedly neurophilosophical work of neurobiologist Humberto Maturana (1985), who developed his own theory of the organization and embodiment of reality in autopoietic systems.[19] Maturana is the founder of neurobiological constructivism, which is a mixture of radical constructivism and the theory of autopoiesis. In the following I will restrict my discussion to this theory.

2.2.1 Maturana's Neurobiological Radical Constructivism   Humberto
Maturana's approach is interesting for at least four reasons. First, it is
genuinely neurophilosophical. He is a neuroscientist, he developed
his original ideas from neurobiological findings, and he calls himself
an experimental philosopher. Second, his fellow student Varela sophisticated the theory of autopoietical systems and brought it into the realm
of cognition research, where it has developed a certain efficacy (Varela
1985; Varela, and Thompson 1991). Third, the theory of autopoietical
systems is being used increasingly to found a new psychotherapy,
so-called systemic therapy (mainly in Germany) and has thus had a
strong influence on popular opinion (cf. Glatzel 1995). Fourth, it will
become obvious that autopoietic cognition theory serves well to explain
intentionality, even though its epistemological aspect reveals it as
inconsistent.

Which elements are basic to radical constructivistic theories? Briefly,
constructivism is meant to be the opposite of any kind of realistic theory
of knowledge. All knowledge, it claims, is only a construct in the mind
of the knowledge-seeking subject and therefore cannot claim to represent objective truth. The titles of the relevant books and articles makes
this evident: "Constructing Realities," "Reality Invented," "Controlling
Perception and Constructing Reality."[20] It is exciting to think that reality
could just be an invention. If it should prove to be true, it would have
consequences not only for epistemology, but also for politics, sociology,
and psychotherapy—for our entire view of mankind. At least that is the
position of the protagonists—and it is their claim.[21]

In order to formulate his idea Maturana uses abstract and unusual
terms he invented just for this purpose. It's like reading Heidegger on
biology. So, in order to test his arguments, we first have to understand
his language. I will explain the relevant expressions. Maturana's starting
point was his work as a neurobiologist. As a student of J. Z. Young[22] in
London he found interest in the connection between biology and language. His early works deal with color perception. Based on his experiments he set up a theory of relative color coding in the retina of primates.
The most important philosophical result of this study was the finding
that colors characterized by their wave lengths do not correlate with the
activity areas of retinal ganglion cells. But color *names* did correlate to

ganglion cell activity. Evidently the correlation does not exist between the things in the world (physically defined color) and the brain (ganglion cell activity), but it does exist between the subjectively experienced color perception (which is expressed in color *names*) and brain activity. The brain is in a context with the outer world, but its activity does not merely mirror that world.

As Maturana himself concedes, many of his results were not reproducible and some were even proven to be wrong.[23] But as a result he retained two insights. First, the nervous system is an *operationally closed* system, which means it is basically busy managing its own activity. Second, we must distinguish between a system *as* a system on the one hand and the functioning of this system as a unit within an environment on the other (Maturana 1985, p. 19). Maturana generalized these insights and developed a general theory of cognition. It is based on the assumption that the brain is an operationally closed system within a living organism and that cognition is only part of the biological nature of organisms. For Maturana organisms are sophisticated systems characterized by the fact that they create their parts themselves in a continuous process and thus keep themselves alive—they "make" themselves, they are *autopoietic* systems. Their concrete material design is their *structure*, but what characterizes them as individuals is their *organization*. Despite structural changes the organization of a living system remains constant; it is continually reproduced.[24] Of course living systems require building materials and energy from their environment, their milieu, but the maintenance of the organizational form is purely an internal task of the system. This way it defines itself: "Living systems are self-generating systems, . . . which define and set up their own limits." (Maturana 1985, p. 280). The reciprocal effects of the system's component parts, its internal *interactions* are solely (!) defined by the current structure of the system, all reciprocal effects are purely local and depend solely on the "present state." Autopoietic systems are *state* or *structure determined*. Their state at time t_2 depends entirely on the state of the system at time t_1.[25]

An autopoietic system is operationally closed. How is it connected to its milieu? Traditional theory of cognition assumes that internal system states *represent* external things. These representations contain information about the outside world. Maturana finds this idea entirely wrong. He concedes that the system and its milieu mutually effect each other. But for the system such *interactions* are merely disturbances—*perturbations*. Whatever such perturbations might cause depends entirely on the structure and organization of the system. Either the organization remains intact, or the system dissolves, it "dies." External disturbing influences thus *select* organized structures in a certain way, but they do not *instruct* it, they relay no *information*. More than any other, it is this point that distinguishes Maturana's theory from traditional cybernetic models. *There is no information relay from outside into an autopoietic system*; there are only active, self-preserving systems that either can or cannot handle disturbance.

Since a perturbation can cause structural changes and an autopoietic system is connected with its environment via perturbations, Maturana calls this relationship *structural coupling*. Structural coupling is the temporal coordination or correlation between environmental influences and structural alterations of the system. "Environment" is a concept relative to a system. A system can only be structurally coupled with areas with which it can also interact. Thus the environment of a system corresponds to its realm of interaction. For example, a system that has receptors only for certain wave lengths has a realm of interaction different from that of a system that has receptors for other wave lengths. But then again, isn't it obvious that neuronal activity contains information? Isn't neuroscience occupied with decoding just this data? No, for the theory of autopoiesis applies to all living systems and thus also to the nonparticipant (scientific) observer. It is only from the view of the observer that information relay occurs; his "observation" is nothing more than the interaction of a sophisticated autopoietic system (the observer himself) with two interacting autopoietic systems. His "objective observation of information transfer" is merely the result of his state-determined brain, that is thereby "perturbed." But don't both slipper animalcules (paramaecium) and mosquitoes live in the same objective environment? According to Maturana they do not. The "objective" environment that the observer postulates corresponds solely to his own realm of interaction, his own subjective, system-relative cognitive realm.

It is obvious how the theory of autopoietic systems becomes radical constructivism. We cannot know anything about objective reality, only something about our own cognitive realm, and that knowledge is not determined by the environment, but only by the state of our own brain. How can we communicate? The structure of living beings is fairly similar. When two living beings repeatedly interact with one another, their state changes begin cooperating, they become *coordinated*. This coordinated group of state changes is now common to both living beings; they have a *consensual* realm. This common realm, in turn, can now be coordinated with other consensual realms. We then have *recursive coordination*. This results in a consensual realm of a higher order and this is the sphere of language. After this sphere has been generated, this realm of higher order can again be coordinated through mutual interaction. The result is theories, facts, and insight.[26] But caution is advised! According to Maturana these theories gained through recursive coordination are not the things themselves! We know nothing about the things themselves. We have merely coordinated our own states with the states of other autopoietic systems. The result is a radical constructivistic conclusion for the theory of knowledge. We can know nothing about the world *because* we are autopoietic systems.

So much for exposition. Maturana presumably employs peculiar terminology in order to avoid using concepts based on representational theory. That is thoroughly legitimate, since it would be counterproductive to use theoretical concepts inappropriate for one's own theory. Keeping this in mind, by replacing his lingo with familiar concepts we *can* concisely describe his theory as follows.

Humans are living systems consisting of parts that produce themselves. Biology teaches us that much. This is also true for partial systems such as the brain. Reciprocal effects in the brain are determined solely by local physical and chemical laws. In order to survive, living systems must maintain balance. This is also true for the brain. The brain's machinery just keeps going, but it is constantly disturbed by foreign forces. Under that pressure, some of the "machines" break down. Some reproduce themselves again, because their procedures have become so adjusted to the environment through contact with it, that they cannot disintegrate themselves. But still the brain does not "represent" its environment, it is merely occupied with maintaining stability. When several brains do this together they are so well adjusted to one another that it would appear to someone observing the system as if they were exchanging information among themselves. But this alleged objective knowledge is nothing but a further adjustment, namely the adaptation of the observant system to both other systems. This is why we know nothing about reality, we only know about our own constructs. They are merely adjustments that result from repeated collisions of blind systems.[27]

2.2.2 Critique   What should we think about this theory? We must distinguish two parts. One consists of the epistemologically radical thesis that the world cannot be known; the other consists of an empirically oriented theory of cognition, which is genuinely neurophilosophical. We may call the first part radical constructivism and the second part an autopoietic theory of cognition. Looking at radical constructivism: This is the aspect that attracts so much popularity for the theory. Everything is relative to the observer! Doesn't this remind us of the central and peculiar role of the observer in fundamental theories in physics? Since they are all subjective constructs, all theories are equal! Isn't this scientific evidence against the reign of rationality? It is impossible to know anything at all about the world! Doesn't this open channels for marvelous speculations about how the world really is? It enables us to reinstate the magic and mystery of which our world has been deprived over the last two centuries, doesn't it? The general public is fascinated by wild ideas, but we must direct our attention to the validity of the arguments behind this position.

To begin with, we can say that it is not merely a new rendition of the old saying "we can know nothing about the world." Neither is it simple idealism or a naive solipsistic position, such as in the claim "the world is as I see it" or (more radical) "the world exists only in my subjective idea." Solipsism of this kind is consistent and irrefutable, which does not mean that it is true. Maturana himself resists such an interpretation: "Unfortunately philosophers and scientists normally think that acknowledging the subject-dependency of cognition leads to idealism and solipsism. I do not believe that that must be the case" (Maturana 1985, p. 301).

Maturana's aim is different. *Employing neuroscientific knowledge* about the brain as a closed system, he attempts to show why knowledge is radically subjective. This makes his theory worse than solipsism, which no one seriously advocates anyway, because it is inconsistent with itself. It is self-contradictory because the reasons it uses are exactly what it denies. Maturana summons empirical biological knowledge, particularly from neurobiology, as the reason for why we can know nothing about the world: "My research on color perception lead me to an extraordinarily important discovery: The nervous system operates like a closed network of interactions" (Maturana 1985, pp. 18f).

His theory, claims one of his followers, is "a consequent extrapolation of 'hard' scientific facts" (Glatzel 1995, p. 56). The radical constructivistic party answers the reproach of being self-contradictory with the argument that there would only be self-refutation at work if they were using a theory of truth derived from correspondence theory (Schmidt 1987, pp. 39–41). Only if they were to assume that propositions are true solely when they correspond to reality would they have a contradiction. In the most detailed critique of radical constructivism, Nüse et al. (1991) have shown that, for the sake of argument, even when we forsake a correspondence theoretical concept of truth, there remain at least three self-contradiction arguments against radical constructivism, which all make reference to the thesis of alleged inaccessibility to the external world. First if an organism has no access to its environment, then it cannot know that it does not have that access. Second, if everything is purely a construct, then there is no foundation on which this can be claimed. Third, if radical constructivism were true, it would be contradictory and false (Nüse et al. 1991, p.326). According to Nüse et al. all three self-refutations arise because findings on the object level (neuroscience, biology) are transferred to a meta-level (observer). The central aspect of arguments contra Maturana is that it is the *reasoning behind* radical constructivism that leads to contradiction, not individual claims. Taken by themselves those claims are not contradictory (which does not imply that they are true). But the reasoning of radical constructivism that "we cannot know anything about the world *because* we are autopoietic systems" is self-contradictory.

How can a radical constructivist deal with this annihilating criticism? He has basically two options. He can present his theory as a whimsical invention on a par with palm-reading, fortune telling, and magazine horoscopes. That is not satisfying, although some constructivists do chose that route. He could also say that his theory offers no *reason* at all for the fact that we can have no knowledge of the world, but that it is simply a heuristic method for developing a theory of cognition. If the constructivist does not select one of these strategies, then he will find himself tangled in self-contradictions at some point. Ultimately, that is the consequence of the epistemological insight that the only true alternative to solipsism is some kind of realism. Even among radical constructivists some realistic tendencies continually resurface: "There are living systems." (Maturana 1985) "There is someone who would like to write a theory of how the brain functions. None of us doubts that he must have a brain in order to be able to write this theory" (von Foerster 1985, p. 135). The fact is that an environment that is not identical to the interacting autopoietic system in question is a requirement for consensual coordination of the first degree. The fact is that language is consensual coordination of the second degree with *another* autopoietic system. And the fact is that the structure of the brain is similar in varying organisms. All these facts demonstrate that the radical constructivist is saying something about the world, at least that there is an environment, that there are other autopoietic systems, and that human brains resemble one another. A radical constructivist is thus a realist on these points. Yet with blatant contradiction radical constructivists firmly maintain: "that one cannot mix radical constructivistic with realistic claims. A constructivist must be 'wholly' constructivistic, must be purely 'radical,' otherwise he foregoes just that potential for innovation, that ensues by dissipating the dilemma of the realistic theory of knowledge" (Schmidt 1987, p. 40f).

In contrast, I maintain that radical constructivism ends either in solipsism or includes an inherent inevitable self-contradiction.[28] This has not gone unnoticed by constructivism's opponents. In countless conferences excited "radical constructivists" argue with indignant "realists" about whether the brain does or does not really exist.[29]

However, we should not wantonly reject the theory of autopoiesis from neurophilosophy solely because it is inherently self-refuting. The truly interesting aspect of radical constructivism is not that it is radical, but that it is constructivism. The theory of autopoiesis unfolds its relevance within a certain mixture of constructivistic and realistic elements. We *do have* access to objective reality, namely through the structural linking of our central nervous system to the environment via the receptors and effectors of our bodies. And we have a subjective phenomenal world that emerges from the operations of the brain itself. But we should not expect that our individual and subjective conception of the world, as we experience it through our senses, discloses nature to us as it really is. We should also not assume that intersubjectivity is always possible, nor that we could think or imagine anything at all if we only had the appropriate information. My point is that the theory of autopoiesis offers us a well founded approach from biology for understanding how communication and language can evolve, although internally our brain is concerned with nothing more than the maintenance of its own states.

The resulting picture appears thus; in one's head there exist numerous neural processes that are the condition for the whole abundance of one's subjective phenomenal experiences. This subjective experience is connected to the non-neural world through the structural coupling of the brain, via receptors and effectors, and to a great extent via other mediating body parts. If we want to understand how we can know anything, we must first come to understand how this structural coupling is designed, particularly how variable and flexible it is, that it can be connected to the non-neural world in such a way that it generates useful images of the world. Radical constructivists know this, too. But they won't concede it, because renouncing radicalness would ruin the mystique of the theory.

If we preserve the constructivistic part of the theory as relevant for neurophilosophy we obtain a scheme of autopoietically active systems that are busy coordinating their consensual spheres. Something like communication evolves. If we take autopoietic theories seriously we can perhaps begin to imagine how something like intersubjective meaning can evolve from purely neurophysiological processes and interactions. It is not surprising that, purged of its popular radical character, the theory of autopoiesis is employed by neurophilosophers for constructing neurosemantics (Kurthen 1992).

The theory of autopoiesis has become part of a comprehensive research program titled "Theories of Self-Organization" (an overview is given in Mainzer 1994). This designation is so general that it at once includes historically heterogeneous schools and also attracts public attention. The theory of autopoiesis is distinguished by the fact that it emphasizes the biological and self-referential character of brain processes without losing sight of the communicative aspect of language that is invaluable for human intelligibility. Incidentally, it shares this merit with so-called teleosemantic theories of intentionality (cf. chapter 3). The radical constructivistic aspect has presumably played a substantial role in making biological principles of communication interesting for a group of people who would normally find the adjective "biological" pejorative. But, despite all its deserts, this does not alter the fact that being radical evoked the most criticism. And rightly so.

2.3   From Eliminative Materialism to Connectionism

2.3.1   Eliminative Materialism   Eliminative materialism can be most simply expressed as follows: There are no mental states in the traditional meaning of the word. In its contemporary form, eliminative materialism arose as an answer to problems of type identity theory. Type identity theory had been rebuked for making nonsensical statements for identifying mental with physical states—statements like "my C-fibers are overly active" instead of "I have strong pains." The reply came quickly. Authors such as Herbert Feigl, Paul Feyerabend, and Richard Rorty developed a response in the 1960s along these lines: "If we intuit that it is nonsense to say something like this, that is because of our speaking habits, we just do not know better." The difficulty arises because we want to identify existing things (neurophysiological states) with non-existing things (mental states). No wonder it doesn't work!

From a scientific standpoint we should abandon our mentalistic vocabulary and replace it with neurophysiological terminology, even though we might continue to use it in everyday life for reasons of convenience, just as we carelessly continue to say—in spite of knowing better—that the sun rises and sets. Paul and Patricia Churchland entered the stage of philosophy flagrantly making this demand. "The one to one match-ups [among mental and neurophysiological states] will not be found, and our common-sense psychological framework will not enjoy an intertheoretic reduction, *because our common-sense psychological framework is a false and radically misleading conception of the causes of human behavior and the nature of cognitive activity*" (P. M. Churchland 1984, p. 43).

This is a radical and provocative standpoint that we can, perhaps, better apprehend when we consider that philosophy of the preceding decades had lost itself among increasingly intricate and abstract debates on language use, conceptual analysis, identity problems, category mistakes, and so on, and entirely ignored exciting discoveries in neuroscience. The argumentation of eliminative materialists was of decidedly scientific theoretical nature. The essential premise consisted of viewing *folk psychology* as a *theory*. If we then examine how the theoretic concepts of this theory are related to theoretic concepts of neuroscience, we find that we can *eliminate* most of the former concepts, because they do not correlate to anything real. Neuroscience, on the other hand, offers correct explanations and concepts.

Thus neurophilosophy ultimately positioned itself at two opposite poles. On one there is interactionistic dualism, advocated by famous neuroscientists, on the other eliminative materialism, advanced by philosophers who—disappointed with philosophy—turned with curiosity to the neurosciences. Eliminative materialism in its strict form has not found many adherents (Bickle 1992, 1995; Stich 1983; Ramsey, Stich, and Garon 1991). The reason is mainly that scientific psychology and cognitive science assume the existence of mental states. Someone swearing allegiance to eliminative materialism would have great difficulty in executing research because the chasm between physiology and psychology is quite wide. Thus the Churchlands' recourse is often to project their conception as a vision for *future* neuroscience. As a matter of fact, during the past decade they have more than once modified their standpoint to a more reductionist position based on a hierarchical order of the world displaying various levels.

Insofar as I am trying to discover macro-to-micro explanations, I am a reductionist." . . . [B]y "reductionistic research strategy" I do not mean that there is something disreputable, unscientific, or otherwise unsavory about high-level descriptions or capacities, per se. . . . High-level capacities clearly exist, and high-level descriptions are therefore needed to specify them. . . . Here, as elsewhere in science, hypotheses at various levels can coevolve as they correct and inform one another. Neuroscientists would be silly to make a point of ignoring psychological data. (Churchland 1995, pp. 100, 102)

This much more moderate statement can certainly be shared by many scientists. But what remains of the standpoint of eliminative materialism? "The possibility of nontrivial revision and even replacement of high-level descriptions by 'neurobiologically harmonious' high-level categories is the crux of what makes eliminative materialism *eliminative*." (Footnote): "Or, as we have preferrec but decided not to say, 'What makes revisionary materialism *revisionary*'" (P. M. Churchland 1995, p. 103). Changing eliminativism to revisionism extirpates only the polemic focus of the debate. The persistent issue for philosophical and scientific discussion is still; which concepts require revision, which can be eliminated, and which endure? The discussion centers around three major themes: so-called qualia (phenomenal consciousness), intentionality (propositional attitudes of *belief-desire psychology*), and the reality and structure of representations. Meanwhile eliminative materialism has found another mighty ally within science: connectionism, also known as the "theory of neuronal networks" (Rumelhart, and McClelland 1986; Rojas 1993; Spitzer 1996). Connectionism questions some of our deeply rooted convictions about the structure of mental states and quickly drew interest from philosophical specialists (Horgan, and Tienson 1991; P. M. Churchland 1989; Bechtel, and Abrahamsen 1991; Clark 1991). Although not all connectionists are eliminative materialists, the idea of eliminating or revising basic concepts about mental states is obviously a regulative aspect of connectionism. This is due less to conceptual analysis than to empirical findings and theories about neuronal nets, and the way their functions are guided by how the brain works. Connectionism caused a change of paradigms in cognitive science, with profound influence on our understanding of the human mind; its basic ideas pull the naturalization of intelligibility within reach. For this reason I would like to discuss the basic ideas and some of the difficulties.

2.3.2 Connectionism Connectionism is a theory for information processing in neuronal nets.[30] Neuronal nets are mathematical constructs of information processing systems that are designed to imitate the way the brain functions. They consist of many simple and similar units, which are roughly designed as neurons and have a specific activation value. The units are interconnected by various links corresponding to synaptic connections. Activity flows through this type of network from one active unit to one or more other units. The amount of activity transmitted is a product of the activity value and the so-called weight of the connection, which determines its strength. The output activity of each unit is determined by the summation of all entering input activity according to a certain function (linear or threshold value function). Normally neuronal nets are ordered in layers, in which activity flows from an input layer to an output layer. There may also be some hidden layers in between. In networks like this, information is represented as a pattern of activities distributed across the neurons. Information processing occurs by the activity expanding throughout the network.

What can connectionistic nets accomplish? Initially, they can only generate a specific output for a specific input. This, however, merely follows the general principle of biological information processing. It is vital for organisms to react to various stimuli exciting their sense organs (input) with certain behavior (output). Basically, it is pattern recognition. In contrast to serial information processing, the advantage of networks organized parallel to each other is that they can process complicated input quickly and are less prone to error. The loss of one or more units in a network is less dramatic than in serial information processing, where the incorrect execution of one single step can cause the whole process to go haywire. Swiftness and error tolerance can be a great advantage in a biological setting. In a network as enormous as the brain, however, all of the weights cannot possibly be determined genetically, for reasons of calculation. It would not even be an advantage to be so because the environment of organisms contains variable patterns that must be recognized. For highly developed organisms with a need for flexible behavior adapted to the conditions of the environment, it would be an advantage to have synapse weightings adjusted according to experience.

Neuronal nets possess exactly this ability to learn. They are adaptive, which means that the pattern of activation strengths and connection weightings adapts itself to external conditions through alterations. It develops from an initial state—which can be configured in any way—through learning processes. A distinction is made between self-organized learning (learning without an external trainer) and guided learning. In guided learning links are gradually reweighted through certain error correcting procedures, so that with each repetition the synapse weightings approach the desired state. Both exciting and inhibitory mechanisms are at work, which are not only simulated in networks, but which have also been shown to exist in biological brains.[31] The "desired state" is a network with synapses weighted such that they produce the desired output pattern for every input pattern. But self-organized learning is more interesting.

In self-organized learning the system properties of the network and the input signals lead to spontaneous learning phenomena. Most of the discoveries in this area have been made with computer simulations of networks, but in the meantime equivalents have been revealed within the brain. So-called Kohonen networks are characterized by the fact that they have a high degree of connection and inhibitory connections exist among the neurons in the output layer. When a network of this type is repetitiously confronted with a multitude of input signals similar to one another, the brain, on its own, develops so-called self-organizing property maps. On these maps the *similarity and frequency of input signals are represented in an orderly manner*. The more frequent a signal is, the larger the number of neurons it recruits; the greater the similarity is among entrance signals, the greater their proximity. Such maps have been found in the human brain. The most well known are presumably Penfield's and Rasmussen's sensory motor homunculi. Special abilities are related to the enlargement of the cortical representations of sensory motor capacities: tactile sense of cat and mice whiskers, the olfactory capacity of pigs, and the lip taction ability of sheep and goats. Genetic determination alone is not decisive for the development of these maps. The stimulation of the corresponding tactile organs in an early critical period is just as important. These types of maps have also been found in humans. And there is a surprising finding. Previously, it was assumed that the structure of the human brain can hardly change (nerve cells cannot regenerate themselves). But new methods in experimental research on brain maps have shown that this notion is false. In brains of persons who have undergone amputations, the size of the maps changes subsequent to being *used differently*. When blind persons learn Braille, the cortex surface that represents the index finger enlarges, the cortex surface representing the left hand becomes larger for people who play the guitar and the violin as they practice. This adaptive process is known as neuroplasticity. It is important for chapter 3.

As yet I have hardly mentioned the intermediate layers of neural nets, but they are crucial for understanding representation in those nets. Networks consisting of only an input and an output layer can only fulfill very limited functions. Intermediate layers make intricate input-output relations possible. Learning—reweighting synapses through experience—does become increasingly difficult. Special learning algorithms have been developed for this problem, the most well known is the *back propagation* algorithm.[32] One example is the network NET-Talk (Sejnowski, and Rosenberg 1987). The job of this three-layered network is to generate sounds (phonemes) from the input of alphabet letters. The goal was to have a textual input that the network could then read aloud. The net must be trained for this in thousands of sessions. The input is a sequence of seven letters each, each letter is to be converted into a phoneme, depending on the three preceding and the three successive letters. The output layer consisted of 26 neurons representing a total of 54 phonemes (these were generated physically by a language decoder). In order to allow the conversion of context-independent letters into phonemes, an intermediate layer consisting of 80 neurons was built in. The interesting aspect was that a cluster analysis of the activation states of the intermediate levels shows that regularities are reflected that develop spontaneously as a result of training. Classes of similar patterns within the intermediate levels correspond to vowels and consonants. Thus the net has performed an abstraction. The representation of these classes is distributed across the intermediate layer. It is not the case that one individual neuron represents an abstract class; this is done by a pattern of activity of a portion of the intermediate neurons. Higher level representations are thus *distributed*.

The Net-Talk experiment is concerned with guided learning. But such abstractions could evolve spontaneously in self-organizing networks with intermediate layers. Abstracta are not learned by neuronal systems *as* abstracta, as if rules had been explicitly programmed into the system. They are brought up spontaneously. The prerequisite, of course, is that regular input-output relations are the basis of the training. There are further variations on the architecture of neuronal nets, such as the introduction of contextual layers with feedback loops. These kinds of networks have been used to simulate understanding language. I will wait to discuss these findings in chapter 3. For the moment we should keep in mind the characteristic features of networks. They have parallel information processing and are fast; they are tolerant of error; there is no dualism of data on the one side and rule based operations on the other; data are "active" and the system behaves in an ordered manner, without being controlled by explicit rules. Representations do not exist as discrete physical values of a state. They are dispersed and can only be identified at an abstract level, for example, as activity patterns of units with fuzzy boundaries (distributed, subsymbolic representation functions).

Naturally, enthusiasm for connectionism also attracted gainsayers. Although it is splendid for solving perception and categorization problems, it does have profound difficulty in coming to terms with certain features of human language. Accordingly, among the critics of connectionism we find mostly scientists and philosophers whose views on the human mind rest on language: the linguists and advancers of symbol processing theory.[33] Besides the discussion on the importance of rules,[34] the connectionism debate mainly pivots around a dispute on the composition of representations. The following exposition describes this critical controversy, which I will attempt to solve later in chapter 3.

2.3.3 The Problem of Compositionality A harmless interpretation of the word "composition" would be that it is a technical term designating the manner in which a complex representation consists of individual parts. However, the question of the degree to which mental representations actually exhibit compositionality has instated embittered controversy between connectionists and advocates of the theory of symbol processing.[35] We have seen above how connectionism conceives of representations. So now we must very briefly go through the theory of symbolic representation.

On the symbolic representation view propositional attitudes—such as the belief that there is beer in the refrigerator—are relations among subjects and representations that express propositions. Mental processes are sequences of single events, or *tokens* of mental representation. Mental processes are computational; this means that they are concerned only with the formal and syntactic properties of mental representations, not with their semantic properties. The causal relation between mental processes is only warranted by the fact that internally they are structurally isomorphic to the sentences that they represent. This is because causal properties only apply to syntactic properties. Thinking has some important features that are similar to language: It is productive, it is systematic, and there is coherence of inference. Thinking is *productive* because it can generate an infinite number of combinations from a finite number of elements. It is critical for the theory of symbolic representation processing that elements retain their meaning even in new combinations. Thinking is *systematic* because we can automatically think a thought of one kind, once we have had a thought of another kind. For example, if we can think "Gaby loves Stephan," we must also be able to think "Stephan loves Gaby." Finally, the *coherence of inference* means the ability to make syntactically and semantically plausible inferences. From the knowledge that something is a brown cow, we can infer that it is a cow. From the knowledge that things get wet when it rains we can conclude from "it's raining" that things will get wet. Cognitive systems can only have these features when the structure of their constituents have the properties that classical theory demands. They must be (a) symbolic, (b) context independent, (c) open to semantic interpretation, and (d) be involved in input-output functions (MacDonald, and MacDonald 1995, p. 17).

In an often quoted article Fodor and Pylyshyn thus contend that connectionism is inadequate as a foundation for a theory of cognition. Their premise rests on the following two assumptions: "Thinking is systematic. Thus internal representations must also be structured (strong compositionality)." Unfortunately, the representations found in connectionist models are not structured. Therefore, connectionism is not an adequate model for human cognition. If however, connectionists would recognize the necessity of structured mental representations at *any* level, then classic theory would be correct to a great extent and in the best case scenario connectionism would only be left the office of providing an implementation theory, that is, explaining how symbol processing mechanisms are implemented in the brain. This would greatly reduce the significance of neuroscience, because then neuroscience would not restrict cognitive models more than any of the other theories concerned with implementation, for example biophysics, biochemistry, or even quantum theory. In a nutshell, the argument is, either connectionism cannot explain any systematic cognitive operations or it is merely an implementation theory of the classical approach.

How do connectionists respond to this attack? Bechtel and Abrahamsen (1991, pp. 226–252) distinguish three different positions. First, there are compatibilists who accept the thesis that the task of connectionism lies in explaining implementation. Second, there are approximationists, who assert that symbolic systems can only approximately portray connectionistic systems. And finally, there are externalists, who view symbol processing as an ability for processing extraneous symbols that connectionistic systems have learned. The externalist's standpoint will be of significance later. In what follows here I would like to describe the approximationist's position.

An essential feature of connectionistic systems is that their representations are *symbolic*. It is only at the subsymbolic level that the systems' behavior can be described formally, completely, and precisely (Smolensky 1988). If we try to transfer the structure of classical symbol processing to the structure of connectionistic systems, this can only be achieved *approximately*. The base of all cognition lies at a subsymbolic, subconceptual level, which Smolensky names an "intuitive processor." Here we find all those cognitive abilities that are not the conscious application of rules: perception, motor skills, fluent speech, intuitive problem solving and play behavior, in short, practically all "skilled performance" (Smolensky 1988, p. 6). This subconceptual level is the level for activation vectors and their changes over time, which can be described using differential equations. The thesis that connectionism is thus repudiating is that higher cognitive systems can be completely, formally, and exactly described with symbolic algorithms. The relationship of symbol processing to connectionism is not one of implementation, but of refinement; it is more similar to the relationship among classical physics and quantum mechanics (Smolensky 1988, p. 12).

The dispute stirred up by Fodor and Pylyshyn has forced the connectionist side to concede that simple connectionistic nets exhibit no outstanding feature of compositionality that could support systematicity. There are also connectionistic representations, however, which do have an obvious compositional structure, but we do not have to view them as systems in the classic sense of the word.[36] But the connectionists' insistence that "true" processing happens at the subsymbolic level is consequential for the notion of what it is about representations that is causally effective. (This relates to the issue of mental causation, which I will discuss later.) The only thing causally effective is local unit activity, which precise algorithms can grasp and which are made up of constituents with *weak* compositional structure. In other words, causally effective structures have a nonclassical structure. Thus the tentatively last round of the debate between Smolensky and Fodor pivots on the extent to which constituents of cognitive architectures are *real*, that is, the structure of constituents exhibits those elements, which perform the causal work (cf. MacDonald and MacDonald 1995, chapters 4–6).

In chapter 3 I will argue that the approximationists' response to the attack undertaken by defenders of symbol processing theory is insufficient. We cannot deny the evidence that our brains represent information in a connectionistic manner. Language-analogous abilities, such as systematicity, productivity, and inference, however, do require further explanation. A solution to this problem—only to mention it momentarily—is only possible with an externalistic answer. In the next section

I will explain to which extent eliminative materialism has developed toward becoming connectionistic neurophilosophy.

2.3.4 Connectionistic Neurophilosophy The "Bible" of connectionism—two volumes by Rumelhart and McClelland—was published the same year as Patricia Churchland's *Neurophilosophy*. In the ensuing years the major advocates of eliminative materialism turned toward connectionism (Churchland and Sejnowski 1992, P. M. Churchland 1989, 1995; Ramsey, Stich, and Garon 1991). Connectionism is viewed not merely as an implementation strategy for cognitive models; it is considered to be a model of cognition itself. It follows that propositional attitudes as functionally discrete, semantically interpretable states with causal roles *do not exist*:

Beliefs and desires are of a piece with phlogiston, caloric, and the alchemical essences. We therefore need an entirely new kinematics and dynamics with which to comprehend human cognitive activity, one drawn, perhaps, from computational neuroscience and connectionist AI. Folk psychology could then be put aside in favor of this descriptively more accurate and explanatorily more powerful portrayal of the reality within. Certainly, it will be put aside in the lab and in the clinic, and eventually, perhaps, in the marketplace as well. (P. M. Churchland 1989, p. 125)

The basic idea of "new kinematics and dynamics" is that representations in the brain are activation vectors of populations of neurons. Cognition is *not* symbol manipulation that follows rules, it is the *transformation of activation vectors* (P. M. Churchland 1989, 1995). An individual learns something by reweighting neuron connections through confrontation with samples of a class. Within the representing vector space a subdivision develops that represents the *prototype*. Categories are represented in the brain by prototype vectors, which, due to their structure, always contain more than the sensory input alone because they are able to correctly integrate new members of the same category, provided there exists a similarity relation. Vector transformations are ideal for converting perceptions and categorizations into motor programs. Actually, sensory motor coordination is the foundation for all higher cognition, since biologically it precedes all more sophisticated forms of cognition. Knowledge is the result of fine-*tuning* synaptic connections and thus it is stored in these connections.

But not only perception, categorization, motor activity, and propositional attitudes can be theoretically explained in this way. Paul Churchland (1989) also uses it to explain some traditional problems in epistemology and the theory of science. To learn a theoretic concept means to configure synaptic weights in the brain in such a manner that the space of possible neuronal activation is partitioned so that a system or hierarchy of prototypes develops. The explanatory comprehension of an event consists of activating the appropriate prototype vector within this hierarchy. Based on this concept, Churchland draws far-reaching political and ethical conclusions in his most recent publication (P. M. Churchland 1995), upon which we shall not dwell presently.

We want to keep in mind that de facto, eliminative materialism has become closely associated with the research program of connectionism. It is not surprising that today we view this affiliation as revisionism. Revisionistic materialism assaults folk psychology as an insufficient theory requiring modification. Similarly, connectionism attacks traditional symbol processing theory. Both camps attempt to replace long-established terms and concepts for mental functions with new, unaccustomed ones. The link to neurophilosophy is the relevance that neurobiological systems have for validating these theoretic concepts. Connectionism sways quite far away from neurobiology in many respects, but as a model it is unavoidable. Meanwhile the trend in computational neuroscience is to simulate real neurobiological systems with the help of connectionistic models of information processing in order to better understand them (Churchland and Sejnowski 1992). I shall show how this approach can be useful for the debate on free will when I discuss intelligibility in chapter 3.

3 Minimal Neurophilosophy

3.1 Systematic Reflections

3.1.1 Neurophilosophy as an Inevitable Research Program We have now become acquainted with various facets of neurophilosophy. I have portrayed the close association to the mind-body problem, disclosed the significance of the problems surrounding reduction, and explored their basically interdisciplinary and transdisciplinary character. Still missing is a more precise characterization of neurophilosophy as a discipline. In the next section I will introduce the concept of minimal neurophilosophy (Walter 1996b), which in my opinion has the greatest chance of achieving an "approximation, mutual influence and fruition among the disciplines of philosophy and neuroscience." But first some general reflections.

The approximation of philosophy and neuroscience is not only interesting and desirable; in a way it is even unavoidable. The reason lies in the nature of the objects that neuroscience deals with.[37] During their work, scientists come across philosophical questions or happen upon philosophical issues by themselves. The process is similar to developments in physics and biology. Scientific theories about space, time, and the beginning of the cosmos touch upon philosophical questions about the nature of space-time and the commencement of the world. The theory of evolution answers our question of how man originated. In the same way, neuroscientific studies naturally lead to questions about how mental phenomena and brain processes are related—whether we are dealing with information processing in the brain, neuropsychological deficits due to brain damage, dreams, split-brain patients, synesthesia, psychoneuro-immunology, or the neurobiological underpinnings of hallucinations and insanity.

By their very nature, questions about mental phenomena have an interdisciplinary character. In contrast to some other sciences, we also have a special nonscientific access to mental phenomena: subjective experience. By using new methods, science can gain new knowledge about old notions and study abnormal variations. An attempt to reflect and make novel findings compatible to traditional conceptions means that one is doing neurophilosophy, whether or not one intends to do so.

However, a good scientist is not necessarily a good philosopher. Many overly naive theories and argumentative pitfalls could be avoided if scientists would make themselves familiar with philosophical reasoning. Philosophers, on the other hand, often develop a stark aversion to the idea of neurophilosophy, perhaps because they define philosophy as a discipline concerned with what is not empirically accessible, or perhaps because they just do not have the necessary background in neuroscience.

Gerhard Roth points out the presumably largest obstacle: "The biggest obstacle in working together is the problem of status of the sciences involved, followed by a far-reaching lack of awareness of the problem, the conceptual systems, the state of the art and the methodological and experimental procedures in each of the other disciplines" (Roth 1994, pp. 10f). We can consider neurophilosophy as a discipline that moves in on the mind-brain problem from two opposite directions. Either we begin on the empirical side and happen upon philosophical questions, or we set out with philosophical puzzles and need empirical findings to solve them. That is a simple description of neurophilosophy based on Thomas Nagel's conception of philosophy (Nagel 1987, p. 5): "The main concern of neurophilosophy is to question and understand very common ideas about mental phenomena in the neurosciences, or aided by neuroscience, ideas all of us use every day without thinking about them." We are dealing here with an *a posteriori* philosophy of the mental, that is, philosophy assisted by empirical evidence. But neurophilosophy is more than merely integrated empirical science. It is best understood as a bridge discipline between subjective experience, philosophical theorizing, and empirical research. It serves to systematically clear up concepts among the disciplines. It does take empirical data into consideration, but because all findings are tentative, it also allows leeway for general argumentation. It takes the issues from philosophical tradition seriously, leaves room for some speculation and does not shun working on recalcitrant problems. It tests the conclusions and internal consistency of theories. And it attempts to determine the limits for plausible empirical statements. Neurophilosophy, in a broader sense, makes substantial use of psychology and computer science. But it is significantly characterized by the fact that it should throw light on the direct link among the two disciplines it is named after (cf. figure 2.1).

Folk psychology plays an important part. It supplies the intuitions that underlie philosophical concepts, which—incorporated in abstract systems—have helped to shape our commonplace psychological ideas over the centuries. Many of our intuitions are partially cultural prejudices. Neurosciences and philosophy also effect each other mutually. While philosophy can provide critical analysis of the concepts of neurophilosophy, the neurosciences can impose empirical limitations on

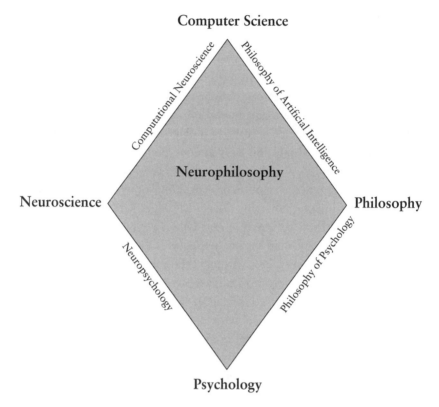

Figure 2.1
Free will and determinism. The four most important disciplines of cognitive science pivot on the bridge discipline neurophilosophy.

philosophical theories. If this mutual process is conveyed openly and in a way that can be understood by all, it could—in the end—lead to revising our intuitive commonplace psychological notions. In this way neurophilosophy has the potential to change our world view.

It is useful to distinguish between general and specialized neurophilosophy. *General neurophilosophy* can be considered the effort to discover a neuroscientifically inspired solution for the mind–body problem. This includes variations on identity theory, interactionistic dualism, and eliminative materialism. *Specialized neurophilosophy*, in contrast, is the effort to discover a solution for specific problems in the philosophy of mind with the aid of findings from neuroscience, or—as a genuine bidirectional approach—to philosophically enlighten special phenomena or problems in neuroscience, such as the problem of transplanting brain tissue (Northoff 1995).

Radical constructivism and evolutionary epistemology are examples of specialized neurophilosophies that investigate how human knowledge is possible at all. My work is another example of specialized neurophilosophy. I commence with a philosophical problem and use neuroscience to understand it better and thus approach a solution. This method is particularly interesting because it is a way of converting philosophical theses into empirically testable hypotheses. If we can consolidate certain theses by doing so we may find that clarification also has ethical consequences, such as implications for matters of penal law.

Theoretically, this concept might sound attractive. But we must ask whether or not it ends in a vicious circle, for the initial question of (general) neurophilosophy is that of the relation of mind and brain. It would appear that this issue should be solved first, because answers for special problems depend on how mind and brain are related. Now, in a certain sense, naturalistic theories in philosophy are always circular. We have to make some assumptions before we even begin doing philosophy or empirical science. But this does not have to be a *vicious* circle, it could also be a *virtuoso* circle.[38] Or, to use another metaphor; not only circles, but also spirals move in circles. However, I do not want to fight off the reproach of circularity merely with well meant and suggestive metaphors. Instead I want to layout a strategy that enables us to minimize the circular nature of our approach. The concept of *minimal neurophilosophy* assists us in doing this.

3.1.2 The Idea of Minimal Neurophilosophy   There appear to be more features separating variations of neurophilosophy than common ground among them. One variation contains religiously inspired dualism, which locates all interesting mental activities of the brain in a self-conscious spirit; another variation exhibits scientistic "hard core" materialism aimed to convince us that many of the assumptions about the mental that we take for granted are just plain nonsense. Then again, there is tantalizing solipsism, tangled in self-contradiction. And last, but not least, we have integrated science with suboptimal results that, nevertheless, threaten to deem philosophy useless. These differences are so comprehensive that discussion among the various camps more often than not ends in world-view battles, if the parties are still talking at all. This is unfortunate, because in some way all neurophilosophies contribute important material for solving certain puzzles. Revisionistic eliminative materialism has particularly innovative facets. It questions our intuitive commonplace assumptions and forces us to consider whether, in the light of neuroscientific findings, we should still hold on to our pet convictions—disregarding our preference to do so. Radical constructivism draws our attention to the fact that the brain is an operationally closed system, at least in a sense that still remains to be defined. Interactionistic dualism—even though it is a poor theory—serves as a counter position that singles out the weaknesses in other theories, for which it is most difficult to find well founded explanations. And the idea of neurophilosophy as an integrated science makes us aware of the fact that neurophilosophy depends on concepts and theories taken from other disciplines. But in the end, all these approaches have one common denominator. They take the findings and methods of neuroscience seriously and strive to incorporate them in their body of theory. It would be desirable to develop a standpoint that emphasizes what these disciplines have in common and neglects their differences as far as possible.

There are many good reasons for such a strategy, which I call *minimal neurophilosophy*, and here are three. First, it is generally agreed that some critical metaphysical issues cannot be solved definitely, but are met with statements that rely on world-view convictions, which themselves rest not entirely on arguments. Such statements are often introduced as unfounded premises. Second, there are pressing questions in specialized neurophilosophy that are too important to wait for total agreement on mind-body issues. Third is an aspect that is persistently ignored in the philosophy of the mental, but which, in my opinion, is most consequential. There is a whole bunch of mental states that differ from one another in several respects and thus should not be all lumped together (cf. figure 2.2). It is not at all obvious that different kinds of mental states all follow the same metaphysics![39] Every mind–body theory (identity theory, functionalism, eliminative materialism, dualism, etc.) normally

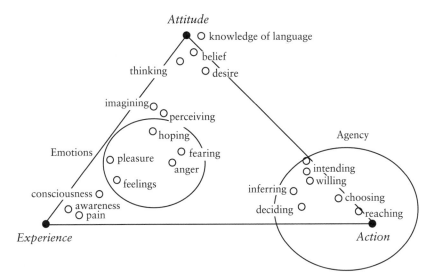

Figure 2.2
The diversity of mental activity. The many kinds of mental activity, taken from Guttenplan (1994a, p. 24). The figure resulted from a list made up by philosophy students. Guttenplan sorted these into three main categories (to have an experience, an attitude, and to act). They are shown here on a kind of map displaying the main categories in a landscape. The differences and similarities of individual activities are symbolized by the distance and relative direction toward one of three corners. The criteria for ordering mental activities within the map were the five dimensions of observability, accessibility, expressibility, directionality, and theoreticalness. Experience, for example, is the peak of the summit for every mental activity that is wholly accessible, not observable, not expressible, not directional and not theoretical. Pain, on the other hand, is quite near, but not exactly on the corner point, because pain is not pure experience. Other mental activities have been entered in the diagram after the same fashion. The mental entities significant for the issue of free will are mainly on the right side of the triangle. This is one reason why the question of ontological status of phenomenal consciousness as a pure form of experience plays only a marginal role within the context of this work. For further details, see Guttenplan (1994a, pp. 6–27).

presupposes that there is exactly *one* special relation among mental states. But why should this be true?

Why should mental states or processes such as thinking, feeling, and deciding all be related to physical states in the same way? Of course it is more elegant to explain *all* mental phenomena with one *single* theory. But I have been unable to find one single convincing argument for why this should be so. Most people don't think it is even necessary to find arguments for this assumption! It just stands for itself. I find this problematic, because it is probably wrong. For example, there are pertinent reasons for thinking that type identity theory provides the right metaphysical solution for the problem of qualia (Hill 1991), or that for the issue of intentionality a functionalistic metaphysics such as that of teleofunctionalism (Millikan 1884) is correct. Some other authors also share this opinion. David Lewis (1989), for example, suggests species specific identity theory. David Chalmers (1996a, 1996b)—who can certainly not be considered a classic substance dualist—suggests that we think of conscious experience as a novel kind of fundamental property that can be understood scientifically, but not deduced from physical properties and laws. He therefore advocates a dualist property theory of consciousness, while simultaneously denying that it is necessary for intentional states (Chalmers 1996a, pp. 82f).

Mental states are not all the same. They can be very different (cf. figure 2.2) and philosophy has by far not yet sufficiently discussed them all. Emotions, for example, have been terribly neglected by the philosophy of mind.[40] We just do not know enough to be able to say which kind of metaphysics is appropriate for which mental state in the end. I will call my idea of sorting different mental states into different metaphysical categories the *thesis of differential metaphysics.*[41] Another way of stating this is, theories with metaphysical statements quantifying over mental entities (Such as: *All* mental states are identical with brain states.) are bound to fail. An approach that promises success would say: *Some* mental states are ... (such as, qualitative states like human pain are identical with a type of neural state, intentional states on the other hand are teleo-functional states). Below is a list of possible relationships:

Some mental processes could be
- in principle not explainable,
- processes of a mental substance,
- correlated one-to-one with brain processes
- emergent processes,
- supervenient upon physical processes,
- mereologically supervenient upon brain processes,
- understood as causal roles of brain processes,
- type identical with brain processes,
- token identical with brain processes
- abstract descriptions of brain processes,
- linguistic interpretational constructs,
- brain constructs, or
- nonexistent.

A comprehensive theory of mental states would have to consist of a disjunction of varying theories about mental states. I cannot say presently what a comprehensive theory like this would look like or should look like. Naturally, a single theory for all states would be more elegant. But I believe that this is just not the nature of mental states. Our theories should be guided by the desire to describe nature correctly, and not whether they fulfill our aesthetic needs.

So what do they have in common? *Minimal neurophilosophy*, let me emphasize this once more, is not yet another metaphysical theory on the mind-body problem, but rather a metaphilosophical strategy of naturalistic provenience for working on a theory of the mental. "*Neuro*" means that we are limiting our work to understanding the mental processes of biological organisms with brains. It is *minimal* because we aim to have the smallest possible number of metaphysical background assumptions— a kind of minimal consensus. What does the framework look like? It can be outlined with three theses as they are shown in table 2.2. These three central theses are advanced by all neurophilosophers. Or, rather, whoever does not share one of them cannot be called a neurophilosopher in the sense mentioned above. I will now more precisely explain the meaning of these theses, but first add a general note. Table 2.2 uses the term "mental *processes.*" Relevant literature uses the terms "states," "properties," or "events." I have chosen the term "process" for two reasons.

Table 2.2
Core Theses of Minimal Neurophilosophy

(T1) *Ontology*: Mental processes of biological organisms are realized by or with the aid of neuronal processes.

(T2) *Constraint*: Philosophical analysis of mental processes should not contradict the best currently available brain theories.

(T3) *Heuristic Principle*: Knowledge about the structure and dynamics of mental processes can be gained from knowledge about the structure and dynamics of neuronal processes.

First of all, it expresses the fact that a mental procedure is a dynamic occurrence over time. This connotation corresponds to the significant characteristics of mental occurrences as we shall see. Second, because it is less familiar in these contexts, it is easier to view the term "process" as a variable. However, the three central theses stated above can be just as well formulated—if one has an ontological preference—using states, properties, or events. Let us now turn to those theses.

(T1) is certainly the least minimal thesis, since it does imply an obligation to ontological monism. This is at least true for the contemporary reading of the word "realization" (cf. Beckermann, Flohr, and Kim 1992, pp. 14–20; Beckermann 1996). It is difficult to see how a dualist could subscribe to thesis 1. He has two options. First, he could have a different meaning for "to realize." Eccles writes of the self-aware mind that uses the brain the way a pianist plays the piano. When he claims that a piece of music can be "realized" on the piano and that mental states are analogous to music or melodies, then going by his meaning for the word "realize" he can say that mental states are realized in the brain. This is a fuzzy use of the concept of realization and I want to avoid it. But we can also understand dualists as saying that the self-aware mind realizes mental states with the help of the brain, it merely uses the brain and the "real" mental entities exist in another world. By saying that, however, the dualist is once again creating all the problems discussed earlier in chapter 1, section 6.3. The motivation for leaving the phrase "with the aid of" in T1 is another. That phrase is needed by those theories that view certain mental states as not solely realized through brain states, but also realized in their relation to the environment or in their ontogeny.[42]

At first glance, it also appears that an eliminative materialist would have difficulties with (T1). How can a mental state be "realized" if there are no mental states? But the eliminative materialist's claim that there are no mental states means merely that there are not mental states as they are described in folk psychology. So, she can read "mental processes" (T1) as meaning those actually existent, revised subsequent entities she has in mind. In a certain sense, then, (T1) is a thesis that can be shared by different neurophilosophers.[43] In any case, it is decidedly and intuitively understandable that because of (T1) it is worth it to use our knowledge about the brain.

For T2 we could also presume that at least interactionistic dualism drops out of the category of neurophilosophy. But a closer look proves the contrary. Modern interactionistic dualists do strive to reconcile their theory with science, even though they have yet to be successful. They are still searching for a gap in which to locate the self-conscious mind or its power to interact, often turning to quantum physics to find it. Contemporary (monistic) libertarians also make reference to quantum physics. In the next chapter we shall closer inspect and criticize that strategy.

(T3)'s meaning becomes apparent when we examine functionalistic and parallelistic metaphysics. The argument for multiple realization[44] is often engaged to demonstrate that restricting realization to purely neural realization weakens the generality of the theory of mental in question. The assumption is that a theory of the mental should be independent of any substratum. A functionalist convinced of the importance of neuroscience is in a dilemma. If he limits himself too much to the brain, he is considered a neuro-chauvinist (Block 1980). If he formulates his theory too generally, he is considered *too* liberal. Because then he would also have to attribute properties to systems with states functionally equivalent to those of the brain—properties that he intuitively would not attribute to those systems. Block uses the Chinese nation example. If the whole Chinese population were to simulate the functional relation of individual neurons (simulate a brain), we would have to attribute mental properties to the population of China as a whole. Minimal neurophilosophy strives for an intermediate position, which—without changing the metaphor—we could call *neuro-patriotic*. Even though neurophysiological properties possibly provide only one of the many options for realizing mental properties, up until now the human being and some earthly animals with brains remain the only actually existing recognized examples of systems with mental states. But, for the moment, we do not know whether other systems besides humans can also exhibit mental properties, and minimal neurophilosophy only claims to unfold a theory of mental states in biological organisms. Of course, it is possible to learn something about the dynamics of mental state alterations in general by studying the dynamics of state alterations in biological brains (the special case). Generalizations are by no means to be excluded. As a heuristic principle, (T3) is also important for the very reason that by studying brain sciences we come closer to philosophical answers—even for questions still unimagined. (Neurophilosophers, however, should know the questions because they have studied the philosophical issues.)

In summary we can say that minimal neurophilosophy is based on the assumption that mental processes exist in biological organisms. A variety of relationships between mental processes and physical or brain processes is available. This selection of metaphysical presuppositions is not necessarily needed by the thinker who has already defined his position on the mind-body problem. But often people are still in the dark. Modifying the bon mot "How should I know what I think, before I hear what I say?" we can almost claim that one is often unsure of one's own metaphysical convictions until one works on solutions for specific problems. A list like ours can then serve the purpose of discovering which prerequisites underlie one's own claims. But it is also useful for hardboiled metaphysicians, for testing the abovementioned thesis of differential metaphysics.

Even though I advocate differential metaphysics, it wouldn't help much to demand that we clarify the nature of all kinds of mental states before we get around to working on specific problems. We would never be able to commence research on them. Instead, and for pragmatic reasons, I will throw all mental states together and plead the cause of using a *default* option for the relation between mental and physical states—well aware of the fact that in special cases this might necessitate correction. The most appropriate concept for such a default or standard option appears to be the idea of supervenience. This we shall examine in the following section.

3.2   Supervenience, Emergence, and Mental Causation

3.2.1   Supervenience   The concept of supervenience (Latin *supervenire*: *super-* in addition + *venire*, to come) is suitable as minimal neurophilosophy's point of departure for at least three reasons. First, it is logically and conceptually well drafted. Discussing it increased precision in portraying various issues in the philosophy of mind. Second, supervenience is a basic principle of naturalism, but it remains neutral on the issue of reductionism and is therefore attractive for various metaphysical positions. Third, supervenience's central concept is covariance, which is also a central methodic instrument in cognitive neuroscience.

The concept of supervenience originated in ethics. It was further developed, however, in order to serve the purpose of describing the relationship between mental (psychological) and physical properties.[45] Stated very generally, supervenience describes the relationship between two classes of properties. Using examples, I will first explain the fundamental idea, which includes three constituents (covariation, dependence, and nonreducibility), before saying why only covariation is uncontroversial. In a nutshell, *supervenience* means: "no difference of one sort without differences of another sort," (Lewis 1986, p. 14).

If there is a difference in one respect, then there is also a difference in another. That is *covariation*. But if there is a difference in the second respect, this does not mean that there is necessarily a difference in the first: Covariation is asymmetric. One of the groups of properties is fundamental—that is the nature of dependence. If we observe two classes of facts, let's say physical and biological, we can say that the class of physical facts is fundamental. Biological facts depend on physical facts, but not vice versa. If the *entirety* of physical facts is determined, that means that all biological facts are also fixed, for example, which objects are living objects. In other words, biological properties supervene upon physical properties.[46] In this example physical properties are called *subvenient*. They form the subvenient base. Generally, supervenience is the name for the relation between two classes of properties, which in the following I will call B-properties (intuitively these are complex properties, higher level properties, macroproperties) and A-properties (simple properties, properties at a basal level, microproperties).[47] In the case of the mind-body problem the A-properties are physical[48] and the B-properties are mental. But before we turn our attention to this application I would like to explain the third constituent, namely *irreducibility*, using an example of the relation between moral (B) properties and natural (A) properties. For this we must make a brief diversion to ethics and the question of just what it is that makes someone or something "good" in a moral sense.

Moore (1912) was convinced that the predicate "good" (a normative predicate) cannot be defined by descriptive predicates, because for any descriptive definition of the term "good" we can further ask why this or that particular descriptive predicate is "good." Moore called this the *argument of the open question.*[49] Converted into the terminology of properties this reads that moral properties are not reducible to natural properties. For Moore *irreducibility* is analogous to *being indefinable.*

Consider St. Augustine, the best example of a (morally) good person (assuming there are members of this species). According to Moore we can claim that the property of being (morally) "good" attributed to St. Augustine cannot be reduced to natural properties (such as his conduct—he doesn't smoke, drink, or gamble—or his psychological properties—generosity, charity, and piety), because for each of these natural properties we can ask why it is that they are prized. In spite of this kind of irreducibility, natural and moral properties are connected by covariation and dependency. Assuming that in a parallel world there also existed a St. Augustine who can be distinguished from our earthly St. Augustine by the fact that he is *not* morally respectable.[50] Because of covariation and dependence the natural properties of St. Augustine's double *must* differ from those of the original St. Augustine, they cannot be exactly the same. In other words, although moral properties do not lend themselves to reduction to natural properties, there can be no difference in the moral constituents without there also being one in the covariant natural constituents. Vice versa this means that if the natural properties are exactly the same, then the moral properties must also be exactly the same. (Due to the asymmetry of dependency that is not true the other way around.)

Believing that all three elements constitute the relation called supervenience, Donald Davidson (1970b) used this concept to characterize anomalous monism. Mental events supervene on physical events. There can be no change in mental events without a change taking place in the underlying physical events. Physical properties are basal, they determine mental properties. Mental properties thus depend on physical properties, although they cannot be reduced to them.

Davidson gave the term "supervenience" a severe formal meaning. In subsequent decades Jaegwon Kim (see 1993, 1994) analyzed the supervenience concept in detail and distinguished various differing concepts of supervenience. There are two main kinds: weak and strong supervenience. If one class of properties weakly supervenes another class of properties the following is true for *all* the individuals of a possible world. If one individual can be distinguished from another in one respect, then both are also distinguishable in another respect. In other words, when in a particular world two individuals of a possible world have the same physical properties (they are physically indistinguishable), then they also have the same mental properties (they are mentally indistinguishable). This model of supervenience, however, allows for the possibility of another world in which certain individuals are indistinguishable from terrestrial individuals, yet they have no mental properties whatsoever. This is possible because on the model of weak supervenience individuals are only compared within a particular world, it is an *intra-world* relation. Technically, the quantifier *all* is applied only to individuals, not to worlds. If we quantify over possible worlds, on the other hand, we are using the concept of *strong* supervenience, which no longer permits an identical world without minds.[51] Strong supervenience means that for *all* individuals and *all* worlds (double quantification) it is true that, if an individual in one world is indistinguishable in a certain respect from an individual in another world, then both are indistinguishable in another respect. Formally, the strong supervenience of a family of properties B unto a family of properties A is defined as follows.[52] B supervenes strongly over A if and only if it is necessarily true for any objects x and y in any worlds w_j and w_k that: If x in w_j is indistinguishable in terms of A from y in w_k (i.e., x in w_j has exactly the same properties as y in w_k), then x in w_j is indistinguishable in terms of B from y in w_k.

Applied to the two examples mentioned above, this means that, in the moral example, x is St. Augustine and y is his double, B is the family of moral properties and A is the family of natural properties. For the example with the mind-body problem, x is a person on earth and y is his equivalent in another possible world; B is the family of mental properties and A is the family of physical properties. By entering the variables we can now formulate the supervenience relation for both examples. For the following passages we are always assuming strong supervenience.

Even if there is a strong supervenience relation between physical and mental properties, that does not at all determine *which* physical properties are the ones on which mental properties supervene. From the perspective of neurophilosophy, we tend to think that subvening properties can only be brain properties. But that does not follow logically solely from the supervenience relation. Which properties are included in the subvenience base depends on how mental states are individuated. It is thoroughly conceivable that states of the peripheral nervous system are needed for individuating mental states. Various theories also assert that the embodiment of a nervous system is mandatory. In that case the subvenience base would have to be extended to include body properties. Still others regard the relation of the brain to its environment as a mandatory factor for individuating representational properties of mental states. If this is true, we have to extend the subvenience base to include this relation or perhaps even properties of the "outside" world. The subvenience base becomes even more complicated if we regard the history of mental systems as a factor necessary for individuating mental content; then we would also have to include temporal properties. And what about the linguistic, social, and cultural environment? At a later point I will argue that for *intentional* states we must widen the subvenience base to include aspects from the history of a system with a brain. Presently I aim simply to demonstrate that a supervenience relation alone does not tell us which theory of the mind is right.

Is the supervenience relation suitable as a mind-body theory? Considering these remarks, we might suppose that the answer will be negative. But the crux is not only that the class of subvenient properties is difficult to determine. Jaegwon Kim and many other theorists of supervenience have come to believe that supervenience is nothing more than an asymmetric covariation thesis. In other words, from the three elements—covariation, dependence, and irreducibility—the definition above contains only covariation and a weak kind of dependence. This dependence is *too* weak, however, to count as a mind-body theory. Strong supervenience is compatible with various varieties of dependence. It is compatible with eliminative materialism, with reductive materialism, with monistic property dualism and even with dualistic epiphenomenalism (cf. Kim 1994; Chalmers 1966a; Grimes 1988). In order to defend one of these positions one must also make additional assumptions, which are not contained in the relation of supervenience itself. This is what the newly popular emergence theories try to achieve. In addition to assuming (mereological) supervenience they also include further premises for the definition of emergence in order to gain a strong form of supervenience, which the relation of supervenience alone does not imply. I will explore emergence theories in section 3.2.3.

The alleged defect disqualifying the supervenience relation as a mind-body theory happens to be an advantage for differential metaphysics. If the supervenience relation were not already available, we would have to invent it for the program of minimal neurophilosophy. Neurophilosophical work can be founded on asymmetric covariation. By no means should our selection of a particular mind-body theory be arbitrary; there are supportive and destructive arguments for each position. But this basis allows us to begin and continue to work without compelling us to first untangle or even cut the Gordian knot of the mind-body challenge. In addition, the concept of supervenience is instrumental in clarifying the ambiguities and formulating possible solutions. We now turn to the question of how the relation of supervenience serves to more closely examine the puzzle of mental causation.

3.2.2 Mental Causation as Supervenient Causation There is a perplexity that holds for every monistic philosophy of mind that is not an identity theory. If the mental is not identical with the physical, how can it be causally effective? Colloquial speech has no trouble with mental causation. We want to go swimming, so we drive to a lake. We'd like a radio for Christmas, so we write "radio" on our wish list. We are frightened when we have to walk in the dark, so we change our route. All nonreductive materialists claim, however, that the realm of the mental is somehow autonomous. How can something mental be causally effective in the world of driving, writing, or strolling? Normally we suppose that the physical world is causally closed; no nonphysical things can be causally effective in it. This complication is not identical, but it is related to the puzzle of interaction in dualism. Monism is not concerned with differing substances, but instead with events or properties. The interactionistic dualist is in trouble because he violates the law of energy conservation in physics, a law that is generally recognized to be true. The situation is similar for mental causation. We have to allow for violation of a fundamental principle, such as the hypothesis that the physical world is causally closed, if we want to consider mental entities as causally effective, in the normal meaning of the word. That is not the acknowledged law of conservation in physics, but it is a basic principle shared by all materialistic theories. In a monograph titled "Mental Causation," Godehard Brüntrup (1994) formulated the challenge of mental causation as a trilemma, that is, as a set of three suppositions, of which at least one must be false:[53]

1. The physical world is completely causally closed.
2. From the causal uniformity of the physical world we can conclude that mental events are not causally effective.
3. Mental events are causally effective.

In order to escape this trilemma, we must drop at least one of the premises.[54] It would seem unsatisfactory to drop the first or the third premise. Questioning whether the physical world is causally closed means questioning our entire scientific world view. It is a generally accepted conviction that we would have to adopt an interactionistic dualistic position in order to warrant premise (3). So if we reject interactionistic dualism, we no longer have that option. Of course, instead we could forfeit premise (3) and maintain that mental entities are causally ineffective. This solution is suggested by epiphenomenalism, eliminative materialism, as well as abstractionism (instrumentalism). The most interesting strategy in Brüntrup's opinion is an endeavor to surrender the second premise. Identity theorists disclaim it, since in the end mental and physical events are (either type or token) identical. Brüntrup sees a further tactic for repudiating premise (2) (or perhaps 3) in the theories of supervenience and emergence. Let us now direct our attention toward mental causation as it is seen in these two theories, disregarding Brüntrup's further reflections.[55]

Let us review what mental causation means. In the broadest sense, it not only means that mental states have an influence on the physical world (mental-to-physical causation), but also that mental states cause other mental states (mental-to-mental causation), or (although seldom mentioned) that a physical state issues a mental state. Jaegwon Kim (1984) has suggested that we conceive *mental causation* as *supervenient causation*. For mental-mental causation (for example, one desire causes another desire) this means there is supervenient causation by B properties if the subvenient A properties are causally related to each other. This type of causation preserves the principle of causal completeness of the world.

Figure 2.3 shows in a graph how mental causation can be thought of as supervenient causation. A properties therein are physical, B properties are mental. Figure 2.3a shows the unproblematic case of normal, physical causation.[56] Certain physical properties P (brain states plus x) cause (uninterrupted line arrow) other physical properties (other brain states plus x). Figure 2.3b shows the supervenience of mental properties M on physical properties (wedge). The wedge symbol indicates that the supervenience basis is fundamental (wider at the bottom) and that it is not easy to move from the top to the bottom, that is, to make a reduction (the line becomes thicker). Figure 2.3c combines both ideas. The dotted line arrows signify the three kinds of mental causation; the most important case—mental-physical causation—is shown as a thick arrow. This illustrates "how mental causation is possible." Any kind of mental causation moving in the direction of a solid line arrow or on a wedge is valid due to the existing supervenience relation and is unquestionably compatible with a causal world view. If there were no supervenience relation we would have to assume *downward* [mental] *causation*.

Have we thus solved (or, as Peter Bieri 1993 would say, "dissolved") the problem of mental causation? Hardly. It has just begun to get interesting. For, as we have said earlier, by itself the relation of supervenience

(a)

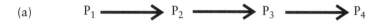

(b)

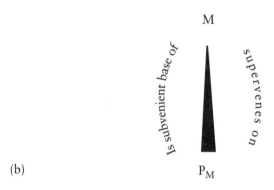

(c)

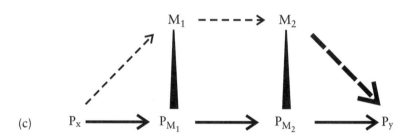

Figure 2.3
Mental causation as supervenient causation. (a) Normal, physical causation ($\rightarrow$); (b) supervenience relation (upward wedge); and (c) mental causation ($\dashrightarrow$) as supervenient causation. See text for explanation.

as defined above says nothing whatsoever about the issue of reducibility or irreducibility. Faced with proponents, Kim asserts that mental causation can only be explained as supervenient causation from a reductive or eliminative standpoint. (This is at least true if we exclude interactionalistic dualism from explaining mental causation.) Kim offers the following reasoning, sketched very briefly here.[57] It rests on these additional principles, which he holds to be true:

The Principle of Causal Completeness (PCC): The physical universe is causally closed. This means that for every physical event that has a cause there is one complete causal explanation in terms of other physical events. (Kim 1993, pp. 239, 250ff)

The Criteria of Reality (CR; a.k.a. Alexander's Dictum): To be real is to have causal powers. (Kim 1993, pp. 287, 348, 350; 1992, p. 135)

The Principle of Causal Exclusion (PCE): No event can be given more than one *complete* and *independent* causal explanation. (Kim 1993, pp. 239, 250)

Kim argues as follows (the principle is given in parentheses). Each physical event (for example, purposively raising an arm) has a complete and independent cause (PCC). If a physical event has a physical cause, it can not have a mental cause *different from that* (PCE). Thus mental events[58] must either be reduced to certain physical events (identified with them), or they have no causal influence in the physical world and are therefore not real (CR). If there is a relation of supervenience, then there is a complete and independent explanation for the supervenient causation in question, in the form of the causal relation among the subvenient events. Therefore, the supervenient events have no independent causal power. They issue their apparent causal effects only in virtue of subvenient properties. The thesis of supervenience alone cannot help a materialist (or physicalist) to explain mental causation. There are two options. Either one must reduce mental events to physical events after all (PCC and PCE), or they must be eliminated because they are not real (CR). If we cannot accept this result, we will have to accept dualism.

It is apparent that in Kim's arguments the concept of supervenience no longer contains an aspect of irreducibility. On the contrary. If we do not want to profess dualism or eliminativism, we must accept reducibility of the mental to the physical (Kim 1993, p. 267), at least, if we think of mental causation as supervenient causation. Nonreductive materialism is nothing but a *myth*—as claims the title of Kim's impressive essay of 1989 (reprinted in Kim 1993, pp. 265–284).

So the opponent in terms of arguments is obviously nonreductive materialism. Currently, interest in this standpoint is quite prevalent, without it being thoroughly clear, however, just which kind of reduction is actually being excluded. In recent years several nonreductive materialists of various shades have employed the concept of emergence to justify irreducibility. Since this concept is widespread and also closely connected to notions of "macro-determination", or "*downward causation*" I will deal with it separately.

3.2.3 Is Emergence Theory a Real Alternative? The concept of emergence is quite old, going back at least to John Stuart Mill, it was later involved in evolution theory, and is now once again an issue in modern philosophy's conception of the mind-body problem. A survey of the entire historical development of the concept would be too bulky for our present purpose.[59] Therefore, after giving a condensed introduction, I shall use a distinction made by Achim Stephan, discriminating between a weak and a strong concept of emergence. We will find that emergence and supervenience are close kin. Then I shall lay out the problem of macrodetermination and that of downward causation. In conclusion, we shall see how contemporary supervenience and emergence theories help reveal a clue to the puzzle of mental causation. (I will suggest a solution in chapter 3.)

To "emerge" means literally "to come forth from immersion"; this is a provisional allusion to the nature of emergent properties. Such properties were hitherto not apparent; they emerge for the first time. Their newness is either diachronic or synchronic (Stephan 1999, pp. 26–32). To be diachronic signifies that an emergent property comes forth for the first time within a temporal perspective.[60] An example would be the characteristic of "living," which "arose" at some point during the course of evolution. By contrast, synchronic observation concentrates on the relation between the properties of a system and the properties of its parts and their organization, regardless of time.

We find the expression "emergence" first used by Lewes (1875). Following ideas of John Stuart Mill, he distinguishes "resulting" from "emerging" properties. A *resulting* property of a system is a consequence of a quantitative summation of the properties of its parts, for example, resulting from simple addition (such as the total weight of a body), or from the addition of reciprocal values (electric resistance), or a vector addition (velocity). *Emergent* properties, in contrast, are qualitatively new kinds of properties that the system exhibits, without the individual parts exhibiting those qualities. Examples are the liquidity of water, oscillation behavior, and the odor of chemical compounds, the catchword being the whole is more than the sum of its parts.

Today the emergent properties of systems discovered by Lewes are simply called systemic properties. Just about all emergence theorists have been and today are materialists, they assumed, and still assume that the entities of the world are made up of physical components. They share the view of supervenience theorists, who insist that there can be no difference in systemic properties without there simultaneously being differences among the properties of the system's parts or the way they are organized (this is the thesis of *mereological* supervenience; *meros* means "part" in Greek). In order to express the dependency of the supervenient on the subvenient properties, emergence theorists speak of *synchronic determinedness* (Stephan 1999, pp. 26–32) or *microdetermination* (Hoyningen-Heune 1994, p. 172), instead of mereological supervenience. The properties and the behavior of a system are completely determined by its components and their organization (the system's microstructure).

Now we have all the criteria for a *weak concept of emergence*:

1. physical monism,
2. the existence of systemic properties, and
3. synchronic determinedness or microdetermination.

No one will deny that emergent properties in this (weak) sense of the word actually exist. They are compatible with reductionistic materialism. Mario Bunge (1984) and Gerhard Vollmer (1992a) make use of them. They are also used to characterize systemic properties in cognitive science, in connectionistic theory, and in the theory of self-organization. So the question is, are there emergent properties in a stronger sense?

Achim Stephan (1999) investigates this from a philosophical perspective. His goal is not to determine whether emergent properties actually exist, but to first establish a concept of emergence that is suitable for distinguishing emergent properties other than merely weak emergent properties. He examines various criteria for a stronger concept of emergence. Throughout its history, the following characteristics have been suggested: originality (newness), hierarchy of existence levels, being in principle unpredictable, being nondeducible, being irreducible, and *downward* causation. Stephan develops a typology for emergence theories and distinguishes a total of six subspecies. Synchronic emergence is the most important among them, because it is relevant for the debate on mental causation. Synchronic emergence is weak emergence plus an insistence on *irreducibility*.[61] Thus we have the fourth characteristic for a sufficiently strong concept of emergence:

4. irreducibility.

In this context to be irreducible means "not deducible from the micro level."[62] This predicate can apply to properties or laws (Hoyningen-Heune 1994). A property or law at the macro level is *irreducible* if it cannot be deduced from complete information about the properties and the organization of the system's components and the laws pertaining to the micro level. Stephan (1999, p. 36) adds, "which these have alone or in simpler systems." This supplement is not negligible because it introduces an epistemic facet in the definition of irreducibility. This is evident in Hoyningen-Heune's work, where he subordinates being deducible (along with being unexplainable and original) to being unpredictable, and then says that knowledge of states of the system cannot be gained by "knowledge of the lower level alone, but exclusively empirically post factum, after the occurrence of the emergent phenomenon itself."[63] The criterion of irreducibility thus once again returns us to our familiar predicament: the problem of reduction. I will not reiterate that problem here (cf. section 2.1.3), but would like to remind the reader that the reductionism problem and the concept of explanation are entwined. This is evidenced by the fact that it is possible to advocate a theory relative concept of emergence, as the founders of the reductionist program, Hempel and Oppenheim (1948), have done. They considered certain properties to be emergent *relative* to a particular theory. Thus, for example, the macro property of being superfluid is emergent relative to classical theory: The first cannot be deduced from the latter. The reason is because superfluidity is a quantum effect; a quantum mechanical description of fluid, in contrast, does allow the deduction of a possible superfluid state. A typical emergence theorist claims more, however. He claims namely that emergents are also emergent relative to a complete and final theory. The trouble is that this claim cannot be tested and the reductionist can always excuse nondeductiveness by the deficient state of his basis theory (cf. Hoyningen-Huene 1994, pp. 185f).

Does the synchronic concept of emergence make progress when compared to the theory of supervenience? For starters we must remember that the original idea of supervenience and the notion of emergence are closely connected. The original idea of supervenience included the three properties of covariance, dependency, and irreducibility. But, unfortunately, it turned out that the formal definition of supervenience only contains a claim of covariation, taken together with an inadequate form of the dependency claim. The synchronic concept of emergence now explicitly reveals those elements that the modernized concept of supervenience no longer contains—strong dependency (3) and irreducibility (4). It also emphasizes the mereological facet, that is, the fact that real systems are made up of components and exhibit various levels of hierarchy.[64] Synchronic emergence is therefore simply a "dressed up" version of mereological supervenience.

Second, I would like to clearly point out that proof of emergent properties is not an *argument* supporting a nonreductive position. The existence of systemic, weak emergent properties is perfectly compatible with reductionism. Claiming that something is synchronically emergent is doing nothing more than *saying that* a weak emergent property is irreducible. Synchronic emergentism is thus only the *expression* of a nonreductive stance. If we want to justify that position, it does not suffice to simply assert the existence of emergent properties. We still require extra arguments for irreducibility.

Nevertheless, these concepts do aid us in examining certain problems. Let us return to the problem of mental causation.

3.2.4 Is Mental Causation Directed Downward? Many emergence theorists postulate causal effectiveness at the macro level. Kim (1992, 1993, pp. 336–357) insists that due to their premise of irreducibility they must necessarily conceive of mental causation as being directed downward. *Downward causation*, also known as macrodetermination, means that emergent (mental) properties (properties of the upper, macro level) can cause something on a lower, micro level; this means that mental properties can somehow have direct causal effects on physical properties.

In fact, many early emergence theorists (like Lloyd C. Morgan, Roy Wood Sellars, but not Samuel Alexander) defended the idea of *downward* causation.[65] But it is also prevalent in the later phase of the discussion on emergence. The term *downward causation* resurfaced in the work of David Campbell (1974), after similar ideas appeared in that of Mario Bunge (1977) and particularly in the 1960s writings of the neurophysiologist Roger Sperry, who we could also call a neurophilosopher.[66] Sperry supports his version of macrodetermination with the example of a wheel rolling down a hill. The course the wheel takes determines the spatiotemporal properties of its components and, in the same way, mental events determine physical processes.

This conclusion issues as a result of blending Alexander's dictum with the thesis of irreducibility: "To be real, Alexander has said, is to have causal powers; *to be real, new, and irreducible, therefore, must be to have new irreducible causal powers*" (Kim 1993, p. 350). Kim, in contrast, is convinced that individual mental events inherit their causal powers from those physical properties that instantiated them. He calls this the *Causal Inheritance Principle*. But we can only have this, if we first accept reduction (Kim 1993, p. 355). How do emergentists react to such a remonstrance that they must rely on downward causation? Stephan (1999) objects that Kim does not distinguish between ontological and explanatory reducibility. Kim's argument is only sturdy if his concept of reduction is understood as being ontological. An emergentist, however, uses "reduction" in an explanatory sense, as "second level reduction." Properties or causal relations are only explanatorily reducible when we are not only in a position to discover the relation of supervenience, but also to *explain* that supervenience relation itself, which means comprehending why it exists. Horgan (1993) also demands that sophisticated physicalism must be able to explain the supervenience relation. A relation that is sufficiently explained and comprehendible would be, in his words, *superdupervenience*. Borrowing that term, Stephan calls the causal relation among two superdupervenient properties superduper-venient causation. Kim's argument is only convincing if we understand mental causation as superdupervenient causation, meaning that the relation of supervenience itself is susceptible to explanatory reduction. As long as the relation of supervenience cannot be explained (by explanatory reduction), however, the emergence theorist is still left with the option of interpreting mental causation as supervenient causation, without facing the implications that Kim claims he must.

We are beginning to see which direction neurophilosophy must take if it adheres to robust physicalism. We will have to explicate the relation of supervenience itself. In other words, we must attempt to explanatorily reduce certain mental properties (those which appear to be causal) to certain physical properties. I will outline a suggestion for this kind of explanatory reduction in chapter 3.

3.3   The Naturalism of Neurophilosophy

What can we gain from all this for the project of a neurophilosophy of free will? The basic idea is obvious. Neurophilosophy can allow those competent in metaphysics to continue quarreling over which mind-body theory is correct and true. Meanwhile, with minimal consensus on metaphysical issues, we are getting on with our work. Getting to the task at hand means analyzing the individual components of free will using our knowledge in neurobiology and attempting to clear up the matter of whether or not, and in which form, free will exists in our world. For now, many metaphysical questions may remain unanswered. Take, for example, the issue of physical realization. From a metaphysical standpoint, this matter is of central importance because it ascertains one's positional preference on the mind-body problem. So philosophers have set out to formulate an exact concept of physical realization (Beckermann 1996). Others deal with the issue rather nonchalantly behind the banner of NOA—*natural ontological attitude* (see Dennett 1991). Again, others cling to property dualism without disavowing ontological monism, careful not to join the company of dualistic interactionists (Chalmers 1996a).

Neurophilosophy of free will is built upon physical substance monism. Other issues, such as property dualism, certain functionalistic theses, and

so on, remain open. It is possible, even probable, that the notion of differential metaphysics will turn out to be true—the thesis that divergent
mental properties have an assortment of metaphysical underpinnings.
Instead of presupposing any single theory relevant for all mental entities—one that could turn out to be wrong—I work with what we already
have: our philosophical theories about free will and our knowledge of
the brain. Of course, I also make provisions, namely, the three central
theses of minimal neurophilosophy. But these do not bind me irrevocably to any particular metaphysical theory. Naturally, it is possible to
begin with a unified theory, whether because it is attractive, because one
is convinced that it is true, or because it provides direction. That is perfectly legitimate. The crucial point, however, is that we definitely depend
on empirical findings for discovering which theory applies to which
mental processes. It is this dependence of theory upon empirical research
that brands (stigmatism welcomed) my approach to neurophilosophy as
"naturalistic."

Naturalism is presumably as controversial as physical realization or
emergence. It would be too good to be true, if we could offer a clear and
generally accepted definition for naturalism and then acknowledge it.
Though there actually are a few lucid definitions, they are far from being
accepted by all.[67] Therefore, I adopt a position similar to that of David
Papineau. He claims that his book *Philosophical Naturalism* is more a
sample of the naturalistic turn in philosophy and less a discussion of naturalism itself (Papineau et al. 1996, p. 657). Instead of searching for an
answer to the query about what naturalism actually is, he *just does it.*
Some think that naturalism is a continuity of science and philosophy,
others that it is a metaphysical bulwark against dualism, others see it as
externalism in epistemology. Papineau actually shares all three opinions.
But instead of inquiring whether these are characteristic of naturalism,
he asks what justifies them. By applying the concept to real cases, I, too,
try to show what it is that justifies these notions. The first of them
is particularly important for neurophilosophy as an interdisciplinary
undertaking.

I also entirely agree with Michael Ruse's note on the problem of naturalism. He states: "For me 'naturalism' has to do with nature, i.e., with
the realm of experience. And since the methods of science are the most

successful access we have to that realm—the single true access that leads to real understanding—I think that a naturalist is someone who seeks understanding through the methods and findings of science" (Ruse 1996, p. 1). Ruse hurries to emphasize what naturalism is *not*. It is not the exclusion of human feelings from science. It also does not imply scientism—the notion that science can solve *all* problems. A naturalistic philosopher also does not strive to be better than scientists in their own fields. That would be hopeless. Instead, he tries to better comprehend specifically philosophical questions by studying the methods and findings of science.[68]

Another significant mark of philosophical naturalism is a healthy portion of distrust in arm chair philosophy and a priori arguments. To avoid misunderstanding, this does not mean that logical arguments are of little value. It just means that in the end nature is the instance against which we must test the truth or falsity of our theories and the validity of our arguments, not pure rationality, not even purely *logical* thinking.

As I have just endeavored to describe it, naturalism allows us to work on an empirically appropriate theory of autonomy and to discover something about human nature, instead of merely chewing indigestible chunks of history; it opens the way to a "Neurophilosophy of free will." In one of the few papers on this subject Oshana (1994) suggests two criteria for a naturalistic concept of autonomy: First, "The properties which constitute autonomy must be natural properties, knowable through the senses or by introspection (or must supervene on natural properties)." In other words, "claims about autonomy can be established *a posteriori* on the basis of natural facts." Second, "the properties that constitute autonomy must not be restricted to phenomena 'internal' to the agent. . . . [A] completely naturalized account will treat autonomy as, in part, a function of natural relations that are *extrinsic* to the individual" (Oshana 1994, p. 76f.).

According to these criteria the neurophilosophical theory of natural autonomy sketched in the next chapter is naturalistic. Besides the premises of minimal neurophilosophy I found my enterprise also on the principle of supervenience of the mental on the physical. I am not convinced that it is applicable for all mental states (this is particularly due to the status of abstract properties). But much is to be said for working with this principle. It is formally well-formulated and enjoys widespread acceptance. It contains essentially the principle of covariation, a principle capable of broad consensus in philosophy, and which in addition is excellently compatible to correlative approaches in brain research. Above all, it is not too particular; it does not claim supervenience of mental states on brain states (*internalism*). Externalism, such as Oshana suggests, will be of importance. Thus equipped, I shall now employ findings from neuroscience to examine, analyze, criticize, perhaps revise, or reject some philosophical theories and arguments. From the standpoint of minimal neurophilosophy there is no principle objection to doing so. Only the yield will show whether it is worth a try. Not to follow this approach on the grounds of its metaphysical assumptions is to deprive us of a significant potential for innovation. Sooner or later we will have to deal with neurophilosophical arguments. In the long run philosophy has never successfully ignored new scientific views of the world nor escaped integrating scientific findings in some form or another into its theoretic schemes.

3

Successor Concepts: Putting Free Will to the Test with Neurophilosophy

1 Doing Otherwise: Chaos Instead of Indeterminism

Synopsis

We shall now examine the plausibility of the notion of an indeterministic free will using criteria from neurophilosophy. We begin—as libertarians generally do—with a nonvalerian, internalist concept of free will. We will take a cursory look at the oldest and one of the most recent attempts to use quantum theory to support a libertarian version of free will, and reject both on the grounds of implausibility. This is followed by modified version of being able to do otherwise (doing otherwise under similar circumstances) and an examination of whether or not it is plausible in terms of neurophilosophy. The chaotic nature of brain organization makes it at least conceivable. Next, we turn to empirical evidence. Faced with the intelligibility argument, this interpretation is less susceptible to criticism than the libertarian version, because in chaos the same mechanisms generate order as well as instability. The successor concept of free will that we can develop with this method—natural autonomy—is, upon scrutiny, a valerian concept of autonomy. Beyond this, chaos theory—being a special case of the theory of nonlinear dynamical systems—provides a first and basic foundation for developing a neurophilosophical theory of cognition. In addition, the theory of dynamic systems suggests that we should not individuate the semantic content of representations solely in terms of what is internal.

1.1 Quantum Theory and Free Will

Given specific conditions, can we behave other than we actually do? That is the central question concerning the first component of free will. In chapter 1, we found that determinism claims that we cannot. So two options remain. Either the world is, or is not, determined. Depending on the route we choose, we can annex two queries. First, assuming our world is deterministic, is there a modified form of being able to do otherwise, that is in any way relevant to human behavior? I shall reply to this compatibilist question with a neurophilosophical answer. Second, let us assume that the world is indeterministic. For all we know, this appears to be the case.[1] Quantum physics gives us the only means with which we can establish an indeterministic version of being able to do otherwise. So our second question is this: Is indeterminism, as exhibited by quantum theory, helpful for understanding the brain? I shall tackle this matter first. Although a few papers on the subject are available,[2] we will inspect just two theories, the oldest and the most recent. These are, respectively, the amplifier theory of the free will developed by Pascual Jordan and the ORCH OR model suggested by Roger Penrose and Stuart Hameroff.

1.1.1 The Amplifier Theory of Free Will   Quantum theory allows for absolutely random events. It states that there are noncausal events, that is, events that are not causally determined, such as the decay of radio-active atom nuclei. Momentarily, this intuitive notion of quantum theory suffices for our purposes (see also chapter 1, section 2.3.2). It would seem natural to exploit this kind of objective indeterminism for solving the mystery of free will. One of the earliest and most persistent promoters of it was the physicist Pascual Jordan (1932, 1934, 1938, 1943). Impressed by the Copenhagen interpretation of quantum mechanics, which attested great significance to the observation (or measurement) of an event, he sized up the situation as follows: "The claim of determinism is this. . . . From the observable state of a person at time t and the observation of all factors influencing him, we can calculate exactly what his state will be at a later point of time t'" (Jordan 1932, p. 819).

Jordan, unfortunately, did not distinguish between (ontological) determinedness and calculability, but we can hardly scold him for that, since in 1932 this distinction had yet to be recognized as an obstacle. Jordan evaluates determinism from the vantage of quantum mechanics and sees quite correctly that for a determinist

the crucial question [is], whether or not organic systems, such as human beings, may be viewed as essentially *macroscopic* systems: Only in that case can we expect (practically) complete causal determinedness in the reaction of an organic creature *in spite of the noncausal behavior of atomic structures*, i.e., if *the entire causal chain of such* reactions occurs in the macroscopic realm. (Jordan 1932, p. 819, emphasis in original)

Jordan continues to say that no, we *cannot* view humans as essentially macroscopic organisms. So he postulates that quantum processes *are* important for human behavior. In a survey of *The Present State of the Amplifier Theory of Organisms* (Jordan 1938) he collects evidence to demonstrate the importance of atomic processes for living creatures. For example, he mentions, enzymes and effects of toxins, where a few molecules issue great effects. His largest group of examples is taken from the field of radiobiology. These show that individual photons and other elementary particles cause mutations or even death. Finally, ahead of his time, he introduces the idea of "one gene = one molecule." After studying his examples he concludes:

It is characteristic of organic nature that the noncausality of certain atomic reactions is amplified to become macroscopically effective noncausality. . . . According to this hypothesis, the structure and the way an organism functions would be just like that of an *amplifier organization*, . . . for short: an amplification theory of organisms. (Jordan 1932, p. 820, emphasis in original)

He divides organism reactions into two classes: a class governed by macroscopic causality and a class of noncausally determined "directive" reactions. What he modestly called a hypothesis in 1932, he later reformulated, rather sharply:

Individual quantum leaps of particular single molecules within the cell critically control the entirety of the cell's life functions. Without exaggerating, we can claim that the content of the amplification theory of organisms summarized in this sentence is certainly a biological insight as is cell theory or micelle theory." (Jordan 1938, p. 545, emphasis in original)

Without exaggeration, notice that this assertion *is* quite overstated. Even today, we have no evidence that "quantum leaps critically control the life functions of organisms." From the onset, Jordan's theory was subject to hefty criticism from empirical biologists. One of his most stubborn critics was the biologist Erwin Bünning (1935, 1943). After Jordan had published his thesis in 1934 in the periodical *Erkenntnis*, Bünning went to work to demonstrate why microphysical events are rather insignificant for organisms. His claims were essentially three. His first objection was that normally organisms exhibit no trace of an amplification of noncausal microprocesses. To show this, Büning takes recourse to phys-iological phenomena such as the phototropism of oat grain sheaths, enzyme effects, and the radiation sensitivity of intestinal bacteria. But even if we perhaps would agree with Jordan that noncausal events are effective in organisms, his argument is misleading. Bünning's second objection is, therefore, that noncausal events are irrelevant for control and direction: The amplifier theory can be repeated *ad absurdum*. Jordan's theory, he says, would "not even make the characteristic per-formance of an organism comprehendible, because the *falsity* of his theory is straightforwardly (at least normally) necessary for just those performances" (Bünning 1935, p. 346). This is true, because, for an organism, a fluctuation effecting the macroscopic level, would normally lead to illness or death. Bünning's third argument (1934) is that non-causal events occur outside of the body and influence it from without (such as radiation effects), so we can assume that (noncausal) direction is *not an organizational principle of the organism itself.* Thus "directive reactions" are not constitutive of the organism itself. Neither of the authors mentions the neurophilosophically intriguing question of just how the amplification is realized within the brain. Bünning devotes a mere thirteen lines to brain cells. There, he (correctly) refutes Alverode's equation of microphysical processes to microscopically visible processes and confirms: "I will not extensively deal with the processes of brain cells. Numerous performances there can certainly only be understood through rigorous causality. Whether we must proceed to measuring and observing individual atoms in order to research brain processes—we do not know" (Bünning 1935, p. 346). In summary, Bünning's arguments against the amplifier theory can be read as follows (translated into the component theory in parentheses). There may be noncausal micro-physical processes (indeterminism is true), and these may, in some special situations issue effects for an organism (the capacity to do otherwise). These effects are normally detrimental; at least do they by no means explain the characteristic behavior of organisms (a variation on the intelligibility argument), and furthermore, some of them are extraneous events and therefore not an organizational principle of the organism itself (they do not establish agency). All three components are also found here.

One difficulty impeding both Jordan and Bünning's arguments is their diffuse position on a substantial matter. Jordan claims that the human being is not *essentially* a macroscopic system, while Bünning argues that microphysical effects are *normally* detrimental to organisms. But what is *essential* and what is *normal*? Within the scheme of the Jordan-Bünning debate we find no answer, since the question remains of how quantum-physical indeterminism can be effective within the brain.

Subsequent authors, in contrast, do try to locate indeterministic events within the brain. It seems plausible; there is general consensus on the idea that the brain is the control organ for human actions and decisions. Jonas (1981) and Eccles (1990) suggested unlikely solutions; theirs violate the law of the conservation of energy and hence need not interest us further. They are scientifically obsolete.[3] However, one available theory attempts to postulate a role for quantum events in the brain. It is in line with physics, being co-formulated by one of the leading physicists of our time. Can this theory provide a plausible explanation for how indeterministic processes play an "essential" role in the brain?

1.1.2 Penrose and Hameroff's ORCH OR Model   Stuart Hameroff, an anesthetist, and Roger Penrose, a physicist, collaborated in recent years to formulate a theory of consciousness. They claim that quantum phenomena occur in certain structures of those nerve cells that might be pertinent for explaining some peculiarities of consciousness, such as the "unity of self, nondeterministic free will, and nonalgorithmic 'intuitive' processing" (Hameroff 1994, p. 91). Both scientists reject substance dualism as a remedy for the perplexities of consciousness and both acknowledge naturalism. However, they do think that traditional reductionism, which takes recourse solely to traditional neurophysiological properties, cannot explain those mentioned mental phenomena. For this we need extended quantum theory, namely a theory of quantum gravitation.

Penrose and Hameroff (P & H) began their investigations independently of one another. As an anesthetist, Hameroff was interested in how anesthetics induce narcosis. Penrose, on the other hand, sought to understand how human mathematicians find proofs, particularly in cases where no algorithm for finding a proof exists (Gödel). Penrose (1989,

1994, 1995) concluded that human thinking is not algorithmic; and this needed explanation. True, P & H's approaches differ in some details (cf. Penrose 1994a, 1994b, 1994c; Hameroff 1994; Penrose and Hameroff 1995; Hameroff and Penrose 1996), but for the purpose of our discussion we can treat them as *one* theory. It will help explain whether and how quantum events can be at work in the brain.

Their ORCH OR (*orch*estrated *o*bjective *r*eduction) theory runs as follows (Penrose and Hameroff 1995, pp. 104f): Certain aspects of quantum theory combined with the phenomenon of objective reduction of state vectors are necessary for human consciousness. The quantum events in question occur in the microtubules. Microtubules (MT) are cell structures that we can best imagine as being cell skeletons. They consist of subunits (tubulines), which are arranged in rows and build tubes. They are spread throughout the cell and provide stability. They are partially built up and destroyed again (polymerized and depolymerized) and serve as a framework for intracellular transportation processes.

Hameroff is convinced that anesthesia expedients have effects on the microtubules, which clearly would show that the latter are necessary for consciousness. Penrose and Hameroff also posit that microtubules are used in "computation." This supposition is based on the concept of a quantum computer (cf. Deutsch 1985, 1992). Roughly, a quantum computer works like this. The numerous superimposed quantum states, which, in a certain sense, exist simultaneously, and which continually proceed to develop according to the laws of quantum physics, can theoretically be used as parallel computational units that process information. When the state vector is reduced, the abundance of parallel states collapses to a single classical micro state, it becomes a "solution." For a quantum computer of this kind to be realized, however, it is first necessary that quantum states (microphysical states) be generated at all. There should be no reciprocal effects going on between the locus of quantum computation and macrophysical states. This, according to Penrose and Hameroff, is why MTs are good for this task. The fact that they are filled with pure water and have a tubular structure make them a potentially adequate medium for quantum events. The arrangement of MT subunits could be used for computation via "cooperative mutual effects." Thus "quantum coherence" could develop among the MT subunits and an "order" for the water molecules could develop on the MT surfaces, such that phenomena like superradiance and self-induced transparency become possible. During preconscious processing the MTs function as little quantum computers. Their diverse possible conformation states exist simultaneously next to each other (superimposed) until the mass distribution differences among the superimposed states become so great that the wave function collapses and the state vector is reduced. This last step, namely the reduction of the state vector via differences in the mass distribution of superimposed states must first be *objectively* explained by a theory of quantum gravity that remains to be developed. If we had this theory, we could talk of "objective reduction" (OR). The resulting conformation state of the microtubules could be understood as the outcome of a "quantum computation," which can be objectively explained, although it cannot be algorithmically deduced. That was exactly what Penrose wanted to achieve!

The resulting states "implement neurophysiological functions." The proteins associated with the MTs (MAPs) fine-tune these physical processes. This is why Penrose and Hameroff (1995) speak of an "orchestrated" reduction. In the next step Penrose looks at neurophysiological experiments undertaken by Benjamin Libet (portrayed in section 2.5.1). From his experiments Libet arrives at the conclusion that under certain conditions it takes a half of a second for neuronal adequacy of conscious experience to appear. Using the uncertainty principle, Penrose calculates an estimate of how many neurons per temporal unit under these conditions must be in coherent superposition in order for a conscious event to occur. He finds that this must be 500 neurons per second. Quick conscious events would require more neurons, slower ones require fewer. Each OR stands for a single conscious event, a series would result in a "stream of consciousness." Each OR can "bind" diverse other superpositions which happen at other times and places, in order to generate the consciousness of "now." Anesthetics generate a lack of consciousness by preventing quantum coherence in the microtubules via diverse mechanisms. The claim is that the ORCH OR model could thus explain crucial functions of consciousness: "(1) control/regulation of neural action, (2) pre-conscious to conscious transition, (3) non-computability, (4) causality, (5) binding of various (time scale and spatial) superpositions into instantaneous 'now', (6) a 'flow' of time, and (7) a connection to fundamental space-time geometry" (Penrose and Hameroff 1995, p. 104). So this is the ORCH OR theory of consciousness, currently the best detailed neurophilosophical theory of indeterministic mental processes.[4] It is highly speculative, it includes many assumptions and claims for which there is hardly evidence. But it is an example of a genuinely neurophilosophical theory because it is based on the conviction that mental processes must be realized in the brain and it attempts to comply with our current knowledge of the brain. It is, however, susceptible to criticism. How plausible is this theory?[5] I will not discuss, but simply concede points 4, 6, and 7. I will also not particularly deal with point 3, the alleged and very controversial idea that human thinking is nonalgorithmic (cf. commentaries in Penrose 1990; and commentators Grush and Churchland 1995). My criticism is particularly directed at the points 1, 2, and 5. Of special concern are (i) the implausibility of the theoretic premises, (ii) the unlikelihood that quantum theoretic events are relevant to brain activity, (iii) the controversial role of microtubules, (iv) noise objections, (v) the unsolved mystery of neural coding and control, and (vi) the concept of consciousness underlying all of this.

(i) The ORCH OR Model is not inconsistent with physics, but it does have a marked weakness. It is founded on a theory we haven't got yet! The theory of quantum gravitation is an ambitious attempt to combine gravitational theory and quantum theory. Certainly this combination is a desideratum for theoretic physics. But whether it will work is still entirely up in the air. Thus the whole theory is built on sand, especially when it assures us that it can certainly explain consciousness, albeit using a theory we do not yet have.

(ii) To date, there is no evidence that the postulated quantum phenomena (quantum coherence, dynamic order of water molecules, and coherent photons, that is, superradiation and self-induced transparency) actually occur within the nervous system. The only paper that P & H quote on this issue is one by Jibu et al. (1994). It deals with the idea that the profound ability of individual cells to react to weak light, which was discovered by another group of scientists, *could possibly* be explained to the effect that water arranged in a particular way within the cell skeleton functions as a water laser. No proof is delivered, however, and the reader should not be intimidated by the authors' extreme competence in physics and quantitative calculations to think that anything beyond sheer possibility is being discussed here.

(iii) It is controversial, whether microtubules are important for consciousness at all. The effect of narcosis expedients is generally not considered to be due to their influence on microtubules, but to their effects on cell membranes and the way they influence certain ionic channels (Forth et al. 1996, pp. 240f). These are *macro*physical effects in the range of millivolts, which are irrelevant to the postulated quantum events. In addition, microtubules end approximately one micron (10^{-6} m) before the synapse—within the realm of quantum events that is an astronomical distance! P & H do notice this problem. They point out that there are other structures between the synapses and the microtubules, such as the synapsins. Nowhere, however, do they mention to which extent this macromolecule could solve the problem of covering the distance. A further objection to the notion that the MTs are significant is provided by the way colchicin, a remedy for arthritis, works. It is known that it suppresses the polymerization of MTs. Theoretically then, it should also have an effect on phenomena of consciousness. It has not been observed, however, that patients treated with colchicin are normally deeply unconsciousness. Nevertheless, Penrose and Hameroff (1995, pp. 105f) do offer some empirical arguments on the matter, which we cannot entirely shrug off. So—in *dubio pro reo*—we shall not let this point count against them. But one critical point is more striking. If MT were crucial for consciousness, then it would also have to be of importance for other changes in consciousness, such as the cycle of sleep and waking. But there is not a trace of proof for that.

(iv) The noise objection cropped up as early as the Jordan-Bünning debate. To which extent must we think of organisms as essentially macrophysical systems? Once again, it is correct that in our traditional convictions all real systems consist of components for which quantum theory holds. As soon as we move to the macrophysical level, however, those peculiar quantum phenomena no longer occur. They show up only in isolated systems or in an environment that is not "contaminated" by macrophysical objects. This can be illustrated as follows. The reciprocal effects between quantum events and normal macrophysical objects cause quantum events to be lost in thermodynamic noise and become ineffective—unless there is a rigorously ordered medium, for example ordered water. For P & H the cavity of the microtubules presents such a medium. So the question arises: Should we think of the insides of the microtubules as essentially macrophysical objects? The proponents answer:

"*Given the apparently noisy, thermal environment within neurons and the brain, how could quantum coherent phenomena occur: (a) within the neurons, and (b) throughout macroscopic brain regions?* This is the crux of the matter" (Penrose and Hameroff, 1995, p. 106). The answer is, all things considered, coherent quantum phenomena *cannot* occur in the brain. First, there is no evidence of the existence of ordered water in microtubules; and second, it is more than probable that elements (such as salts) dissolved in the inner cellular waters would extinguish quantum phenomena. P & H argue to the contrary that contaminants having molecule diameters smaller than water molecules would hinder the dynamic order of the water and thus prevent a basis for quantum phenomena. Therefore, intracellular ions appearing in high concentrations, such as sodium, calcium, and magnesium would not disturb quantum phenomena. The authors admit, however, that the presence of chloride makes water order impossible. This is why they limit the effect of quantum events to the dendrites (end branches) of neurons (Penrose and Hameroff 1995, p. 108).[6] Naturally, the question remains of how quantum phenomena are still supposed to transport information along the axons. The noise objection is therefore, as it was for the Jordan-Bünning debate, a critical point, but it can, at least in principle, be answered empirically. We can maintain that to date there is no solid empirical evidence that local quantum phenomena play a role in neurons, and that there are good arguments to the contrary.

(v) A further point is related to the noise objection and is equally important. Even if there somehow were local quantum effects in MTs, how can a local quantum effect become a global one? It is supposed to be a strength of the ORCH OR Model that it will some day explain the unity and global character of consciousness. Inconsistencies begin with the fact that microtubules are found in *bundles*, but according to the theory, quantum effects only occur in the cavities of *individual* MTs. How can the MTs synchronize or pass on their quantum phenomena if they cannot bridge the noisy gap? How can neighboring neurons, still separated by cell membranes, synchronize themselves? How shall quite distant parts of the brain ever be able to exhibit quantum mechanical global effects, without exchanging information or drowning in noise? These problematic issues are not addressed, although precisely these are supposed to be solved by the theory. In contrast, traditional neurophysiology does present some well formulated theories about how global phenomena occur in the brain (Koch and Davis 1994). It is not as if we must rely on quantum mechanics because we don't possess any other reasonable explanations. The claim that the perplexity of neural control is remedied by the ORCH OR theory is simply false. It is not discussed even once.

(vi) However, P & H can still claim that one phenomenon, namely the aspect of "now," stubbornly refuses to be explained by neurophysiology. The aspect of "now" that we find in consciousness, that is the fact that at a certain point of time t we are *instantaneously* aware of certain things. Doesn't the collapsing wave function imply "the summary of all superimposed states happening in a single moment?" Note that the idea of consciousness conjured up by P & H for the reader is misleading. This becomes clear when we consider which authority they appeal to. They make reference to experiments conducted by Benjamin Libet, which are meant to demonstrate how long it takes for a decision to become conscious. The import of these experiments, however, is highly controversial.[7] The fact of "being now" that is part of consciousness is certainly worthy of explanation. The best explanation is that it is a *user illusion* (Metzinger 1993; see also Pöppel 1985; and Dennett 1991a).

In summary, the ORCH OR model is based on physical theories that do not yet exist. It claims that there are local quantum effects, which has yet to been proven. If they do exist, we still cannot explain how they can unfold global effects. Therefore, they do not help us to explain the unity of consciousness entailing free will. P & H also summon an incorrect notion of consciousness. And the problem of control (intelligibility)—for our purposes perhaps the most important feature—is not even touched upon. From a neurophilosophical point of view Penrose and Hameroff's is an inadequate theory, not suitable as a background for libertarianism. It is, nevertheless, a scientific theory, susceptible to empirical criticism and falsification. But because it exhibits so many deficits without really being in a position to explain matters, which (at least in principle) traditional neurophysiology could explain just as well, for our purposes we will consider it refuted. Let us now turn to the compatibilistic issue of how we can modify the ability to do otherwise and which neurophilosophical arguments we can find for such an understanding.

1.2   Order from Chaos

1.2.1   Doing Otherwise: A Moderate Version   Even though our world at times appears to be indeterministic, that in itself is not an argument in favor of free will. There are two reasons. First, we have the intelligibility argument, which states that an action or decision cannot be intelligible, if it is free only in virtue of being *undetermined* or in virtue of being essentially due to undetermined events. Second, we have seen that there is little plausibility of local (indeterministic) quantum events in the brain. What does this imply for a theory of natural autonomy? One option would be to skip the first component and consider it irrelevant for a theory of autonomy. I will not take this path, because I am convinced that our intuitions about being able to do otherwise are central for the concept we have of ourselves and that they have a real basis. Another option is to modify the first component. Moore took this route when he interpreted the ability to do otherwise as "a person would have done otherwise, had he wanted otherwise." I will also not travel down that compatibilistic road either, but instead I shall ask: Can we less drastically modify the ability to do otherwise in a way that at least partially satisfies our intuitions? In order to investigate this I will counterfactually first assume that classical determinism holds in our world. If we can establish a weaker form of the ability to do otherwise in a deterministic world, then it should indeed be possible to do so for an indeterministic world.

In a world fully determined in the classical sense there can be no personal ability to do otherwise if by this is meant that under identical circumstances and valid laws of nature a person could do something different from what he or she actually does. But identical constraints and initial conditions never occur twice or even more often! True, people often do act under comparable or similar conditions, but never under identical conditions. If the brain is sensitive to the smallest changes in constraints, we can formulate a weaker version of alternativism, which could be true in a deterministic world. Then a person can do otherwise (act, decide, choose, desire otherwise) when in spite of very similar circumstances and under the smallest changes in constraints and initial conditions she could act, decide, choose, or desire otherwise.

What have we gained by this modification? Are we not simply subject to random direction, are we manipulated by tiny deviations in physical processes? Doesn't the intelligibility argument prevail? That depends on *how* the brain is sensitive to the valid constraints and initial conditions. If we are dealing merely with stochastic deviations that are amplified, then the intelligibility argument does triumph. What we need are real processes, which despite being sensitive can continue to generate stability, order, and control. Pascual Jordan had already observed this challenge. He wrote that "the conspicuous stability of organisms, expressed by the 'teleological' character of their reactions, cannot be understood solely using amplifier theory" (Jordan 1932, p. 820). Since minimal neurophilosophy assumes the supervenience of mental states on brain states, we can study the dynamics of brain states in order to discover whether processes occur in the brain, that generate stability on the basis of quasi-indeterminism and to which extent they constitute a basic principle of brain organization. So-called chaotic systems are good candidates, as we shall see in the following. The chaotic system is a special case of dynamic systems, so first we must introduce a few fundamental concepts from the theory of dynamic systems, using the example of a chaotic system (1.2.2). Next I shall present neurophysiological evidence that at diverse levels of complexity the brain is essentially a chaotic system (1.2.3). Then I will introduce some samples of modeling psychological and cognitive phenomena after dynamical system theories. In closing, I finally examine how the chaotic organization of our brain and our behavior contributes to making the modified version of the ability to do otherwise one of the essential elements of a theory of natural autonomy (1.3).

1.2.2   Basic Concepts of the Theory of Chaotic Systems   In everyday conversation we use the term "chaos" to denote disorder, total confusion, or the unraveling of all order. Mathematical chaos is something else. It means a certain form of nonlinear behavior. Chaos, to be precise *deterministic* chaos,[8] is stochastic behavior in a determined system (Elbert et al. 1994). Apparently random behavior is actually based on an order that is not readily observable. Typical specimens of chaotic systems in nature are the weather and biological populations. Everyone knows how imprecise weather predictions tend to be, although they are better than their reputation. But no serious meteorologist would make a scientific prediction for the weather a week in advance. The reason is simple. It is simply impossible. Discovering an explanation for this is credited to Edward Lorenz, who in 1960, using a Royal McBee—a very primitive computer—tried to calculate a global weather model based on twelve rules. The results were astonishing:

> On a winter's day in 1961 Lorenz wanted to keep an eye on one of the sequences in a longer print-out. He found a short-cut. Instead of starting up the whole procedure again, he started in the middle of the system. In order to set the machine at a starting position he entered the numbers as they had appeared in his last print-out. Then he went down to the cafeteria to escape the noise of the machine and to drink a cup of coffee. When he returned an hour later he noticed something unexpected, something which would become the seed of a new science. The new curve should have exactly copied the old one. The number input had been identical both times. The program was unchanged. While he stared in fascination at the print-out he discovered that the new course of weather was so much different from the previous one that within just a few months [of simulated weather; H.W.] all similarity disappeared. He compared the previous series of numbers with the new ones. He could just as well have drawn two lists from a hat at random. His first thought was that one of the tubes must be broken. But then he realized that it was not a functional error. The problem was the numbers he had used as input. Six decimal places were stored in the computer's memory: 0.506127. The print-out had only room for three: 0.506. Lorenz had decided to use an abbreviated, rounded series of numbers. He had assumed that a deviation in a ratio of one to one thousand had little impact. (Gleick 1988, quoted in Paslack 1991, p. 120f)

This extreme dependency of the weather on the smallest changes became well-known as the "butterfly effect." The movement of a butterfly wing in Brazil could in principle initiate a tornado in Mexico.[9] Where does this extreme sensitivity toward minute deviations originate? Lorenz recognized immediately that it was due to the combination of being non-linear and iteration (repeating the same step using the outcome of the previous one). Within a short time it was noticed that other systems also exhibit chaotic behavior: convection patterns in liquids heated from below, the pulse of chicken heart cells, and oscillating concentrations in chemical reactions. Computer simulations of prey-and-predator systems, star oscillations, and stock market patterns also display this type of behavior. What do all these chaotic systems have in common?[10] They exhibit feedback, they behave in a nonlinear manner, and are extremely sensitive to changes in constraints and initial conditions. Even if two almost identical systems are only minimally different when they begin, their states can be very much different from one another after just a very short time. The crucial point is that those differences may be infinitely minute.

This sensitivity involves some interesting features. The most important one is that the system's behavior becomes basically unpredictable. A chaotic system is unpredictable, *even though* it is strictly deterministic. Many chaotic systems can be generated with simple, deterministic, recursive equations. The only way to know something definite about a system's state at time t is to observe the system at that time; in the case of computer simulations, this means running the program up to that time. This feature of nonpredictability can lead to differentiation in the concept of determinism from a physicist's vantage. We are confronted with deterministic behavior, according to Thomas and Leiber (1994), when the state of a dynamic system at any particular point in time in principle unequivocally and completely determines the further development of that system. *Weak* determinism then means that the same initial states lead to the same final states. (Expressed mathematically, there are deterministic equations of movement.)

In contrast, *strong* determinism claims that similar initial states also lead to the same end states. (Mathematically expressed, there is topological stability in the phase space.) We will return to discuss phase space later. At this point I have just two brief remarks. Instead of strong and weak determinism we often read of strong and weak causality. These concepts are intertwined. Even if the terminology we have thus far introduced allows us to say that chaos violates the principle of strong determinism, we merely mean by this that *in principle unpredictability is given when we have strongly divergent developments*; but that a *strict ontological determination* of succeeding states by their preceding states remains untouched (at least in a deterministic world). None of the arguments listed in chapter 1 are invalid. However, this is exactly what we were looking for: a theory supplying justification for a weak form of being able to do otherwise in a determined world.

Concerning phase space: The phase space of a system is an abstract space in which every alterable feature of a system is described in a dimension of its own. If a system is described by n state variables, the state of the system is unequivocally determined by a point in n-dimensional space. For example, if the behavior of a pendulum is described by its location and velocity, its state can be clearly defined by naming a point in two-dimensional space. A so-called phase portrait geometrically represents the behavior of the system. When every state of the system has been defined by a point in the phase space a line results describing the behavior of the pendulum. This line is called the state *trajectory* or path curve. An ideal, frictionless pendulum, for example, has a circle as a state trajectory, since it continues to swing indefinitely. But real dynamic systems are subject to friction. A pendulum without a motor will stop swinging at some time because of inevitable loss of energy due to friction. In phase space its spiral-like path continues to approach one specific point, no matter where the starting point was. Metaphorically speaking we could say that this point "attracts" the pendulum; it is a fixed point attractor. Generally speaking, an attractor is a set of points in a phase space in which the trajectory of the system, commencing from a limited pertinent realm, flows to the so-called attractor basin. Phase space can also be modeled on scenery of hills and valleys, in which a fixed point attractor is a valley into which a ball will roll, sooner or later. (A pointed hill is a repellor, a spot that repels the system.) Naturally phase space can contain several attractors and repellors. Another attractor is the border cycle. A battery-driven pendulum clock, for example, will always regain a specific oscillation frequency, even if we knock or stop the pendulum, its trajectory will always return to a specific closed curve in phase space. In nature, predator and prey systems exemplify border cycles. A more complicated attractor form is a torus—a surface having the shape of an doughnut. It is generated when a pair of oscillators are coupled, like two motor driven pendulums, two planets, two oscillatory electric circuits, or two predator and prey systems (such as a trout-pike and an insect-frog cycle).

Such attractors correspond to formations in classic physics: they are stable and predictable. But what are chaotic attractors like? Recall Edward Lorenz's system of equations for predicting the weather. The trajectory of prognosticated weather is not closed. Once the system has been started up at a particular point, its trajectory never returns to that point.

If the system commences twice at two separate but proximate points, within a short time the trajectories diverge and become increasingly distant from one another. There no longer is stability within the phase space. This is what Lorenz found so surprising. How can we imagine this geometrically? Since there is a limit to phase space, the two trajectories cannot continue to diverge exponentially without end. The attractor must therefore fold back onto itself. Generating a chaotic attractor can be thought of as a series of stretching and folding the phase space, the way we knead dough. Geometrically this results in lines resembling turned-in folds. In other words, the geometry of chaotic attractors is fractal. Every zoom-in reveals new details.[11] The idea of folds also supports our intuition about why trajectories drift apart in unpredictable ways. It is simply impossible to predict where any two little tangent bits of dough will be, once the pastry has been thoroughly kneaded.

Due to these features, such attractors are called "strange" attractors. Although unpredictability is true, the idea of attractors offers a bit of order in the midst of chaos. We know at least something about the behavior of the system. Diverse parameters can characterize chaotic systems: metric entropy, fractal dimension, and the Lyapunov coefficient. These not only characterize known attractors, they also help determine whether a certain system with observable behavior is chaotic.

A dynamical, chaotic system can also very well exhibit stabile patterns. Briggs and Peat explain this vividly using the example of the population size of insect larvae (Briggs and Peat 1990, p. 80–85). Imagine a population of larvae that is subject to some form of hatching control, such as being sprayed with insecticide. The population will only increase if the hatching rate is greater than 1, that is, if more larvae are hatched than already exist. The growth of the population at hatching rates >1 can be described with a modified Verhulst equation:

$$X_{n+1} = HX_n(1 - X_n)$$

The essential features are being nonlinear and displaying iteration (repetition of the same step with the outcome of the preceding step): X_{n+1} is the size of the population for the subsequent year, X_n is the size of the current population and H is the hatching rate, which is influenced by many extraneous factors.[12] If we select a hatching rate of 1.5, the population will increase in the following year. In the year after that, however, it will decrease because of the nonlinear Verhulst factor. Finally it will settle around a value of 0.66, or 60% of the original size of the population. In chaos terminology we have here a so-called fixed-point attractor, which determines the development of the size of the population for a hatching rate of up to approximately 3.0. If the hatching rate exceeds the critical value of 3.0, the resulting population size will oscillate between two stable values. This is qualitatively comprehendible. A small population (value 1) reproduces heavily and deposits many eggs. Next season, the area is overpopulated (value 2) so that only few insects survive to reproduce, and in the season after that, they are back to value 1. Represented in graph form this drifting apart resembles a fork or bifurcation of the trajectory. (A bifurcation is a sudden transitory phenomena, in other cases it is called a phase transition.) What happens when the rate of hatching continues to increase? If it reaches a value of more than 3.4495, the population oscillates between four stable values, a forking of the bifurcation itself has occurred (see figure 3.1). Every four years there is a difference in population size. At a hatching rate of 3.56 there are eight stable values (attractors), at 3.5969 there are 16 attractors, and when the hatching rate reaches 3.56999, the number of different attractors has become infinitely large. Although the development of the population follows a simple, deterministic, recursive equation, it has become impossible to predict that size. This path that chaos can take is also known as the "period doubling path."

Using phase space we can display this development in a graph (see figure 3.1). The way in which the points repeatedly fan out from the left and the right implies that filling up the phase space chaotically has become a peculiarly ordered process. Not all of the phase space is completely filled up until the hatching rate reaches a value of 4.0. Below that, we do see some order. First, the system oscillates within the value range of hatching rates between 3.56999 and 3.7, at first between four and then between only two "chaotic" ranges, before they melt down to a single one. Second, there are parabolic dark lines, along which the system can be found to be located with a high degree of probability. Third, in the expanding shaded area there are white bands, ranges, or windows, in which the system once again becomes stable and predictable, there it

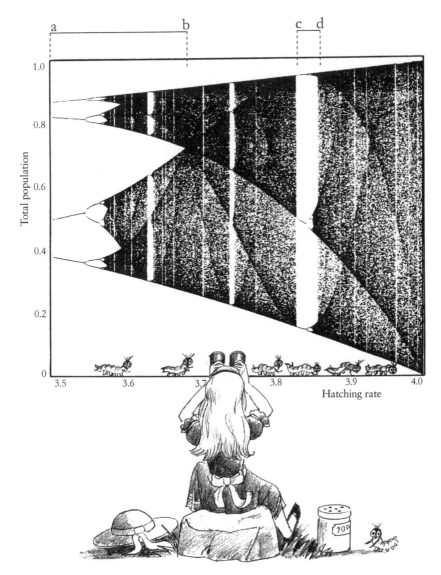

Figure 3.1
The path of period doubling to chaos. From Briggs and Peat (1990, p. 85).

oscillates between a mere few values. These areas of stability and predictability occurring in the midst of apparent random oscillations are known as *intermittence*.

Intermittence is intriguing. Normally we think that we live in a stable world and that chaos reflects a disturbance. But the opposite could be true: Perhaps we live on "islands in the midst of chaos" (Waldrop 1993), in realms of intermittence, which only appear to us to be stable because crucial control parameters exhibit corresponding values.

A control parameter is a variable that can be used to control a system's behavior. In our example, food supply, amounts of insecticide or even the hatching rate itself can be control parameters; in an oscillating electric circuit it could be the voltage, or the setting of the variable condenser. *Control* in this case does not mean that the effect resulting from altering parameters is predictable, but only that that effect critically influences the system's behavior.

Chaos not only exhibits some order, it also exhibits universality. This means that it has properties that are independent of being concretely instantiated. In 1975 Mitchell Feigenbaum discovered a universal series of numbers describing the behavior of chaotic systems with the property of period doubling. The equations he examined are independent of any specific case and applicable to quite different systems. The transition from periodic to chaotic behavior always occurs at the same value of a variable, which regulates the maximum. This value is Feigenbaum's number 4.99920. . . . The universality of this number is so impressive that it is sometimes considered a new constant within nature. Chaos also exhibits a relation to the world of fractals (Peitgen, Jürgens, and Saupe 1992). Fractals are structures similar to themselves in various aspects, such as a coastline or a Mandelbrot set in mathematics. As I mentioned earlier, they are marked by the fact that the same structure is repeated in large and small aspects; mathematically this repetition is infinite. They are generated by iteration, which is presumably why they are akin to chaotic systems.

In summary we can maintain that, first, chaos is generated by a combination of iteration and the property of being nonlinear. Second, certain chaotic systems exhibit bifurcations, that is, sudden, nonlinear discontinuities. Third, chaotic systems do exhibit a certain degree of order, crucially determined by how certain state variables are adjusted. And fourth, stability does not imply a lack of chaos; it can be found in the midst of chaos, in realms of intermittence.

1.2.3 The Chaotic Brain   We have seen that chaotic systems pose some interesting questions. Heeding a neurophilosophical standpoint, the query is this: Is the brain a chaotic system at all? Although still relatively new, research on the brain using methods of dynamical system theory delivers increasing evidence that it is, perhaps, true. Chaotic systems are characteristically nonlinear, recursive, and exhibit discontinuity and chaotic attractors. There is evidence that those features also apply to the brain:[13]

1. The brain's functional cells, neurons, behave particularly nonlinearly. On various models of isolated neurons it has been shown that neuronal firing behavior, which can be very simply demonstrated in a two-dimensional phase space (frequency and amplitude) does indicate chaotic behavior when it is represented in a graph. Albeit, few of the studies employed quantitative methods. Chaotic behavior of some of the elements of a system does not prove that the system itself is chaotic; it is remarkable though, that chaos shows up at a level exhibiting such low complexity.

2. A general structural principle, namely the extremely high degree of networking with positive *and* negative feedback loops, makes it mathematically very probable that chaos occurs. Feedback loops are the empirical correlate to recursion in mathematical equations, which generate chaotic images. They are particularly present in the neocortex, the part of the brain that is indispensable for cognition and consciousness.

3. There are certain phenomena that can be measured by electroencephalography (EEG) and magnetencephalography (MEG), which can count as evidence that the bioelectric activity of the brain is brought forth by nonlinear system dynamics. For one, there is proof of amplitude-dependent frequency behavior. Slow waves have high and fast waves have low amplitudes. Occipital alpha-rhythm that emerges when visual input is blocked by closing one's eyes can also be understood as a border cycle. Third, there are bursts in EEGs, that is, intermittent, sudden outbreaks of electric excitation, for example spike-wave-complexes during epileptic seizures or in the form of K-complexes during sleep. Fourth, it is known that in nonlinear systems periodic stimulation not only generates frequency of stimulation, but also a special behavior

around the resonance frequency, such as the harmonic doubling of periods. This corresponds to what can be observed during periodic light stimulation in EEGs (photic driving). A similar phenomenon is observable with the 40 Hz steady state answer in acoustic systems. Fifth, and finally, the presence of discontinuity phenomena has been proven, for example in the EEG correlates of bimanual coordination (Zanone and Kelso 1992).

4. Experimental tests on animals also indicate chaotic phenomena. Chaotic behavior could be proven for single cells: in the motor and visual brain areas for apes and in the hearing system of cats. One of the best researched fields is the olfactory system in Leporidae (Skarda and Freeman 1987; Freeman 1991, 1995; Elbert et al. 1994, pp. 30–32). Highly irregular activity patterns of the olfactory nerve play a part in scent recognition. Computer simulation of the relevant processes make it appear plausible that strange attractors are involved when rabbits are trained to recognize scents. In a relaxed state, brain activity is chaotic. It is complex and appears to be random, but it is controlled by hidden ordering principles. During perception of a learned scent while inhaling, an EEG shows a state ordered with more sophistication, that is, the attractor is of a lower dimension. Throughout the smelling process and with constant stimulation, chaotic activity patterns stabilize. When the rabbit learns to recognize new scents, a new kind of attractor develops. All others are slightly modified. This indicates a certain holism within the physiology of perception. Repetitious disorder brings an advantage for Leporidae. Under natural conditions they must be sensitive to the most minute stimuli and recognize scents as quickly as possible. In terms of electrophysiology, a rabbit's brain must quickly generate different activity patterns. In terms of chaos theory, that activity must "fall" into a certain attractor. Repeated recognition does not require a comparison of all scents stored away, nor a search in a catalog. Instead, it is a process of pattern recognition via temporally extended pattern generation. Incidentally, previous to revealing chaos, these experiments revealed temporally coherent oscillation processes. It seems that there might be a connection between this currently very popular concept of coherence (a survey can be found in Singer and Gray 1995; and Engel et al. 1997) and chaos theory.

5. In recent years the electric activity of the *human* brain has also been researched using mathematically developed tools, and there have been findings. In contrast to investigation on individual cells, this research not only employed graphic tools, but also quantitative instruments, such as fractal dimension, metric entropy, and Lyapunov exponents. The calculation of these, however, depends on certain assumptions, and therefore

it remains controversial whether their outcomes really indicate chaos in the brain. In order to calculate whether brain activity actually is based on nonlinear dynamics, it would need to be measured over a longer period. For it is theoretically possible that many different variables could determine that activity *linearly*. But because brain activity is not stationary, we just can't say. So we must rely on indirect methods. Periodic series are analyzed with special methods, based on the supposition that measuring individual variables supplies information about the dynamics of the entire system. The subjects of research were phenomena such as the effects of closing one's eyes, the effects of touching, of seeing, of imagination and word processing, of sleep and hypnosis, as well as pathological states like buzzing in the ears, epilepsy, and schizophrenia (Elbert et al. 1992, 1994; Lutzenberger et al. 1993). Although much is still obscure, the following sketch is beginning to develop. The electric sum activity of the brain (EEG) can be viewed as a deterministic chaotic system brought about by a nonlinear system with four to six variables. Model calculations show that an EEG can be understood as the result of coupled oscillations of neuronal populations (Basar and Roth 1996, p. 309). This coupling limits the dimensions of the activity as a whole; normally it is limited to a four- to five-dimensional attractor.

Variation of dimensional complexity in humans under varying conditions is quite complex. At rest a human EEG normally has a low fractal dimension. Of course, we must note that being at rest is a poorly defined state. In their project, Lutzenberger et al. introduce a verbal alliteration task as a control condition. This allows control over what the test persons are thinking—at least better than when the condition is merely described as being "at rest." It turned out that the greatest numbers of dimensions were found in creative, less controlled tasks requiring imagination (pondering, having fantasies, day and night dreaming), followed by tasks of touching, then tasks of observation, and finally, the alliteration control condition. Closer examination reveals, however, that the number of dimensions increased only in those areas not effected by solving the task, while the quantity of dimensions in the active participant brain areas decreased. We need more research that quantitatively records chaotic states before we can outline a more exact idea of brain dynamics. Metric energy and Lyapunov exponents are better than determining dimensions, because they reflect temporal development, that is, the dynamics of brain activity (Elbert et al. 1994, p. 19).

1.2.4 Synergetics and the Theory of Dynamical Cognition We might get the false impression that chaotic systems are the only dynamical systems around. But systems theory includes much more (cf. Jaeger 1996). The spectrum ranges from Ludwig von Bertallaffany's "General System Theory" to cybernetics, to various theories of self-organization in biology, physics, and mathematics. In the present context I would like to discuss two theories that relate to the chaotic organization of the brain and have become important for cognitive science: synergetics and dynamical cognition theory.

The theoretical counterpart to Anglo-American chaos theory, namely synergetics, was developed by German physicist Hermann Haken (1983, 1995). While chaos theory tries to explain how apparently randomly effective processes actually result from an underlying order (hidden para-meters), the theory of synergetics (cooperation) tries to explain how well-ordered structures spontaneously arise in unstable systems through processes of self-organization.[14] The classic example suggesting the idea of synergetics is the transition from normal light to laser light. In a subcritical state the atomic micro-oscillators in laser light oscillate in disorderly fashion with varying frequencies. When the energy supply increases, a critical threshold is exceeded and one frequency becomes dominant; all other micro oscillators adjust themselves to it. The final result is coherent laser light of one single frequency. According to Haken, it is the amplitudes of the light waves that bring order into the light. He calls these "order parameters." In the process of creating laser light, a light wave with the amplitude of an order parameter "forces" the atoms to emit light of its wave length (*stimulated emission*).[15] Speaking anthro-pomorphically, Haken calls this the *principle of enslavement*.

The enslavement principle is at once an original yet controversial contribution to synergetics. Basically it states that in an environment of instability a few collective variables, the order parameter, determine the macroscopic state of the system by enslaving all the other possible forms of movement. The principle of enslavement is said to show up in extremely different kinds of physical and biological phenomena of self-organization. One example is the rhythm of clapping heard in concerts when the audience requests an encore after a performance. One person begins to clap and then more and more applause follows. At first the claps are unordered, but soon the whole audience is clapping in rhythm. One of the clapping frequencies "enslaved" the others, guided the others to join it. The value of this theory is that merely finding ordering parameters allows us to study systems at a level above the chaotic sublevel, using just a few parameters. The theory's deficiency is that system variables, which are actually only descriptions, are taken as causal variables. From a mathematical stance the principle of enslavement says only that the solutions of the differential equations describing the system depend crucially on slowly changing variables (ordering parameters), while quicker variables can be neglected (Stephan 1996). The fact that phenomena are describable with synergetic concepts does not mean that those concepts explain them in terms of causation. While causal relations in laser physics can be understood with Haken's often cited "circular causality," that notion does not help to understand examples taken from other sciences, like the social sciences (cf. Haken 1996).[16]

As we have seen, synergetic's instruments are particularly useful for studying complex and unstable processes exhibiting phase transitions. Understanding system dynamics by using just a few parameters serves to compress information (Haken 1996, p. 588). In cognition this includes metastabile perception processes such as the perception of toppling figures (Kruse et al. 1992; Kruse and Stadler 1995) or the psychological phenomena of suggestibility (Kruse et al. 1992).[17] Hansch (1988) outlined a program for the "psycho-synergetics" of emotional and motivational processes. Höger (1992) studied perspectives of chaos research in the psychology of stuttering. Schiepek (1996) applied chaos-theoretic methods in psychotherapy research. Stadler, Kruse, and Carmsin (1996) even sketched a theory of schizophrenia based on it. The thesis of synergetics is that cognition is "the generation of order within a balance of stability and instability." (Stadler, Kruse, and Carmsin 1996, p. 351).

All things considered, while synergetics does offer a set of fine-tuned instruments related to chaos theory, it is also true that the central role of the principle of enslavement attracts criticism that this theory is purely metaphorical. That becomes particularly conspicuous when order parameters are understood as mental events: "Let us consider an extreme case, namely the brain. We treat the neurons, including all their links, as subsystems. Chemical and electric activities can be described by a myriad of microscopic variables. But in the end, thoughts act as order parameters. Each part is a condition for the other" (Haken 1983, pp. 15f).

What is a thought? And how does it *influence* the brain? Via its mental content? In order to answer these questions we need neurosemantics, that is, a theory that explains how neuronal states can have meanings (see below). Achim Stephan (1999, pp. 232–238), who harshly criticized the principle of enslavement, remarks, just for the sake of fairness, that Haken—albeit with restraint and in a remote context—does acknowledge the trouble with interpreting ordering parameters as causal:

> Laser waves are something material, and we feel directly how they play their role as informers by physically . . . effecting the electrons of the atoms. But later on we will meet examples in which the informer is not tied to anything substantial. It is then a conceptual (thoroughly mathematically comprehendible) variable, which reflects the consensus of the individual parts of the system. (Haken and Haken-Krell 1989, p. 57)

Naturally, conceptual variables can also be effective, namely, when they are represented neurally—and that is considerably facilitated by a symbolic public language (see below).

Synergetics and chaos theory make use of similar mathematical instruments. In recent years a branch of research beyond chaos theory and synergetics found its place in cognitive science, applying just these instruments. The purpose is to design quantitative models of cognitive processes that are formulated mathematically in such a way that they remain susceptible to experimental testing. It is called dynamical cognition theory[18] and is meant to be a theory midway between symbolic and connectionistic cognition research. In some respects, it is superior to both of the other theories because models of symbolic and connectionistic systems are special cases of dynamical systems. Do we need a dynamical theory? The main argument in its favor is that the models it builds necessarily include the *time* factor, a feature that both symbolism and connectionism have neglected.

Cognitive dynamical systems are situated (they exist) in an environment with which they are directly coupled. States change in a parallel way, without being previously algorithmically calculated by the system itself. Changes within the system can best be described using mathematical instruments such as differential equations. Dynamical systems flow, they change with time. Overall, temporal patterns and the recognition of those patterns are a major part of this approach. The program claims *It's about Time* and *Mind as Motion* (both by van Gelder and Port 1995). The latter book describes various fields of application that exhibit quantitative models. These deal with the development of movement and pace patterns, language articulation, language itself, decision making, recognizing visual events, and psychotherapeutic interviews. In the next paragraphs I shall take a closer look at one of these models, based on the example of *decision field theory*.

Pasemann (1996) studied the neurodynamics of internal representations with the help of dynamical systems theory. Beyond the time factor, he particularly examines the link between a cognitive system and its environment. If it is true for the dynamics of cognitive systems that they are typically coupled to and embedded in the environment, then it is obvious that the internal state of the system, particularly its function of representation, cannot be understood disregarding that environment. Thus Pasemann writes:

Representation should be thought of as something fleeting, something that comes and goes in the form of dynamic brain activity patterns. It is an expression of the coherence between internal neurodynamic processes and the external environment, which is reflected in changes of receptor activities. . . . An inner representation is stored nowhere as a semantic configuration, it unfolds via and in the global dynamics of a cognitive process. . . . As such it gains, or better: it generates meaning only in that fleeting moment, in which it is effective, i.e., in which it can be used to execute some task relevant for behavior. (Pasemann 1996, pp. 82f)

In Summary we can say that dynamical systems theory is a serious theory of cognition. Heed of the environment, fleetingness, and dynamic representations are of central importance for naturalizing intelligibility. Chaos theory is particularly relevant for the ability to do otherwise. Though it employs the same mathematical means as dynamical cognition theory, there is no "essential connection between the two" (van Gelder and Port 1995, p. 35). Not every dynamical system necessarily has a chaotic organization. The brain is organized chaotically—at least we have fairly convincing evidence for this hypothesis, as we have seen.

Now we shall explain the role that chaos plays in the notion of natural alternatives.

1.3 Natural Autonomy and Alternatives

1.3.1 Natural Alternatives   Instability and unpredictability, combined with a peculiar order and mathematical universals such as the Feigenbaum number and the Mandelbrot set have mislead some scientists to think that a chaotic system can somehow rescue us from determinism and give us a *mysterious* kind of freedom (*Chaos frees the universe*, Davies 1990). The renowned scientist and journalist Robert Wesson wrote in his book *Chaos, Chance, and Natural Selection*:

> Although it is subject to psychic laws, the mind has its own type of causality. Conditioned reflexes, a favorite example given by psychologists because they are clear and apparently simple, say nothing essential about the mind. Whatever relation may exist between mental states and states of the brain or mutual effects of neurons, it remains vastly incomprehensible and complexly chaotic. As far as we know, the mind does not at all behave contrary to physical or physiological laws; but within undetermined and turbulent brain activities it is free. The mind, much more so than the weather, cannot be simulated. It is a controlling and order-generating essence above a chaotic substrate, the unlimited complex mutual effect of elements in the brain. (Wesson 1993, p. 332)

This description is not particularly informative. It brings gusts of dust, but little content. When the dust has settled, nothing substantial remains. Wesson contrives an imaginary opponent (the psychologist who is also a reflex theorist), makes some concessions to naturalism (the mind is subject to laws, and does not behave contrary to laws), and makes some unfounded claims (the mind is subject to its own kind of causality), some of which remain unexplained (what it means to be free) or are simply false (the mind cannot be simulated). The idea that freedom can be founded on this type of interpretation of chaos is hopeless.[19]

Nevertheless, chaos is important for our naturalistic project, because "alternative possibilities must be rescued from libertarians" (Waller 1993, p. 74). A crucial aspect of natural alternativism is spontaneous variability. Paths remain open; they are ready and available when we need them. This type of alternativism is real and we can observe simple versions of it in lowly mammals. Waller's example is the white-footed mouse. Although white-foot mice know exactly which way to go to find food, once in a while they spontaneously detour from the right path; some researchers would say that this is incorrect behavior. Yet this behavior is vital:

> Thus if the white-footed mouse never strayed from the one true path, it would be unlikely to discover the benefits that might subsequently appear along other routes and would be ill-equipped to respond rapidly should its most beneficial route be closed off or run dry. By occasionally taking alternative paths, the white-footed mouse keeps its options open. (Waller 1993, p. 74)

Of course, the mouse naturally is unaware of autonomy in the *human* meaning of the word. Alternativism characteristic of human autonomy, nevertheless, does exhibit a very similar pattern to that of the mouse. Success—in learning, solving problems, or doing experiments—rests on a behavioral pattern similar to that of the mouse. We follow a certain path because it guaranteed success in the past, but we do not stop exploring alternative paths. If the once successful pattern of behavior loses its effectiveness, *we have an alternative ready and waiting.* And, like the mouse, we do not entirely give up the previously successful pattern of behavior, we return to it even when we know that it is no longer efficient. If, under different conditions, it should once again prove to be expedient to our purposes, it is less likely that we will overlook the advantages it offers. Now certainly rationalists will protest that in contrast to the mouse, people possess *reason*. This is correct, but it does not effect the characteristic feature of naturalistic alternativism. The white-foot mouse explores its paths with an excellent sense of scent, keen eyes, and agile feet. People explore their options using reflective, analytic intelligence. Without those we would be poorly equipped to deal with the myriad of routes and behavioral patterns that confront us, just as the mouse would be lost without its olfactory and visual senses. Reason, according to Waller, is necessary for human autonomy. However, it is *not* expedient to finding the one and only correct, reasonable way to go, but rather, it is used to keep alternative options open.[20]

If chaotic processes actually play a part in our actions and decisions—and there is plenty of evidence that they do—then we have discovered a mechanism for the variability we require. *In spite of similar* conditions, humans do not always follow the same patterns, they (sometimes) act differently.[21] The crucial deviance from determinism and the amplification of noise effects is that stability and variability are two sides of the same coin, namely the chaotic organization of the brain. Depending on the value of certain order parameters a chaotic system is sensitive to changes and thus variable, or it is stable, linear, and predictable in its behavior. The phenomenon of intermittence shows that the latter is possible *in the midst of chaos*. The switch from chaotic to stable behavior can often be achieved by altering a single ordering parameter, such as the frequency of an oscillating system. Chaotic behavior is adaptive. Using chaotic behavior, a cognitive system retains the option of reacting quickly, flexibly, and sensitively to relevant stimuli, changes in the environment, or ideas. This does not mean that it cannot be determined in a strict sense of the word. The vital difference to the libertarian model is that quasi indeterministic behavior is generated by a mechanism that also generates order.

1.3.2 The Nature of Decisions Now I would like to more closely examine how chaos contributes to those decisions, which we would traditionally denote as being free. One option is obvious. We have seen that chaotic systems exhibit bifurcations. These are points of instability, at which the further behavior of the system takes either of two directions. In terms of chaos theory, two trajectories are "possible," each leading to a different place, distant from the other in phase space. Formally, this has the following in common with decision situations. A person goes through a thought process until he reaches the point where he must select one or the other option. Is it not also possible to characterize real decision situations (or their cerebral correlates) as forked states? Couldn't chaos theory approximately solve the issue of what it means to decide (cf. Walter 1996a)? A solution like that seems obvious, but, in fact, the matter is more complicated.

This model suggests the following problem. If it were correct, wouldn't we be constantly astonished about people's decisions, *including our own*? Doesn't chaos end in epistemic and *auto-epistemic* indetermination? We spoke about the concept of epistemic indetermination in chapter 1. A system is "epistemically indeterminate" when we cannot know how it is determined, even though on an ontological level it is strictly determined. "Auto-epistemic indeterminacy" makes a double reference to the knowing subject: He *himself* cannot know, how *he himself* arrives at a decision. If chaotic brain processes are the neurophysiological substrate of decisions, why don't we persistently find our own decisions and actions surprising? Why do we seemingly often know why we decided as we did? Does the intelligibility argument hold here exactly as well as against the libertarian?

Although it is naturally not so seldom the case that we actually are surprised about our own decisions, this objection can be met by adhering to a diachronic viewpoint, which means that we take the temporal development of decisions into consideration. Decisions are not processes that occur at a point in time, they are *events extended through time*. This fact is usually ignored in philosophical debates on free will and autonomy. The classic model of a decision runs like this: "A self finds itself at a time T with a certain battery of mental states (beliefs, memories, desires, fears, goals, values, and so on.) Free will consists in a rationally controlled transition to a condition at T + 1 that contains a choice." (Double 1991, pp. 38f)

This description suggests that decisions occur at a particular point in time. Under this assumption it is hardly imaginable how a chaotic process could produce such a rationally controlled transition. For even the smallest change could guide the decision in either one or the other direction. A chaos theory analysis of decision-making processes would have to replace this misleading notion of decision-making with a realistic one. Real decision situations are more like the picture that William James, the father of American psychology, sketched almost poetically in *Principles of Psychology*:

The deliberation may last for weeks or months, occupying at intervals the mind. The motives which yesterday seemed full of urgency and blood and life today feel strangely weak and pale and dead. But as little today as tomorrow is the question finally resolved. Something tells us that all this is provisional; that the weakened reasons will wax strong again, and the stronger weaken; that equilibrium is unreached; that testing our reasons, not obeying them, is still the order of the day, and that we must wait awhile, patient or impatiently, until our mind is made up "for good and all." This inclining, first to one then to another future, both of which we represent as possible, resembles the oscillations to and fro of a material body within the limits of its elasticity. There is inward strain, but no outward rupture. And this condition, plainly enough, is susceptible of indefinite continuance, as well in the physical mass as in the mind. If the elasticity give way, however, if the dam ever do break, and the currents burst the crust, vacillation is over and decision is irrevocably there. (William James, *The Principles of Psychology*, 1890, p. 529)

Of course, not all decisions take weeks or even months, and not all are made as consciously as James describes. But what is true for *all* decisions, whether conscious or subconscious, what is true for all decisions *without exception*, is that they are extended over time. Perhaps there is a lower time limit, beneath which we would only speak of reflex reactions. The exact definition is unimportant. Significant for our purposes is merely that by introducing a temporally extended decision process the strength of chaotic systems develops its full potential. For now the fluctuation of stability and variability is fully developed. To achieve that we must change the traditional notion of decision-making.

Models of human decision-making used in psychology and in the economic sciences today normally are based on the idea of subjectively expected utility.[22] A person examines alternatives, allots a certain value to each one, and then in one step she calculates the best alternative and acts accordingly. But a realistic theory of human decision-making must also reflect the temporal aspect of the decision-making process. I would like to mention two such models.

Dörner (1996) describes decision-making processes as "antagonistic dialogues." Using the example of how a woman arrives at the decision to get a divorce, he demonstrates the development of such a decision-making process. At first there is an impulse to take action, which arises in a certain situation, such as an argument at the breakfast table. Immediately opposing impulses turn up, such as the fear that the couple's daughter will lose her father. The result is an appetence-aversion conflict. A divorce would be rewarding, but also threatening. In the inner antagonistic dialogue that ensues, various reasons for and against the decision are brought forth within the system. These, in turn, taint the present situation and how it is experienced and allot a greater or lesser preference to the intent to divorce. Dörner offers a formalized model in which he introduces abstract variables such as the strength of motivations, which can change over time. He details different options for elaborating the structure of decision-making and how motivation strength changes. In principle, such a decision-making process could go on indefinitely, but in reality it terminates at some point. It ends either "as it should" with a decision (one motive is significantly valued and leads to action), or it leads to a meta-conflict (increasing anxiety that no decision has been made), which in turn may or may not terminate "as it should." Interrupting the regress or coming to a decision can also result from changes in other parameters, such as the importance of the conflict in comparison to other issues (a child becomes ill) or the urgency of the decision.

Dörner's formalization, however, is still a classic symbol processing approach. In contrast, *Decision field theory* (DFT) (Busemeyer and Townsend 1993; Townsend and Busemeyer 1995) lays out a real dynamical theory using dynamical systems theory. As a model for decisions it begins with a system of defined preference states related to defined decisions. The state of the system *develops over time* and can be described with differential equations that depict the relationship between factors such as motivational value and the actually anticipated value of a defined choice. Because central variables in DFT can change with time, it can account for temporal oscillations, shifts, and changes like those described by James and which presumably also occur in other, faster decisions.

The two theories have no need for notions from chaos theory. For our purpose it is important that both deal with decisions as something extended through time. The chaotic nature of the brain could be useful for executing this kind of antagonistic dialogue in the first place, that is, not merely being pushed to action by an impulse. This type of self-organizing process is not unusual in certain nonlinear systems. A decision is a process during the course of which the trajectory of the system, beginning at an unstable state (an impulse to act which has not yet been heeded), "visits" various places in phase space and finally moves toward a stable state. This stable state corresponds to the attractor basin and can be nonchaotic (as with irrevocable decisions) or chaotic. In the latter case a residue of being able to do otherwise remains. In contrast to the amplifier model, the transition from the search phase to a stable decision phase is guaranteed by one and the same mechanism.

This weak form of an ability to do otherwise is part of a neurophilosophical theory of natural autonomy. To a certain degree we must remain sensitive to changes in constraints, whether they consist of rain (in which case the mouse will chose a different path), a noncontrollable occurrence of memories (which can change the intent for divorce), or a sudden idea for a mathematical proof (which can then be formalized using appropriate tools).

1.3.3 Controlling Chaos I have shown why chaotic alternativism as an element of natural autonomy is not felled by the intelligibility argument in the same way that the intelligibility argument knocks down indeterministic alternativism as an element of free will. Free decisions and actions are extended through time and thus provide room for chaos and order. Nevertheless, many questions remain, or—we should say—need to be *rephrased*. Not a deficiency, this is but a normal and desired effect of any innovative theory. Novel answers have new problems in tow. A central query is the extent to which it is actually plausible to assume that abstract descriptions of neuronal states (attractors) are the subvenient basis of mental representations. We will return to this question on a later page; presently I will simply assume that we can accept this notion.

Is a chaotic decision-making system actually controllable? It is a feature of chaotic systems that minimal and often random influences can produce dramatic changes in behavior. Even though decisions are temporally extended and thus allow room for "capturing" chaotic transitions, can we really control chaotic systems in any relevant way? Lack of predictability is a given principle, not merely a condition of our limited ability for introspection. But control is, in fact, possible.

Ditto and Pecora (1993) have shown how to "master chaos." They present two models: Synchronized chaos and the OGY method (Ott, Grebogi, and Yorke 1990). We will discuss the latter.[23] The key to understanding it is the idea that a chaotic attractor is a combination of infinitely many unstable yet *periodic* trajectories. The trick is to stabilize the chaotic attractor at any one of those periodic attractors. This happens by collecting limited, but informative data about the current state of the system. In a second step, using this restricted information, either a few or only one of the control parameters is slightly altered. This process is then repeated. Technically speaking: The result is a periodic sequence of points in the state's space, which can be represented in a Poincaré diagram, and allows the system to run until it approximates the desired periodic orbit. Then the system's parameters are changed so that in the next period the trajectory is most likely to meet the same point again. Naturally this slightly moves the chaotic attractor, so that in the following iterative step we are again dealing with a slightly altered, new attractor. In the most favorable scenario the attractor coaxes the system to follow the desired orbit. Otherwise the parameter is changed anew and there is a novel attractor, which perhaps exhibits the desired properties. Expressed intuitively, you turn a few knobs and vary the processes by trial and error until you get a stable outcome. The process is similar to balancing a ball on your head. The ball tends to fall off (the trajectory drifts away). In order to keep the ball in a stable position one must move back and forth (adjusting parameters), which in turn changes the direction in which the ball will roll (altered attractor). The movement outside of the ball is not pure reaction, it is anticipatory and requires a good feel for the ball (implicit knowledge about the attractor), as well as some practice (trial and error with feedback). We can imagine the chaotic trajectories of neuronal representations along these lines (see also Eiser 1994). Through practice and experience we learn in the course of time to stabilize our chaotic brains. So we behave in a stable manner and nonetheless maintain an ability to do otherwise in a more subtle sense.

Naturally the question remains: Who controls the control parameters? Who is the lord of the manor? These questions are close kin to our intuitions about agency. We shall not here anticipate the third part of this chapter. So for the moment we must do with an answer that seems wanting: The head of the household is *the system itself*. A crucial element of *self* control is that collecting data about the state of the system happens introspectively, via feelings and sentiments. This explains why only the system *itself* can achieve control. However, this control is not cognitively transparent for the system *itself* (it does not explicitly know the attractor). Above all, control is not teachable, it is only learnable. The system itself strives during experience to achieve control, or stability. In the course of time one learns which signals one must heed. Later we shall see that there is good neurobiological evidence for the idea that decisions are often guided by such introspective sentiment processes. Feelings are not the opponents of intelligible behavior. On the contrary, they are a necessary ingredient. But more on that later.

1.3.4   Natural Alternatives and Ascribing Responsibility   Looking at some examples we now want to examine how a weaker form of alternativism is related to the challenge of responsibility. Instead of asking whether we *are* responsible, let us ask the more modest question of the degree to which a weaker version of the ability to do otherwise—if it were to correctly describe us—would *justify attributing responsibility*. Once again, my perspective is diachronic, albeit for a wider time period. The extent to which we are chaotically organized presumably changes during the course of our lives.

As adults we are—to a certain extent—"calculable," but children are not. Children are often unpredictable, spontaneous, and unsteady—even in their own eyes. They can be deeply involved with or concentrated on doing something, and yet their attention can be diverted by small external influences or spontaneous inner events. In the course of development this changes, but it is for this reason that we rightly consider children only partially responsible for their behavior. If this were due to the chaotic nature of children's brains, it should be possible to prove that empirically, for example, by examining children's EEGs. At the behavioral level Esther Thelen (Thelen 1993; Thelen and Smith 1994) interprets psychological development research using tools of nonlinear systems theory. She sketches a general dynamical theory of development. It is particularly interesting that in her theory natural fluctuations, which means natural variability, are not noise, but necessary elements of adaptive and flexible behavior. Children's behavior is strongly chaotic. Children are not in a position to act sufficiently autonomously, self-determined, according to stable principles. As they develop, they can deal with increasing awareness and more responsibility with disorderly spontaneous processes. This is a social learning process. In the course of growing up—a time in which rules and norms formulated in language play an important part—children learn to control the ordering parameters of their chaotic brains, so that they can demonstrate predictable and stable behavior. If control becomes *too* habitual, however, and they behave similarly in similar situations, then they no longer have alternatives available in the weaker sense. They become overly predictable, calculable, inflexible, in a word: obstinate. We do not hold elderly obstinate people responsible for their behavior to the same extent to which we hold flexible people responsible; *they just can't help it.* Even the best schooled mind makes no difference. If a robot were programmed to obstinately obey Kant's categorical imperative, we would not be swayed to attributing responsibility to it.[24] Only flexibility and the capacity for adaptive behavior in changing situations and the principle option of not following a maxim under altered conditions—which means abandoning the attractor—gives meaning at all to the idea of appealing to one's responsibility.[25] There are thus two opposing developments. In the behavior of children, candor, flexibility, and chaos are large factors that decrease as they grow up and create stable attractors. Then controlled, predictable behavior increases and can even reach the point of elderly stubbornness. The greatest degree of being able to do otherwise, which is still compatible with controlled behavior, lies somewhere in between. There, order and regularity are part of chaos itself. Only a certain degree of the type of being able to do otherwise, which we have discussed, can be combined with control.

Finally, a naturalistic version of alternativism is not only expedient to understanding free will, but also useful for understanding other issues and phenomena. It aids in explaining how genetics and environment cooperate in human development. If the instantiation of maxims were too rigid, namely if it followed only genetics, and were not sufficiently sensitive to influences (i.e., the instantiation of stable, nonchaotic attractors), then people would not be *flexible enough* for an ascription of responsibility to be justified. And if the environment had not provided for the instantiation of those maxims in the form of controllable chaos, then we would not be *stable enough* for the ascription of responsibility to be justified. Once again, observe, children. Parents know that in some situations children are not chaotic, but actually pretty predictable. By repeatedly confronting a child with a certain situation one can constantly provoke fear or joy. These behavioral patterns are genetically determined and presumably fixed in structures of the nervous system. They follow stable attractors. In this respect children are not "free," they are genetically committed in a way that the principle of strong causality is once again valid.[26]

The issue of fault related to acts of affect can also be dealt with from this perspective. Fabian and Stadler (1992), for example, attempt to explain the behavior of wrongdoers in psychologically stressful social situations by introducing chaos theory. There is evidence that acts of affect are often kindled by slight causes that lead to exaggerated reactions. An explanation might be that psychological stress in social situations induces instability in the motivational field and leads thereby to fluctuations at points of instability (bifurcations), a drift towards stable, deeply anchored attractors (such as flight and attack attractors acquired phylogenetically). Perhaps this is why such wrongdoers afterward usually cannot rationally explain their behavior manifested in affect.

Phenomena like compulsion can also be explained in principle. An irresistible coercion to act in a certain manner could be caused by the existence of a stable—even overly stable—attractor, which is no longer flexible and cannot be adequately influenced. At least it is not sensitive to small changes in the constraints in a way which is true for "free" actions. But they also cannot be changed by appealing to reason, because an attractor is not a proposition. It is necessary to *unlearn* such activity patterns. Interestingly enough, behavioral therapeutic approaches are particularly successful in treating compulsory disturbances (Hand 1992).

These examples are meant to illustrate how the ascription of responsibility is related to dynamical system behavior. Attributing responsibility is a social strategy for defining and maintaining balance between chaotic, unpredictable behavior and rigid, regulated, automatic behavior.[27] Naturally, not all has been said on the issue of responsibility. We have not discussed the extent to which decisions can rightly be *attributed to persons*. But we have achieved this: Contrary to the normal compatibilist strategy of entirely uncoupling responsibility and alternativism, I have tried to show that our intuition about being able to do otherwise has real roots and also that a weaker version of it very well has to do with the fact that—and how—we hold each other responsible for our acts.

At this point it is probably time to admit that for a while now I have been dealing with the more speculative side of neurophilosophy. That is thoroughly legitimate. Well-founded speculation *is* the program of neurophilosophy and distinguishes it from other interdisciplinary neurosciences. But from time to time we must remind ourselves that occasionally such speculations have feet of clay. Undoubtedly, there is evidence that the brain is organized chaotically. And *if* chaotic processes are an important factor in decision-making, then it is understandable that we intuitively believe that we can do otherwise. But the exact role fulfilled by chaotic processes in the brain remains controversial and unknown. In addition, I have made some fairly strong assumptions. The notion, for example, that attractors—being mathematical abstractions—could represent behavior-guiding ideas (maxims), does appear quite far-fetched. A maxim can be reflected upon, weighed, evaluated, or brought into play with other reasons and motives. How is that possible? My neurophilosophical analysis of the ability to do otherwise is hard to believe, until I can present a plausible theory about how mental representations of reasons and maxims can be recategorized as brain states. In other words, without being anchored to the ground of the philosophy of mind by a theory, of representation neurophilosophy of the free will floats in thin air. We shall next remedy this deficit.

2 Biological Roots of Intelligibility

Synopsis

We begin this section analyzing why determinism as well as indeterminism pose a problem for the component of intelligibility. How can actions controlled by the past be intelligible; how is intelligibility compatible with chance? The solution requires a theory about what it *means* to act for reasons. We get there via a theory of intentionality. This will be a detailed, biologically founded theory of intentionality, namely teleosemantics. It proves useful as a neurophilosophical theory of representation. It offers a naturalistic explanation for the semantic content of neuronal (thus mental) states and suggests a concept of intelligibility in terms of biology. In the next step I will extend teleosemantics to become what I call *adaptive neurosemantics*. This is achieved by also applying the theory—according to its prerequisites—to non-evolutionary selection and adaptation processes, so important in brain processes. Next, I discuss how *externalizing* language and the introduction of written language explains why we can make use of its symbolic structure, *although* we are connectionistic systems. Finally, I join up the results to the problem of intelligibility. I offer a solution to the problem of intentional causation by expanding the subvenience basis of intentional states and establishing a super*duper*venience relation using teleosemantics. We must abandon the traditional notion of *direct* intentional causation. I also conclude that determination by past events does not threaten the intelligibility of intentional states. A welcome by-product of those reflections is the conclusion that standards of rationality can at least partially be explained by following them up from biological standards. I will then discuss Benjamin Libet's famous experiments on free will and consciousness and criticize the conclusions he draws as seen from the standpoint of adaptive neurosemantics. I complete this section with a discussion on the participation of the frontal lobes in intelligibility.

2.1   Analyzing the Intelligibility Problem

Intelligibility is an important part of free will. I formulated this intuition as the second component of my working definition. Every theory of free will must inquire just what intelligibility is (see chapter 1) and how it relates to indeterminism and determinism. I call this *the problem of intelligibility*. It looks different for each position. For libertarians it is stated: How can an act be *simultaneously* undetermined and intelligible? Psychological determinism denies that it can (see chapter 1). In contrast, the determinist must ask: Can intelligible actions be controlled by past events, without losing their specific feature of being intelligible? Self-refutation arguments deny that they can. The emphasis of the argument was that beliefs, judgments, and arguments cannot be reduced to causally determined relationships if they are to maintain their specific character. To meet that argument the determinist must plausibly explain a naturalistic theory of reason or rationality, in other words, what a theory of intelligibility would have to encompass in a deterministic world.

I claim that libertarians also must rely on such a theory. Contemporary libertarians profess determined action for reasons just as deterministic theories do. So although we have a specifically libertarian problem (compatibility of indeterminism and intelligibility), the "intelligibility problem" is the same for the libertarian and anti-libertarian alike! The libertarian is forced to use an explanation strategy that he himself introduces against determinism in the self-refutation argument and which he would rather circumvent: making a decision or action intelligible by explaining it with the use of past events. Let's explore two prominent examples.

Robert Kane (1985, 1988, 1989) suggests a thesis of dual rationality for solving the specific libertarian problem. He says that a choice is *rational* if the person has *reasons* for choosing as he does, the choice *is made* for these reasons, and the person considers them more important than reasons for an alternative course of action (Kane 1989, p. 232). *Dual* rationality is when the choice is *rational, no matter which of the two alternatives is chosen.*[28] For Kane the indeterminism so crucial to a libertarian position is not located in reason or in reasons. Where else? He says that his theory is only valid for decisions preceded by an inner struggle. In his opinion, the *amount of effort* spent in inner struggle is undetermined (Kane 1996, p. 128). He believes that by this he can reconcile indeterminism and intelligibility. Such decisions are dually rational because both possible options are explained by reasons. To be precise, *weak-willed* decisions (in which the effort was not great enough) are explained by character and motives, *strong-willed* decisions are explained by character, motives, and *additional* undetermined effort. Once instantiated, one can find a rational explanation for either alternative for action, since both result from reasons.

At this point, I wish not to reiterate the discussion of whether having some undetermined aspect about them really makes actions free in the desired meaning of the word. Presently, it is more significant that Kane's theory also allows for the intelligibility of actions that are entirely determined by reasons.

This is also true for Peter van Inwagen, another prominent libertarian. He concedes, as Kane does, that actions entirely determined by reasons are intelligible. This, in van Inwagen's opinion is not the exception, but rather the rule. Free-willed actions are much rarer than is generally thought to be the case and only occur where reasons do not unambiguously determine that action (van Inwagen 1989, pp. 233ff). He distinguishes three classes of possible free acts: those in which reasons for alternative acts weigh equally (cases like Buridan's donkey); those in which there is a conflict between duty and propensity (between long term interests and momentary desires); and those in which one must choose between incompatible values. According to van Inwagen, most of our actions do not all belong in one of these three categories; this means that they are strictly determined and nevertheless intelligible, since they result from reasons.

Both Kane and van Inwagen at least partially acknowledge the psychological determinist's argument, since they consider free acts and decisions to be the exception to the rule. Intelligibility is not reduced to an empirically unfathomable and unexplainable instance of reason as it does for traditional libertarians. A causal conception of actions, which views reasons as determinate causes, does, however, pose a problem.

The debate on the causal conception of action (Röska-Hardy 1995) takes either the form of "reasons versus causes" (Lennon 1994) in the theory of action or the form of "mental causation" in the philosophy of mind (see chapter 2). For our purposes the term "intentional causation" would be more appropriate. Disregarding dualist arguments, there are basically two camps. *Causalists* view reasons as traditional, albeit very special causes. As neurophilosophers, we can tentatively think of acting for reasons as acting with intent, whereby intentions are realized as neuronal states. *Intentionalists*, in contrast, claim that actions resulting from reasons exhibit a semantic dimension that physical processes lack and can only be grasped by an understanding attitude.

Hence, this debate is about the relationship of intents, beliefs, actions, and a causal component. The causal theory of action advocate has a problem. In determinism even intents are determined by events in the distant past. This is intuitively implausible, because purposeful action appears to occur wholly in the (conscious) present and the aspect of meaning or reason involved seems to be disconnected from the past. Another difficulty is that intentional causation has a *normative* aspect. An example of the "misdirected causal chains" (Davidson 1973) demonstrates this well. It can happen that a person intends an action and the intended result ensues, but does so *in the wrong way*. Imagine that one man wants to kill another with a rifle; he shoots but does not hit him.

His shot frightens a herd of wild boars, who then trample the victim to death. The man did set off a causal chain, that even lead to the desired result, but not in the intended manner. Not every causal chain that terminates in a desired result is suitable for a causal theory of action. The distinction between correct and incorrect causal chains is a *normative* distinction, which has no place in causal explanation.

In my opinion, both problems can be solved at once. In one way the first difficulty (How can an intelligible action be controlled by the past?) even holds the solution for the second complication (the normative aspect of distinguishing "correct" causal chains). Reference to the past provides the normative element of intentional attitudes, which are the basis of intelligible actions. If we could formulate an acceptable theory for intentionality, we would already be halfway toward a theory for intelligibility. The concept of meaning is central to both theories. A theory of intentionality deals with what we mean when we say that physical states of a system *have* meaning; a theory of intelligibility deals with how a system *grasps* and utilizes meaning for its own purposes. The role human language plays in this puzzle is essential. Another crucial step is to make plausible how a system with intentional content is able to understand abstract and general principles and use them in behavior. For understanding the intelligibility problem it is important that this capacity for using highly complex semantic content does not contradict being determined by past events. As I have mentioned, the solution lies in a theory of intentionality founded in biology.

In order to move on from intentionality to intelligibility we must pass through the intermediary phase of representational theory. In previous chapters we have already gathered up some essential parts for such a theory. From cognitive science we adopted connectionism, which better models human cognition than does symbol processing theory. I assume that the subvenient basis for representational states consists of neuronal activation vectors, which can be thought of as attractors. At the beginning of the last chapter we saw that dynamical systems theory, of which chaos theory is a special case, can describe mental processes more realistically, because it views cognition as a process happening in real time. But the question was not answered of why or how it is that neuronal states mean anything *at all*, how they can have representational content. We proceed toward a neurophilosophical theory of cognition by exploring teleosemantics.

2.2 Teleosemantics

2.2.1 Evolutionary Philosophy and Biological Intentionality   "Teleosemantics" denotes a group of theories that interpret "intentionality" using the biological concept of function. Organs and behavior can have biological functions. It is the heart's function to pump blood, the eye's function to make vision possible, the function of skin pigment changing color is to assimilate a chameleon to its environment for protection from predators, and the function of the bee's dance to indicate a place of nectar.

In the following the term *intentionality* does not stand for a property of *consciousness*, it stands only for bare semanticity (aboutness) (Kurthen 1992, p. 13). This usage also encompasses unconscious states and the nonmental, such as sentences in a language, signs, symbols, artifacts, and so on. Teleosemantics isolates the question of intentionality from that of consciousness. Conscious states *also* exhibit intentionality, but not qua consciousness.[29] What then, is the origin of intentionality? The source of intentionality, according to teleosemantics, lies in the history of the development of structures that exhibit intentionality (organs, sentences in language, mental states, neural structures). The idea of selection is central to it. An example from biology illustrates this.

Why do cows have udders? So that they can nurse their calves—a reasonable answer. Yet this answer is *teleological* (Greek *teleos*, complete, final, from *telos*, completion, end, +logy), it implies "in order to" (nurse their offspring). Teleological explanations refer to the future. If *future* events are causally important for teleological explanations, then they can never be equivalent to traditional causal explanations, unless we presuppose an effect from the future. That seems undesirable. In biology, teleological explanations are transformed into causal ones by introducing evolutionary causes. Cows that had udders, with which they nursed their offspring, reproduced on average more successfully than cows

without udders. Contemporary cows have udders, because their ancestors did.[30] Teleological explanations in biology are thus *abbreviated
causal explanations.*[31]

The situation is analogous for intentional explanations. Intentional
explanations are also abbreviated causal explanations. Just as biology
gives evolutionary explanations for the functions of organs, so can
teleosemantics (basically) give evolutionary explanations for the intentional content of structures found in biological systems. To that extent,
it belongs to a group of *evolutionary philosophies*, which hold that evolution theory is the correct empiric foundation for their philosophical
theses. Closest kin is evolutionary epistemology (EE). It claims to have
an empirically founded answer to the question about how we can know
anything about the world: "Our instrument for knowledge is a result of
evolution. Subjective knowledge structures are suited to the world
because in the course of evolution they developed through adjustment to
the world. And they (partially) correspond to the world, since only a correspondence like that would make survival possible" (Vollmer 1975, p.
102). The chasm between "biology of knowledge" (Riedl 1980) and
more sophisticated human performances in knowing is still rather deep.
"Evolutionary psychology" has just arisen within recent years (Barkow,
Cosmides, and Tooby 1992; Wright 1994; Buss 1995; Tooby and
Cosmides 1995). A crucial advance in the development of the human
capacity for knowledge was the skill of designing, acquiring, and using
argumentative language. We urgently need a theory that closes the gap
between perception and language.

Ruth Garrett Millikan's *theory of proper functions* (TOPF in the following) is an ambitious attempt to find an evolutionary foundation for
intentionality and semantic content in language and thinking.[32] I discuss
her theory as a paradigm for teleosemantic intentionality theories.[33] Millikan begins with the uncontroversial existence of meaningful structures
in language. No one would claim that their *meaning* is solely a result of
their inner structure. That is not the case for mental states. Philosophers
and cognitive scientists alike claim that mental states have meaning
because of their intrinsic structure. Meanings of thoughts are introspectively accessible via consciousness, and it is just by having this
access that we know what we think. Wilfried Sellars put it this way:

Intentionality is *given*. Millikan calls this traditional standpoint meaning rationalism,[34] and she is not particularly fond of it: "My desire is to kill meaning rationalism *dead*, and then beat on it. Perhaps I will succeed in raising one or two more doubts about it" (Millikan 1993a, p. 12). In contrast to philosophers like Kripke and Putnam, she advocates a decidedly realistic, biologically founded theory of knowledge:

> psychology is not at root a science involving laws, . . . explanations in psychology are unlike explanations in the physical sciences, . . . it is inescapably a deeply *ecological* science dealing with *how the organism interacts with its wider environment*. . . . I open the possibility of a naturalist treatment of the nature of knowledge based on a biologically rooted theory of competence. . . . *Reasoning, I insist, is done in the world, not in one's head.* Logical possibility (known a priori) is impossible. And the only hope for intentional psychology is to embrace its biological roots. (Millikan 1993a, pp. 11–12, emphasis is author's)

Millikan's theory is marked by four features:

1. *Biological foundation*: Human intentionality is based on biological proper functions developed during the course of evolution.

2. *History*: Intentionality exhibited by physical entities can be explained only by recourse to their history of selection.

3. *Externalism*: These explanations necessarily refer to the interaction of intentional structures between the systems that exhibit them and the environment.

4. *Normativity*: The normative character of intentional states is traced back to biological proper functions.

The concept of proper functions is a generalized version of biological functions and the single most important theoretical concept in Millikan's theory.[35] In a first approximation we can understand it to mean this: An entity has a proper function if it developed during a process of selection (particularly natural selection) and the exercise of this function by the entity's ancestors is essential for explaining its existence. In short, we can say that this entity is *meant for something*. Thus the udder is meant for nursing calves. Let us look at the concept of proper function and its critique in some detail.

2.2.2 Proper Functions   A heart has several physical and chemical properties. It increases the weight of an organism, it makes sounds, it is red, it consists of muscle cells, and so on. The *proper function* of the heart, though, is to pump blood. That is what it is for, that is what it is *supposed to do*. The proper function of sperm is to fertilize an ovum. The proper function of some mechanism in the goldfish's central nervous system that causes him to draw minute particles floating in the water into his mouth, is to get food. What characterizes a proper function? The causal history of its origin. Hearts exist *because* they pumped blood in the past. To be precise, organisms with hearts fulfilling this function generally proliferated better than those for which this was not the case, and thus contributed to the continued reproduction of hearts.

The causal *history* of the performance of that function is an irremovable element in explaining the existence of entities with proper functions. Such explanations refer to "normal" circumstances. In Millikan's terminology "normal" circumstances are not average or standard conditions, they are *historically optimal* conditions for the real manifestation of that proper function. "Normal" explanations are those that refer to these normal conditions. The concept of normal conditions does not imply that under normal conditions the function in question was always fulfilled or will always be performed. It is entirely sufficient for the proper function to have been exercised in a critical number of cases. Thus a sperm almost never meets an ovum, and the goldfish spits out the majority of particles it sucks in.

The critical aspect of Millikan's theory is that it defines proper function *so generally* that, while biological functions belong to the class of proper functions, so do other items, as long as they satisfy the prerequisites of the definition. One of the prerequisites is the feature of belonging to a family established by reproduction. First, Millikan defines "Ancestors of a member of a reproductively established family" (Millikan 1984, p. 27), and then "direct proper function."

Direct Proper Function

Where *m* is a member of a reproductively established family *R* and *R* has the reproductively established Normal character *C*, m has the function *F* as a direct proper function iff:

1. Certain ancestors of m performed F.
2. In part because there existed a direct causal connection between the character C and performance of the function F in the case of these ancestors of m, C correlated positively with F over a certain set of items S that included these ancestors and other things not having C.
3. One among the legitimate explanations that can be given of the fact that m exists makes reference to the fact that C correlated positively with F over S, either directly causing reproduction of m or explaining why R was proliferated and hence why m exists. (Millikan 1984, p. 28)

In short, a function is a proper function of an entity m, if its existence can partially be explained by the fact that ancestors of m actually performed this function in a critical number of cases. This definition is so broad that it not only includes organs (such as hearts), but also forms of communication (such as bee dances), gestures (such as shaking hands), language tokens (such as names, words, sentences, quotation marks), artifacts (such as automobile parts), or mental states (such as beliefs, desires). *Direct* proper functions, however, are not sufficient. There are diverse kinds of proper functions. An item can have several proper functions simultaneously, temporarily, alternatively, and so on. Millikan goes to great lengths to explain and define diverse subgroups of proper functions.[36] One example can be used to illustrate three of them (namely relational, adaptive, and derived proper functions). I have chosen the bee dance[37] in order to make Millikan's abstract exposition somewhat more graphic. Nevertheless, it remains an extremely condensed version (practically summarizing the entire second chapter in Millikan 1984), which must be reread to be grasped entirely. (In order to read the definitions without the bee dance example, I have separated the two expositions by inserting brackets.)

Relational, Adapted, and Derived Proper Functions (abbreviated version of Millikan's theory taken from *Language, Thought and Other Biological Categories*, p. 49*)

1. An entity A [a neural item in a bee, which lays out the movements in the bee dance] has a *relational* proper function when it is supposed to produce something [the bee dance] that bears a certain relation to something else N [nectar], such that N is "so situated" in relation to A.
2. If an N [nectar somewhere] exists, which is "so situated" in relation to A, then A becomes for the moment *adapted*, and acquires an *adapted*

proper function [to point to the nectar somewhere]. N is now the current *adaptor* for A and for this adapted function of A.

3. Whatever A produces qua performing a merely adapted function is an *adapted device* D [an actual bee dance that indicates a real occurrence of nectar].

4. Functions of entity A [the neural items that generate the actual bee dance] that lie beyond the production of any adapted device D that A produces are *derived proper functions* of D [derived from the real bee dance which indicates real nectar] derived from A's proper function plus, perhaps, A's current adaptor.

5. Some of D's derived functions may be *invariant derived functions* of D [showing other bees the way to the nectar, procuring nectar for the bee population, and so on] of the producer [the bee itself or neural structures in the bee]. Others are merely *adapted derived* proper functions [in a concrete situation guiding the other bees to fly South-Southwest], adapted to D's particular constitution [the concrete features of some bee dance indicating some real nectar] but, originally adapted to A's adaptor [the real occurrence of nectar].

TOPF stands or falls with the theoretical notion of proper functions, so it is no surprise that most of the criticism is directed toward that central concept. We shall examine it and the critique. The three major attacks include the claim of circularity, the Pangloss objection, and the argument of the double (another variation of which is the argument of the archetype). In the following we will discuss and dismiss them (see also Walter 1997c).

2.2.3 Proper Functions in Trouble?   One of the major and most frequent objections, played out in several variations, is that of circularity. Basically it states that the concept of proper function presupposes what it intends to explain. In this sense it is similar to the self-refuting argument of determinism (cf. chapter 1). This objection can be most easily refuted when it rests on a lack of knowledge about the theory. It is simply wrong to claim that Millikan refers to a "dispositional moment which is not captured in causal explanation" (Keil 1993a, p. 99).[38] "To describe the biological function of an item is *not* to describe its dispositional capacities" (Millikan 1993a, p. 171). "I had in mind a '*because*' that was strictly causal. If it is to be causal, the 'because there is something it can do' *must be an elliptical reference to something past* and to something once *actually* done" (Millikan 1993a, p. 33; emphasis is mine, H.W.). More serious is the criticism that the theory of proper functions presupposes intentional concepts such as "explanation" (Putnam 1992, chapter 2) or "causality" (Keil 1993a), since these notions are used in the definition of a proper function. If this criticism implies discovering a *petitio principii*, then it is wrong. The TOPF nowhere claims to explicate the concepts of explanation and causality; it simply uses them to define proper functions. What is the criticism getting at? Let us look first at causality.

In terms of genetics, it is indeed circular. It is undoubtedly true that human effectiveness already existed as a familiar phenomenon before any scientific theory of causality was imagined. Only much later in the development of the human race did anyone begin explaining human effectiveness in terms of causality. But this is only a (trivial) historical idea, for how could it have been otherwise? Presumably more is at the bottom of this criticism, namely that the paradigm of causality itself is a human product and there is no such thing as scientific causality. Scientific causality is a purely "anthropomorphic metaphor" (for the implied general critique of naturalism see Keil 1993b, p. 229–360). This consideration refers to Georg Henrik v. Wright's interventionistic theory of causality. But following up this line of criticism would demand entirely revising the conventional understanding of causality in natural science. We would need some very strong arguments to defend such an anthropomorphic theory of causality and the success of it is questionable. Nevertheless, we can defend the TOPF even without the concept of causality by limiting ourselves to explaining the intentional through the contribution of *factual events*. Naturally, one could claim that past events, too, are only intentional constructs or metaphors. But in the end this leads to radical constructivism, which we already dismissed after lengthy consideration in chapter 2.

How about "explanation?" Explanations refer to something and hence have an intentional element. That is entirely correct. But this type of self-reference only discredits the TOPF as a natural theory when we demand too much of naturalism. Should we dismiss every "linguistically conceived" theory of language as useless, every theory of science that attempts to explain what "explications" are, every theory of definition that defines definition, and every philosophical theory addressing the meaning of "meaning?" Self-reference is unavoidable. It is only fatal when it issues intratheory contradictions or empty circles. No critic has proven that yet for the theory of proper functions. If anything at all, we have here not a *vicious*, but a *virtuous* circle: a proliferate, self-correcting, noncontradictory feedback loop that also includes empirical findings (Vollmer 1985, p. 232–250).

The second significant assault on TOPF is the *Pangloss* objection. It gained attention in biology as critique on the concept of adaptation (Gould and Lewontin 1979; Gould and Vrba 1982), but it is also directed toward evolutionary epistemology (Engels 1987, pp. 155–215) and the theory of proper functions (Lyons 1992, pp. 317f). A TOPF theorist claims that *all* features of an organism testify to adaptation[39] and exist *because* they fulfill functions and hence were selected. But this is incorrect. Neither are all features developed in the course of evolution signs of adaptation, nor are all selected beliefs correct (Whyte 1993, p. 50). Many features arose randomly or without the pressure of selection (this is claimed by the theory of neutral evolution). This objection discredits neither evolution theory nor the theory of proper functions. First of all, the theory of neutral evolution in considered refuted in biology, at least in the pan-neutralist version. Second, neither evolution theorists nor TOPFists defend a Panglossian view; the claim is merely that there is adaptation such that it allows survival under certain conditions in comparison to other varieties of the same species. Third, co-opting a function in the course of history degrades neither selection theory nor the theory of proper functions. Features can exhibit double, several, and serial functions (Millikan 1984, p. 35). For the ancestors of today's birds, feathers probably first fulfilled the function of providing warmth, then weight reduction, then facilitating hopping, and finally making flight possible. Changing functions are not negative for TOPF, they are explicitly taken into consideration as an option and integrated into the theory (Millikan 1984, p. 32). Double and stacked functions and the option of changing functions illustrate how greater changes can occur gradually (Vollmer 1986, p. 24–29).[40] So, this second standard objection can also be dismissed.

The third objection, the *archetype* objection, is directed toward the central position of history in the theory of proper functions. There are two versions of the argument. The first takes the form of a thought experiment (Lyons 1992; Kurthen 1992).[41] Let us assume that by cosmic chance there exists somewhere in the universe a double of myself. Since he does not have the right history, he does not have any ancestors, he does not belong to a reproductively established family, therefore he has no proper functions. That means that the function of his heart is not to pump blood, his sentences have no meaning, his thoughts have no content, his intentions have no goals. This is so implausible and contra-intuitive that the theory must be wrong—or at least needs supplementation. It's obvious that my double's heart *can* pump blood, and if his neural states are identical to mine, then he also has the same thoughts.

Millikan strictly denies that. She insists on the relevance of history because she wants strictly to reduce teleological explanations to causal explanations. Therefore, she avoids recourse to dispositions and propensities at all costs. This creates a dilemma. Either we hang on to the meaning of history and fight off our strong intuitions, or we make reference to dispositions and propensities and let circularity in through the back door. Millikan holds that "proper function" must be understood as a theoretical term for explaining intentionality in our current real world, not in any counterfactual world. Certainly we can imagine that a "functioning" organism is somehow created by cosmic chance, it is actually possible without violating natural laws (due to the probabilistic nature of quantum mechanics); but there are no such organisms under (or above) the sun. The reason why my double has no proper functions is that he came into being *by chance*. If the double came into existence as a *copy* of an original, by tele-cloning or reconstructing from a blueprint, *then* he would have proper functions. This sounds counterintuitive, but perhaps this reflection makes it more plausible: Perhaps my randomly created double—if he has exactly the same brain structure—also has the same phenomenal experiences, and yet his thoughts do not automatically *mean* anything. This reply is compatible with differential metaphysics of intentional and conscious states.

The same objection can also be expressed entirely without any thought experiment, namely as a *first token* argument. New features undoubtedly arise through selection. Does the first sample of a newly established item have the same functions as its (not mutated) descendents? No, not really: Potentially it can perform the same functions, but it does not have the same *proper* functions. How is that? Obviously we must distinguish between two kinds of functions: a function that an item performs or could perform based on the way it is built, and the function that the item *is supposed to* perform.[42] In later publications Millikan distinguishes between mechanofunctions and teleofunctions. Griffiths (1995) analogously distinguishes effects from functions. An example serves to illustrate the distinction. Which function does the nose perform? Among the mechanofunctions (effects) there are those such as supporting eyeglasses, being a focal point for crossing one's eyes, acting as a bumper zone when boxing, a handle for pulling disobedient pupils around the classroom, and so on. But the nose's proper functions are inhaling and olfaction. In order to distinguish these functions, we must refer to history. Naturally, not all effects performed by ancestor noses were proper functions. It is only true of those that irremovably contribute to the explanation of the existence of contemporary noses—via their function in a story of selection. (Dr. Pangloss was wrong!)[43]

Are proper functions thus only a subclass of mechanofunctions? Not necessarily. For it is possible that the proper function changes while the mechanofunction remains the same. In other words, the material constitution and hence the disposition of an item remains the same, while the proper function changes in new environmental circumstances. Imagine that the direct proper function of a red dot on the beak of an island finch is to frighten away a particular predator. Suddenly the predators die out because of an epidemic introduced into the area by female finches that an ornithologist had brought along on his trip to the island. It happens that most of the new finch ladies have two properties: they are more attractive than the female finch island dwellers, and they prefer the color red. The result: As time passes, they replace the native female finches; simultaneously the male finches with red spotted beaks have the best chances to reproduce. What can we say about the proper function of the red dot on the beaks of male finches on the island at the time when the ornithologist first arrived there? First, there is no doubt that the dot caused (had the effect, performed the mechanofunction) the newly arrived finch ladies to pay attention to them. But is this really the proper function of the dot? The theory of proper functions says that it is not. Only after male finches become selected because of this dot would this dot have that proper function. Naturally, the transition is fuzzy. It is not clear, at exactly which point in time a dot like this has a new proper function. But this is not an argument against the theoretical definition of a proper function. Even the meaning of a sentence or a thought can only be *exactly* determined in the fewest cases. So here we have an example in which the mechanofunctions (possible effects) of a spot have remained identical, while the proper function has changed.[44]

If we now insist on sticking to our intuitions and claim that our double's sentences mean something, then we must ask ourselves what it means for something to mean something. We need a theoretical definition of meaning and must demonstrate how it can do better than TOPF. Intuitions alone are not arguments, merely impulses to find some.

2.2.4 Intentional Icons and Three Aspects of Reference   Intentionality interpreted as being meaningful is an attribute that applies to all items with proper functions. In contrast, "reference" is whatever an expression in language or another sign denotes that is meant by it. Millikan thinks that there are three parts to the reference of items that have semantic content: (1) a standardizing and stabilizing proper function, (2) meaning (in Frege's sense of the word), and (3) intension. The most important of these is meaning. Let us briefly explain these three aspects of reference (cf. also Kurthen 1992).

The *stabilizing and standardizing proper function* (SSPF) of a item that denotes something (such as the linguistic device "elm") is to guarantee that in communication situations the use of this device by speakers and hearers is not ambiguous, but exhibits some degree of uniformity. The producer and the consumer of a linguistic device must use it similarly in a critical mass of cases, otherwise usage would gradually decrease and that item would drop out of the language. Its SSPF is an important aspect of the reference of "elm." This is why we can identify certain occurrences of "elm" because of the specific history of its usage and need not wait for an analysis of current usage or an analysis of its syntax. This is also why we can use the expression "elm" meaningfully, without being able to tell the difference between an elm and a beech tree. For if the reference of "elm" depends on its SSPF, it is independent of the explicit knowledge of an individual user.

The second and most important aspect of reference is the sense—or as Millikan puts it—the *Fregean sense* of an item.[45] What does this mean? In one phrase. The Fregean sense is an item's *being supposed to correspond to something*. This clearly expresses the teleological aspect. *This teleological aspect can be reduced to a causal explanation by using the notion of proper functions.* "Being supposed to do" is an abbreviation for the causal history of its origin. Here a few examples. The Fregean sense of a warning screech is that it is supposed to be made, and in the face of danger it is supposed to have a certain effect on other members of a species. The Fregean sense of a bee dance is that it is supposed to indicate a place of nectar and guide other bees to it. The Fregean sense of the imperative "bring me the apple!" is that it is supposed to cause a hearer to bring an apple to a speaker. If a bee dance, a forewarning, or a sentence happen randomly—if they do not have the right history—then they make no Fregean sense. If a chimpanzee toying with a typewriter happened to type the sentence "it is peaceful at the top of the mountain," the written word "top" would not mean top, even if a person reading it might *interpret* it to do so.

Millikan defines a class of devices that she calls *intentional icons*.[46] This class includes all sorts of items that we call "signs," many communicative devices in the animal world, sentences in public languages, and also the class of "representations." Intentional icons must satisfy certain conditions in order to qualify as intentional icons. They stand halfway between a producer and a consumer, they serve communicative functions, and they adapt the user to existing circumstances in such a way that he can perform his own proper functions. The importance of proper functions for the definition of intentional icons is revealed in the following definition. I have put explanations and two examples separated by semicolons in brackets; the example of the bee dance and the sentence of a public language.

Intentional icons satisfy the following conditions (taken from Millikan 1984, pp. 96f):

1. *They* [bee dances; sentences] *belong to* [one or more] *reproductively established families* [such as the class of variant or the class of invariant features of the bee dance; sentences and their elements (words, phrases) belong to the class of invariant grammatical structures as well as to other classes with variant and invariant features (script, phonetics, punctuation marks, etc.)].

2. *They stand midway between a producer device* [the dancing bee; the speaker] *and an interpreter device* [the user, the other bees; the hearer].

3. *One of their essential proper function is to adapt the interpreting device to conditions such that it can perform its own proper functions* [collect nectar, perform an act; draw a conclusion, criticize an argument].

4a. *In the case of imperative sentences* [commanding elements of the bee dance; commands, wishes] *it is a proper function of the interpreter device, as adapted by the sentence, to produce conditions* [flying to the source of nectar and collecting it; following an order, fulfilling a wish] *onto which the sentence will map in accordance with a specific mapping function.*

4b. *In the case of indicative sentences* [conveying information about the location of the nectar; making statements that can be true or false], *the Normal explanation of how of the sentence* [which in turn refers to historically optimal conditions], *adapts the interpreter device, makes reference to the fact that the sentence maps* [correspondence relation] *conditions in the world* [nectar is actually at that place; the sentence *is* true].

Intentional icons are fairly complex items with semantic content.[47] They are usually temporary adaptations to a changing environment. Often they exhibit indicative and imperative elements simultaneously. The proper function of a warning screech is to indicate danger, as well as to stimulate an adequate reaction in nearby members of the species. Thus, a warning screech is both an indicative as well as an imperative intentional icon. It is indicative, because the normal conditions under which it occurs consist of certain circumstances; it is imperative, because its normal conditions prescribe that it cause specific effects that produce certain circumstances. The same is true for the bee's dance. It fulfills its proper function when it correctly indicates a place of nectar *and* causes other bees to seek it. Sentences in a language are also intentional icons. Commands are imperative sentences; statements are indicative. They arose in a language community in order to fulfill certain communicative functions. They exist *because* they fulfill these functions in a critical mass of cases, or their precursors did. If normal conditions for fulfilling the proper functions of indicative configurations of world affairs prevail, then those configurations of world affairs do correspond to them. A traditional way of saying this is to say, "They are true."

So here Millikan is working with a correspondence theory of truth. As she correctly remarks (Millikan 1984, p. 86f), the trouble with correspondence theory is *not* that it shows that there are correspondence rules between true sentences and configurations of world affairs, but that there are *too many* of them—an infinite number of them. Every correspondence theory, whether of truth or of representation, must therefore be a theory about what particularly characterizes correspondence rules that *correctly* correlate representation and what is represented, true sentences and configurations of world affairs. Those special characteristic features are not merely formal criteria, such as coherence, simplicity, or being logical: "The specialness that turns a mathematical mapping function into a representation-represented relation in a given case must have to be some kind of special status that this function has in the real, natural, or the *causal* order rather than the logical order. Thus, any coherent correspondence theory of truth must be part of our total theory of the world" (Millikan 1984, p. 87).[48] Teleosemantics offers such a theory. Based on the theory of evolution it naturalistically distinguishes correct correspondence rules. Correct rules are those to which an intentional icon is supposed to correspond.[49] That is precisely the definition of Fregean sense.

Millikan considers *intension* to be the least important, but most complicated aspect of reference. To her, "intension" first of all has to do with what occurs inside the speaker or hearer of a language. Terms in a public language have an SSPF and a Fregean sense independent of the speaker. Every individual speaker using this tool has developed his own manner of using it, such that he can employ it in accordance with its own proper function. To illustrate this theory of meaning we can simplify and imagine the process of thinking as inward speaking.[50] When a speaker introduces an expression from public language into his own inner idiolect, he must "translate" the external expression to an internal one having the same meaning. For this he needs a procedure that guarantees that the inner expression maps in the same way like the external expression and that this mapping relation remains uniform in numerous repetitions of the expression within inner speech.

What is important is the distinction between implicit and explicit intensions. Later on it will play a part in characterizing rationality. An expression (for example, "apple") has an implicit intension when internal iterations are produced by mechanisms that can be derived *directly* from sense impressions (apple taste, appearance, or smell). An expression has an *explicit* intension when in internal iteration it is *newly* produced from sentences that *do not* contain that expression. An expression can have diverse explicit intensions. We can produce an internal term for "apple" from the thoughts stimulated by reading "fruit, five letters, can be made to sauce" while working a crossword puzzle. But we can also produce it when pondering an overheard sentence such as, "My sister already gave us so many yesterday!" or upon hearing the command: "Give me one of those round things in the bowl!"

Before turning to characterizing mental states in terms of teleosemantics, let us summarize the above. Stabilizing and standardizing proper functions provide that hearers and speakers can communicate, they fulfill social and communicative functions. The Fregean sense connects an intentional system with the world, because "something's being supposed to be for something" can only be explained by special distinguished correspondence rules with the world. Intension is "using a device within a system." In order to have an intension with semantic content, a device must already have a Fregean sense. Intensions are subordinate to an externally individuated Fregean sense. What, then, is the meaning of meaning? The meaning of an intentional icon lies in *the kind of structure that would have to be in the environment of an organism so that the icon suits the environment—according to its mapping function, and the organism can successfully use it in a normal manner.*[51]

2.2.5 From Bee Dances to Rational Thinking We shall now outline how more complex human representations and rationality can be explained naturalistically and without vicious circles. Admittedly, this is a very rough sketch, but it need not fear comparison with alternative naturalistic theories.

Let us begin by characterizing "representation." For starters we can say that a representation is an intentional icon, whose "referents are supposed to be identified" (Millikan 1984, p. 101), and whose proper function is, among other things, to "participate in mediated inference" (Millikan 1993b, p. 103).[52] For this we need merely to use two overlapping intentional icons, that is, icons that share a referent with the same real value.[53] An act of correct identification occurs when a user employs two intentionally overlapping icons in order to perform a proper function and when the normal explanation of this proper function must refer to the fact that the real value of these referents is the same (Millikan 1984, p. 24). If a speaker utters the sentences: "Here's *lunch* for Theresa!" and "Be careful, *it* is hot!" and the interpreter puts the dish on the window sill to cool down, she has used two overlapping intentional icons and correctly identified the common referent with the same real value.

Representations must not be linguistic. Imagine a gazelle with intentional icons in her head, realized as neural maps. Imagine that one map includes the place where she last found water and another includes areas where she last saw lions. Both maps include her own resting place. Now, if she combines both maps, by using her own resting place as a mediating inference, the result is a new, third map showing that lions are near her old water hole. Assuming that the gazelle's brain functioned normally while combining the maps, "normal" meaning that it functions in accordance with its biological "design," then this is a typical example of mediated inference. Two vehicles of information were combined to generate a third vehicle containing new information via a mediating referent.

Although the inferences needed here resemble those for drawing conclusions in logic,[54] such representations must not necessarily be like sentences. Imagine that by combining information gained by *seeing* an object with information gained by *touching* it one arrives at the conviction that a green apple is hard. The premises are percepts, the conclusion is a thought. Nevertheless, the process is an inference and happens via a mediating term. The percepts involved are thus representations, so we can characterize representations as those intentional icons which are supposed to participate in "processes of information transformation between items with semantic content" (Millikan 1993b, p. 104).

Based on this concept of representation we can now ask what "sentences in a language of thought" could look like (see Millikan 1993b). As discussed in chapter 2, the compositionality of language and thinking is an explanandum for every naturalistic theory of intentionality. Any theory should be able to explain why new semantic entities can be generated from a new combination of referents or aspects of older entities. The simplest explanation for this would be that elements that make up entities with semantic content have unchanging meaning due to their syntax and are recombined following certain rules. This strong notion of compositionality is the foundation of symbol processing theory. In Millikan's terminology, for internal representations, this would mean that the meaning of newly "composed" sentences results purely from their intension. But Millikan characterizes compositionality externally. A representation is compositional, if operations or transformations of parts of a representing system can be done in such a way that they correspond to certain reorganizations of things in the world. Semantic composition is nothing more than a mapping between a representing item and a represented matter, which can be transformed. "Sentences in a language of thought," however, do not exhibit strong compositionality. First, element meanings are not independent of context. Second, the correspondence of compositional elements is secondary. In the first instance, true *sentences* correspond to matters, and in the second instance the elements of the sentence correspond to some thing. Third, the meaning of an element is not determined solely by syntax. *Mental representations can be semantically identical, yet syntactically entirely different, as long as they correctly identify their real value.* Likewise, two neuronal representations can have different physical manifestations, yet be semantically identical.

Instead of satisfying two strong conditions for compositionality, "sentences in a language of thought" have two other conditions to meet. First, they must exhibit a *subject-predicate structure*, and second, they must be candidates for *transforming negation*. What does this mean? Let us begin with the *subject-predicate* structure. It must be possible to transform an intentional icon that corresponds to other subjects with the same predicate and it must be possible to transform those that correspond to the same subject with different predicates. This is why bee dances are not sentences, for they exhibit no subject term: Bee dances says nothing more than where nectar can be found. Neither is a rabbit's thumping (a warning signal) a sentence, for at no time nor place does it ever mean anything other than danger. Vervet ape alarm cries, on the other hand, do have a subject-predicate structure. They express times and places, which vary with the times and places where enemies are (subject terms), and there are different types of cries indicating different types of enemies (predicate terms). Unfortunately, they can never be negated. So they are also not sentences.[55]

How can teleosemantics deal with folk psychologies (beliefs, desires, intentions), which are important for information transforming processes of items with semantic content? In outline, as follows: The main proper function of a *desire* is to contribute to its fulfillment, which means to bring about that matter in the world it represents in accordance with a normal explanation. A desire is an *imperative* intentional icon. Another proper function of desire consists of being involved with beliefs in inferences. "Inference," as mentioned, denotes combining icons with other icons via a mediate item, to produce new icons which convey new information. Beliefs are *indicative* intentional icons. They are identified by the circumstances that must prevail so that they can fulfill their proper functions. One of their proper functions is to participate in inferences. Another proper function of beliefs is to support desires in producing their fulfillment. So beliefs are secondary to desires. A representational system that merely reflects, but is not *active* in the world, is not to be found in Millikan's theory. A mirror does not represent anything.

The normal conditions that must prevail so that desires and beliefs can fulfill their proper functions are those that must prevail in a normal explanation of their existence. Beliefs normally only fulfill the proper function of supporting the fulfillment of desires when those beliefs are *true*, which means that the icon-relationship to the circumstances in the world is correct.[56] Oedipus's false belief that Jocasta was not a member of his family did not contribute to satisfying his desire that the prophecy of the oracle at Delphi would not become true, although a true belief, namely that Jocasta is his mother, would certainly have facilitated the satisfaction of that desire. That contribution would result from the fact that Jocasta really *is* his mother (cf. Kurthen 1992, p. 163).

Analogously, desires also have conditions for satisfaction. Those are the conditions that must prevail if a desire is to fulfill its proper function of causing specific effects or producing certain circumstances. But how do we get from desires to intentions? The journey is three-legged: desire–goal–intention. Desires alone do not guide action. One can have many desires characterized by the conditions of their satisfaction (such as getting to a Caribbean Island in ten minutes), which cannot really be satisfied. Other desires compete with one another, like the desire to stay in bed reading and the desire to complete the work on one's desk. Once one desire is victorious over the other, a goal representation is created, like a plan to get up and work for three hours. In order for action to occur, the goal representation must cooperate with various explicit and implicit convictions. Millikan puts it this way:

Desires . . . might be thought of as competing with one another for allocation of resources, which, once allocated, turn them into goals, then perhaps later, when belief in their impending fulfillment is warranted, into intentions. (Millikan 1993a, p. 166)

What is essential about intentional action is that it fulfills a particular kind of biological function, namely, an imperative function, or a goal representation. (p. 168).

Imperative representations are blueprints or plans for what is to be done. (p. 166)

[T]hey are supposed to *cause* the world to vary as they vary" [while indicative representations are *caused* to reflect the variations in the world.] Their job is to guide the organism toward achievement of the ends they represent. (p. 166)

Presumably, the biological point of the capacity to *represent* goals to oneself is to make it possible to vary them, evaluate them, arrive at them rationally, and arrive at rational means of fulfilling them. (p. 166)

Does the capacity for representation automatically include rationality? No. Childish thinking may, more or less, exhibit representational features, without necessarily being rational. Many adult thoughts are also not particularly rational, as we witness everyday. So what distinguishes rational from merely representational thinking?

Both rationality and language are characteristically systematic. Being systematic is the skill of being able to automatically think a thought of a particular kind, if one can think another. It is not identical to inference-making skills. Inferences, can be made from simple intentional items, without those items being *explicit*. Thus, a neural state can represent a predator, from which a beaver infers to issue a screech warning. But this does not mean that the beaver explicitly represents the predator. Furthermore, undoubtedly, it is possible that many inferences are inconsistent with each other. An organism can entertain any number of contradictory representations, either because its cognitive mechanisms function abnormally, or because abnormal conditions prevail. The skill of revealing and eliminating contradictions among inner representations ("coherence of inference") by no means follows from the definition of representation we are using. These two skills are major features of rational thinking (Millikan 1993a, p. 114). So we can set up a preliminary definition of rationality in TOPF lingo; or to be cautious, let's say that this definition expresses at least two necessary conditions for rationality: An organism is *rational* if it can make valid inferences in which all premises bearing information are explicit and if that organism can discover and eliminate inconsistencies among its representations.

Whatever one may think of this definition; it obviously is not a circular definition presupposing rationality just because it uses the terms "inferences" and "premises." Rationality can be explained naturalistically without circularity. Its genesis can be traced through intermediate stages in the animal kingdom; it is applicable to humans; and it is set not in a transcendental realm of intelligibility, but placed within the range of biology, to which man irremovably belongs.

This suffices to demonstrate that the theory of proper functions is also adequate for a naturalistic approach to human, intelligible thinking. In order to be applicable to neurophilosophy, however, it must be formulated still more specifically. In other words, teleosemantics must become neurosemantics. We shall now examine that transition.

2.3   Adaptive Neurosemantics

2.3.1   From Teleo- to Neurosemantics
I now plan to develop a theory of adaptive neurosemantics. Borrowing heavily from Millikan's teleosemantics this theory demonstrates how meaning is generated in the brain.

It is a basis for neurophilosophical approximation to the problem of intelligibility. However, Millikan's theory demands extension, if we are to use it for neurophilosophical purposes. Martin Kurthen, a neuroscientist and philosopher, claims that theoretical neurosemantics might solve problems such as "discovering meaning and semantic content in the brain, or revealing in which sense, under which prerequisites, and whether at all we can say that cerebral states have something like semantic content." (Kurthen 1992, p. 358). This is only possible in a naturalistic way, if semantics are based on nonsemantics (Kurthen 1992, p. 39). In other words; the theory may not presuppose what it intends to explain. We could achieve this if we could trace neurosemantic content back to biological and neurological facts. Obviously, teleosemantics suits this task well.

Kurthen suggests that we should not reify "meaning," not think of it as something spatiotemporal, an object that can be "found." But, if a causally efficient content should repeatedly occur in the brain, then, according to Kurthen, we can define that content as the role and function of cerebral states. We must define neurosemantical content as content *for* the system in which it occurs. In the widest sense, then, neurosemantics is a theory of how meaning is *used*; simultaneously it is *teleological* semantics.

Kurthen designs neurosemantics around four main theses (Kurthen 1992, pp. 420–427, 446).[57] *Monistic cophenomenalism* emphasizes that a cognitive system is interlaced with its environment. The smallest unit in neurosemantic explanation is, therefore, not an isolated cognitive system, but the union of that system with the relevant portion of the world. This notion coincides with an externalistic standpoint in the theory of knowledge. The second thesis (*praxiology*) posits that in order to explain a system's cognitive ability, we must view that system from the perspective of practical reference to the world (the system's actions in the world). Recall that Millikan also emphasizes that representations must be used, if the are to have meaning. Kurthen's third thesis is that of *antirationalism*. The scientist's manner of rational observation is not the fundamental model for cognition. Cognition is based more on pre-predicative, practical understanding. This method is "being open for the relations of a thing with which a system is concerned" (Kurthen 1992,

p. 446). Heidegger's influence is tangible. The idea, though, can be interpreted less poetically by remembering that teleosemantic content is founded on historical development in which individual cognitive systems are in a web of purposes. Man possesses pre-predicative understanding, because nature designed him such that he simply fits into the world and under normal circumstances can move about in it effortlessly, without being constantly explicitly aware of it.

Finally, Kurthen's fourth consideration is *teleology*. Neurosemantic content is content by function. But Kurthen's teleosemantic approach differs from Millikan's teleosemantics in two areas. He feels that reference to history is obstructive and can be dropped. He founds this on the argument of the double, dealt with in several versions (Kurthen 1992). He advocates an unhistorical concept of function similar to that propagated by Bigelow and Pargetter (1987), based on a dispositional *forward-looking approach*. Further, he thinks that an evolutionary groundwork with emphasis on the survival value of adaptation is too narrow. This coincides with the complaint frequently expressed about evolutionary epistemology (cf. Engels 1987), that it is limited to seeking explanation merely for genetically anchored knowledge, particularly functions of perception.

This criticism of teleosemantic content is not justified. Rebuking the evolutionary approach for being too restricted is the result of a common misunderstanding. Any critique on the history-aspect can be weakened by expanding teleosemantics to include a larger time domain. This helps to explain human thinking's directness and flexibility, which allows generating new semantic content within brief periods. Both arguments lead to *adaptive neurosemantics*. Neurosemantic content is generated in the process of adapting a cognitive system to its environment, in which it acts and in which it is embedded. Adaptation is a process that occurs not only on a phylogenetic time scale, but rather on many different time scales, right down to the range of seconds.

2.3.2 An Anti-evolutionary Misunderstanding Millikan correctly states that her theory relies on the validity of evolution theory. Humans and their brains are de facto products of evolution. But this often evokes the following notion. Proper functions may be a useful concept for explaining mechanisms like food gathering, care of the young, proliferation, and mating behavior; but evolutionary teleosemantics cannot explain cultural functions (or beliefs). This is because evolution only happens via gene variations and phenotype selection, and the basic human genetic make-up has hardly changed in ten thousand years. Complex cultural human achievements are much younger. Therefore, evolutionary teleosemantics could not explain new, unique, and complex intentional human achievements.

Although this conclusion may intuitively seem right, it is wrong. Just because my toolbox is ten years old does not mean that I cannot repair anything that was invented recently. Just because our vision apparatus served survival purposes in the prehistoric world does not mean that evolutionary theory could never explain why we can see digital television. Is the telos of bare survival sufficient for explaining the content of the desire to drink water, but insufficient for explaining the content of a belief that Kurosawa is a better movie director than Houston (as Kurthen claims, p. 182)? Now, by no means can I comfort you that this will be easy and unproblematic. I only claim this. The fact that basal brain mechanisms evolved ten or a hundred thousand years ago does not imply that its older functions do not adapt themselves to new ones or that it cannot produce new functions while adapting to a changing environment.

What we inherit, of course, are not concrete semantic contents, but brain structures, which, in the appropriate environment, can make an organism capable of instantiating mental content in processes. We must, however, give up the idea that these are *universal* skills. Our picture of the brain as a learning machine that can be manipulated as we please is getting tattered. *Evolutionary psychology* views it more as an organ consisting of diverse modules of adaptive specialization. *Psychological mechanisms are for solving problems of adaptation.* Academic psychology continues to ignore this adaptive perspective. Its categories of the human mind propagated in all common textbooks (learning, memory, attention, thinking, decision-making, intelligence, motivation, emotion, development, etc.) do not correspond to the categories of evolutionary psychology. If there is anything like modules of the mind, they would be more like a family of instincts that solve problems of adaptation.

These instincts could encompass some of the following modules (taken from Pinker 1996, p. 473; see also Barkow, Cosmides, and Tooby 1992):

1. Intuitive mechanics: knowledge of movements, powers, and changes that objects undergo.

2. Intuitive biology: understanding how plants and animals function.

3. Intuitive mathematics: grasping a small quantity of objects.

4. Mental maps for large areas.

5. Selection of habitat: search for a safe and bountiful environment that generously provides information, basically like a savanna.

6. Danger: fear and caution, phobias for stimuli such as high altitudes, being closed in, dangerous social contacts and poisonous animals or predators, as well as the desire to know the circumstances in which these stimuli are harmless.

7. Nourishment: What is edible?

8. Contamination: aversions, reactions to certain things that appear nauseating, intuitions about contagion and disease.

9. Awareness of present sentiments, such as feeling happy or sad and moods of satisfaction or restlessness.

10. Intuitive psychology: predicting the behavior of other persons based on their beliefs and desires.

11. A mental archive: data base for individuals, with blanks for relations, status or rank, documentation of mutual favors, characteristic skills and strengths, and criteria for evaluating each feature.

12. Self-esteem: collecting and organizing information about the value one has for other persons, and preparing this information for others.

13. Justice: feelings about rights, obligations and retaliation, including feelings of wrath and revenge.

14. Relationships, including favoring close friends, and caring for offspring.

15. Partnership, including sexual attraction and love, loyalty and separation.

This list may be incomplete; some items may be wrong, others pure speculation. But there is some concrete evidence that the brain has specialized modules. This is true for schemes of what is young (Lorenz 1978), for phobias (which are objected, directed fears) (LeDoux 1994), for basic emotions (Ekman 1982; Machleidt, Gutjahr, and Mügge 1989), and for perceiving faces (Farah 1996). A module for social cognition is currently being debated (Raleigh et al. 1996). And there is also evidence of universal patterns in dealing with plants and animals as well as intuitive mechanics (Pinker 1995, pp. 474ff), even though no concrete brain mechanisms have been discovered that serve these functions. As described above, if we understand the mechanisms of the brain as they have evolved to be adaptive mechanisms that help to solve problems and fulfill functions, we begin to imagine what it could mean if Kurosawa is a better movie director than Houston. Both are individuals, who, employing their skills and strengths, have produced things that evoke approval effects in us. We evaluate these individuals by setting up a social ranking order among them, based on criteria that evolution has provided us, or for which we can explain how we learned them in terms of evolutionary development.

2.3.3   Selection Type Theories and Time Spans   In spite of the tool box argument, we are not satisfied. Isn't it beyond all doubt that we can think up new things? Isn't our cultural and linguistic development evidence that we have opened up spheres of meaning that had no part in our evolutionary history? Can't every healthy individual generate novel and creative mental content immediately? Yes, certainly, and it sometimes happens. Even though we presumably follow evolutionarily anchored patterns over long stretches of our lives and in our thinking, and it is questionable to what extent we can really "exceed" them (see Wright 1994), it still seems necessary even to me that neurosemantics claiming to be true must have an explanation for how novel mental content can be generated within a short time span.

   The key to extending neurosemantics lies in understanding that while biological selection can be recognized as the contingent basis for all *human* cognition, it can also be seen as a theoretical special case within a more general theory. This is not self-contradictory. It means that for *explaining* human cognition, reference to biological evolution is unavoidable, but it does not exclude that there could be other forms of cognition that do just fine without biological evolution, like systems of strong artificial intelligence. In addition, it is possible because the theory of proper functions not only explains the teleofunctions that emerged through evolution, but also explains teleofunctions that arise in analogous processes that obey the general criteria formulated by TOPF for systems exhibiting proper functions. A brief characterization of those criteria is *cycling, copying, selection*. There must be material objects that are cursory, copied, and selected. In other words, the principle of natural selection—in an abstract version—is central. And this is where we can begin extending neurosemantics to become adaptive neurosemantics. *If we reduce the time span for selection and thus shorten the adaptation process involved, the history of the circumstances is also abbreviated and we can define neurosemantic content without recourse to the concept of disposition.*[58] Everything pivots on the principle of selection.

The theory of natural selection, so essential for evolution theory, is a special case of the abstract class of *selection type theories*. These theories serve the purpose of solving problems of adaptation (Darden and Cain 1989, p. 104). Darden and Cain, who developed their scheme independently of Millikan, examine three concrete examples for these kind of selection type theories: Darwin's theory of natural selection, the theory of clonal selection in antibody production, and selective theories of higher order brain functions.[59] They begin with the theory of natural selection. After analyzing it, they abstract from constraints of evolution in order to isolate the five most important general features. According to Darden and Cain (1989, pp. 116f) we can specify a "type" of selection theory using five features:

A. Preconditions
    i. A set of Ys exists and
    ii. Ys vary as to whether they have property *P* and
    iii. Ys are in an environment *E* with critical factor *F*.
B. Interaction
    iv. Ys, in virtue of possessing or not possessing *P*, interact differently with environment *E* and
    v. critical factor *F* affects the interaction such that
C. Effect
    vi. the possession of *P* causes Ys with *P* to benefit and those without *P* to suffer.
    vi'. This causal interaction may have the concomitant effect of sorting out Ys.

D. Longer-range effect

    vii. C may be followed by increased reproduction of Ys with P or reproduction of something associated with Ys.

E. Even longer-range effect

    viii. D may be followed by longer-range benefits.

They proceed to show that not only is evolution theory an instantiation, that is, a real example for this type of theory, but other theories are also, like the clonal theory of antibody production mentioned previously. The body can produce antibodies for all kinds of substances, even those with which the individual has never had contact. How is this possible? The simplest explanation is that a foreign substance is presented to the immune system, and using that, it creates antibodies (instructive explanation). This would explain why antibodies fit so well. But the theory is wrong. Every organism already possesses a library of antibodies—billions of them. When a substance penetrates an organism, a suitable antibody is produced from the available selection. In other words, the environment does not *instruct* the body to develop a new antibody, but rather, a suitable object is *selected* from a huge store. Can this principle be applied to other theories?

Looking back into the history of biology, it appears that wherever a phenomenon resembles learning, an instructive theory was first proposed to account for the underlying mechanisms. In every case, this was later replaced by a selective theory. Thus the species were thought to have developed by learning or by adaptation of individuals to the environment, until Darwin showed this to have been a selective process. Resistance of bacteria to antibacterial agents was thought to be acquired by adaptation, until Luria and Delbrück showed the mechanism to be a selective one. Adaptive enzymes were shown by Monod and his school to be inducible enzymes arising through the selection of preexisting genes. Finally, antibody formation that was thought to be based on instruction by the antigen is now found to result from the selection of already existing patterns. It thus remains to be asked if learning by the central nervous system might not also be a selective process, i.e., perhaps learning is not learning either. (Niels K. Jerne, 1967, quotation taken from Calvin 1996, p. 9)

The neurosciences soon followed suit with a myriad of selection type theories inspired by Darwin.[60] I will sketch significant parts of that development. Besides Thorndike (1980, note 213), the English neurobiologist John Z. Young was one of the first to introduce selection theory into neurobiology. In *A Model of the Brain* (1964) he discussed how the nervous system can achieve coordination by weakening synapses. Richard Dawkins (1971) presented a similar thought when he guessed that the "selective death of synapses" could possibly be a mechanism that explains memory.[61] In the meantime it has been empirically proven that shortly after birth an overproduction of synapses (contact points between nerve cells) exists, which diminishes within the course of early childhood development (Johnson 1997, p. 32.39). This elimination of synapses proceeds differently, depending on the cortical area. In his theory of "selective stabilization" Changeux suggested that those synapses remain (are selected) that are actively used by the developing nervous system (Changeux and Danchin 1976). Shortly afterward, Edelman[62] published a theory of neuronal group selection, which Darden and Cain cite as a classical example of a selection type theory: "The basic idea is that the brain is a *selective* system that processes sensorimotor information through the temporally coordinated interactions of collections or repertoires of functionally equivalent units each consisting of a small group of neurons" (Edelman 1978, p. 52). Neuron populations are "degenerated." They are isofunctional. They react identically to identical stimuli, although they are structurally not identical. This degenerative pattern is the source of variations. There are some variants that basically exhibit the same input-output behavior although they differ in structure. The difference in structure causes them in changed conditions to display slightly altered behavior. In the course of repeated stimulation, some particular structural variants of the neuron population will be preferred over the others by, for example, following Hebb's rule of learning.

In 1989 Edelman restated his theory, titling it "Neural Darwinism" (Edelman 1989). This name indicates its close relationship to biological evolution theory. Selection processes in neural Darwinism, however, happen over much shorter periods of time. There are three different phases of selection exhibiting diverse mechanisms. First, there is selection during embryonic development. In this case, crucial local neurochemical processes bring cells into place with the aid of growth factors, and this entire procedure takes place in competition (Edelman 1988). Genetic and epigenetic factors guide the linking of neurons. The second phase is after birth. The originally, slightly undifferentiated links between cells conspicuously change in constellation and strength. Links originally available in great quantity die with a lack of stimulation or usage, only the active ones "survive." Third and finally, there is selective stabilization of neuron populations within the framework of sensory-motor interactions with the individual environment.

Selection provides that from an abundance of already existing variants there are those are leftover which, in a particular environment and under certain circumstances, best fulfill certain functions. The constellation, the links, and the maps of neuronal states are what they are *because* under the pressure of selection they fulfilled certain functions best. Notice how frictionless neural Darwinism fits into Millikan's theory. During the course of learning, so-called "maps" are generated, with the special purpose of categorizing external objects and internal procedures. Edelman and his group designed automatons that, based on the principles of the theory of neuronal group selection, can categorize things via mutual competition among the maps. The critical aspect is the mutual competition among degenerated groups of neurons and the fact that categorizing achievements can be better established within perception, when percepts are also *used* by motor actions.

Mappings like this are also present in the human brain (cf. chapter 2). The reciprocally close networking of maps by *reentrant loops* is the most important prerequisite for categorizing in Edelman's theory. External stimuli activate maps. These activate higher level maps, which, in turn, effect other maps. When an activity state has been generated it is repeatedly fed into the network of maps through the reentrance loops. The interesting thing about these cortical maps is that they can change within the course of a lifetime. This phenomenon is called *neuroplasticity*. "These maps are not static even in an adult organism, they behave *adaptively* to the input. It is as if input signals constantly *compete* for cortical surfaces for information processing: The more frequent and important an input is, the more surface it gets or grabs" (Spitzer 1996, p. 155; emphasis is H.W.'s). If one of a monkey's fingers is amputated and the other four are heavily stimulated, within a few days the proportions in the representations on the map in the monkey brain change. Neurobiology and the modeling of neural networks provide evidence that these maps are the basis for neural representations and are generated by selection processes meant for solving problems of adaptation. This is why they also have proper functions that have emerged in the course of interaction with the environment.

2.3.4   The Explanatory Value of Selection Theories   In a publication in 1987, Calvin, a theoretic neurobiologist, coined the term "Darwin Machine" to denote the brain. In the following years and based on this idea, he sought evidence for his idea that neural Darwinism could be instantiated in the brain. In his newest book *The Cerebral Code*, (Calvin 1996) he argues that any neural Darwinism must be in a position to name the structures that are copied and selected. He thinks he has found their neuro-anatomical basis in the cortex. The neocortex exhibits a hexagonal activity pattern that repeats itself approximately ever 0.5 mm. The neural anatomical foundation for these hexagons could be the cortical modules and the pattern of horizontal links, as they have been described for the visual cortex in various species (see Lund 1988; Rockland 1993; Calvin 1995). Calvin's theory gets fairly metaphorical and I am unsure whether it will prove itself durable. But the valuable idea in his work is that not every process of selection is Darwinian! What does that mean?

Remember the abstract elements of selection type theories. In order for something to be a selection type theory it is not enough that there is an abundance of elements, from which a few are selected. What is crucial is the existence of variants on a pattern, which are reproduced or copied, and that the appropriateness of those variants has an effect on reproduction. Calvin shows that there is no real copy process in Edelman's theory. Thus it is not actually a Darwinian theory. Francis Crick (1989) had already expressed the lack of analogy to Darwin's theory when he suggested that it be called "neural Edelmanism" instead of neural Darwinism. Calvin himself lists six criteria for distinguishing a Darwinian theory from simple selectionism (Calvin 1996, pp. 21, 99–101):

1. There must be a reasonably complex pattern involved.
2. The pattern must be copied somehow (indeed, that which is copied may serve to define the pattern).
3. Variant patterns must sometimes be produced by chance.

4. The pattern and its variant must compete with one another for occupation of a limited work space.

5. The competition is biased by a multifaceted environment.

6. There is a skewed survival to reproductive maturity (environmental selection is mostly juvenile mortality) or a skewed distribution of those adults who successfully mate (sexual selection), so new variants always preferentially occur around the more successful of the current patterns.

Only when all six conditions are satisfied do we have a Darwinian process appropriate for generating structures that creatively adapt themselves to the environment. Besides these, there are additional elements that could make such a process more effective, although they are not necessary. Calvin mentions five: stability arises by "getting stuck" at a local minimum; systematic recombination generates more variants than do copy errors and mutations; a fast changing environment creates additional complexity; parceling, that is, spatial division, accelerates the process; and local extinction also accelerates the process, because it leads to the creation of niches (Calvin 1996, pp. 23ff, 101f).[63]

Whatever the value of Calvin's theory, it seems that from his reflections we can gain that a polished theory of neural Darwinism must comply to certain criteria. His formulation of constraints is related to his research in evolution theory and population dynamics. Even for evolution theory it is true that natural selection is not the only evolutionary mechanism at work. Just as important for the origin of the species are factors like genetic drift, isolation, and recombination. So when are explanations using *selection* particularly relevant?

Amundson stated some general criteria for determining when a selection theory is explanatorily valuable (Amundson 1989, p. 417). First, there must be an abundance of variation. Variation should be spontaneous, inheritable, and available in great quantities, but its effects should be small and continuous. In terms of the environment it should be undirected (random). There should be a sorting mechanism that originates in the environment of variations and causes persistence of those variations that fulfill the needs of the system, although these mechanisms themselves are not purposive. The further a system deviates from these criteria, the less valuable is the explanation of any particular selection theory. This means that as soon as variants are reduced, or if they depend strongly on the environment, or the more purposive a sorting mechanism is, the less we need a selective explanation, because then the whole process can be explained in terms of the underlying mechanisms.

It is important to analyze explanatory value because doing so demonstrates how intentional explanation compliments physiological explanation and vice versa. Selective explanations rely on teleofunctions, physiological explanations can do with mechanofunctions. Once we have discovered the mechanism of visual face recognition, evolutionary explanations for face recognition become less important. When we know the direct, physiological (proximate) causes, we no longer necessarily need explanations relying on distant (ultimate) causes. But if we want to know whether the teleofunction of certain brain structures is to recognize faces and not merely, let's say, recognizing vertical symmetry, then once again we must make reference to the past. Using another example from philosophy, what does a frog's eye tell its brain? Does a frog recognize insects with the assistance of its brain? Or does it only recognize tiny dark moving shadows? Mechanofunctions alone cannot settle this matter. Observing the frog's behavior in the laboratory, where he snaps at every shadow, we would have to say both are true. But when we ask what the semantic content of the frog's representation is, we must reply "insects." Efficiently recognizing those objects at least partially explains the existence of those visual mechanisms. Now, we could suggest that the fact that the frog is so easily duped demonstrates precisely the difference between salientian and sapient thinking. But if you find that convincing, reflect a moment on our attitude toward dolls with faces like human offspring, or how the expressions of men perusing glossy magazines can hardly be distinguished from those observing attractive women. Only reference to the past and the history of the origin of neural mechanisms tells us something about the semantic content of representations.

Adaptive neurosemantics must satisfy Amundson's criteria to a certain point. If our neuronal representations should actually consist of chaotic activity vectors, as our discussion of alternativism seems to imply, then it is easy to see how haphazard variations generate new variations of activity patterns, which in turn get selected. But for such a theory to also explain human thinking and the capacity to quickly create new thoughts with semantic content, we must shorten the time span in selection theory even more.

2.3.5   Ultra Fast Adaptation in the Brain: A New Theory of Consciousness?   Physiological theories about brain functions work with time spans that come much closer to the temporal processes of thought. We are not talking about structural links and their changes, but about physiological activity within the range of seconds and milliseconds. At the beginning of this chapter we have seen how the spatial activity pattern in the rabbit's nose served the purpose of recognizing scents. The activity patterns of a functioning brain can for the moment be considered to be existing structures, whose existence is partially explained by the fact that they were *selected because* they fulfill certain functions. This allows the generation of semantic content within very short time spans, content that is realized by global activity patterns in the brain. Roughly, reciprocally connected neuron populations activate each other and strive for a stable state. During this process, temporary variations of a spatiotemporal activity pattern are generated. Among the constraints that support stability are not only complementary effects within the brain, but also interaction with the external world. Only those states that comply with internal and external constraints are selected. A temporarily stable state can be interpreted semantically *because* the stabilizing process is an adaptation—an adaptation either to an input caused by an external object, or an adaptation to different internal activity patterns that already exhibit neurosemantic content.

This notion of ultra fast adaptation initially implies nothing more than abstractly widening a concept in the time domain. What we need now is research on concrete brain mechanisms that manifest ultra fast adaptations. Calvin's theory of hexagonal activity patterns is one suggestion. But neuroscience offers other approaches compatible with a posit of ultra fast adaptation and which can be taken for indirect empirical evidence.

Mumford (1992), for example, explains the brain's knowing achievements by mutually adaptive influences during the interaction of higher and lower brain regions. The activity patterns of those regions change reciprocally according to a ping pong principle until a stable state is reached that is adapted to visual input. Another example is the phenomenon of coherence in firing rates of neurons and neuron populations (see Singer and Gray 1995; Llinas et al. 1994; Engel et al. 1997). Oscillation rate coherence is considered a phenomenon that makes object recognition possible because it synchronizes diverse neuron populations with differing "tasks" (proper functions!) and their impulse patterns. Synchronization depends on invariance elements in the extraneous environment and is therefore a case of ultra fast adaptation. Crick and Koch (1990) found their theory of visual perception on synchronizations within the range of 40 Hertz. A third example is that of the nonlinear systems discussed earlier. We showed how attractors can be viewed as activity patterns of the brain that—in the process of recognizing—generate an adjustment, that is, correlate a stable activity vector (attractor) with a particular input (Skarda and Freeman 1987). A fourth example is Jason W. Brown's theory of micro genesis. This theory assumes that mental states unfold in the brain within a certain period as neuronal activities of certain spatiotemporal configurations. Cognition is a process-like development in micro sections, each lasting a few hundred milliseconds. The fascinating thing about this theory is that for all cognitive activities it implies passage through phylogenetic older brain sections that can most easily be attributed with proper functions. It thereby couples a current state of consciousness with its own history within a very short period. Brown finds support for his theory in symptoms of neuropsychological deficiencies that bring phylogenetically older functions of the brain to light in cases of brain damage. And finally, fifth, Edelman extended his theory of neural Darwinism to become a theory of consciousness (Edelman 1989, 1992). His idea is that the brain executes a "process of self-categorization" with the assistance of certain cortical systems. Self-categories are created by an adaptation process between past perceptual experiences and signals about internal system states. Via iterative links, self-categorizations are connected to brain regions processing current environment signals. Current perceptual categorization and self-categorization are again correlated with each other by repetitious links. That is the neural foundation of primary consciousness. Consciousness is nothing more than "remembered present." Higher forms of consciousness arise when this process of adaptation includes language regions.

Details of these theories are plentiful in relevant literature. (One last theory, mental Darwinism, will be portrayed at the end of this chapter.) For now a speculative remark is due. Most of these theories (synchronization, micro genesis, consciousness as remembered present) were designed as theories of consciousness. I would like to draw a reverse conclusion and make a neurophilosophical guess. Integrated ultra fast adaptation is a (proper) function of consciousness. Of course, this conjecture mentions nothing of the phenomenal nature of consciousness. But if this or a modified version of it were correct, we would have an amazing finding. A theory of intentionality, designed by bracketing the phenomenon of consciousness, would be able to tell us something about just that consciousness.

But let us postpone the topic of consciousness and turn to language. Edelman might justly demand that language centers must be integrated into mutual adaptation processes in order for "higher" consciousness to exist. But internalistic perspectives are inadequate. We must realize how important externalized, public language is for thinking.

2.3.6 Neurophilosophical Remarks on Language What distinguishes human beliefs from animal convictions? The oldest (and probably best) answer is language. I have indicated several times that Millikan's theory aims not only to explain biological functions, but also linguistic meaning. In fact, her theory is primarily motivated by considerations from the philosophy of language. The human capacity for language raises several empirical and philosophical questions and problems. At this point I would like to express my views on just two issues about the pivotal importance that language has for neurosemantics. The first issue is the extent to which linguistic structures were determined by the structure and functions of the brain as it evolved. The second is the issue of how connectionistic neurophilosophy is compatible with the symbolic nature of language.

Let us address the relationship between evolution and language. Noam Chomsky, founder of generative transformation grammar compares the capacity for language with an organ: "We may usefully think of the language faculty, the number faculty, and others, as 'mental organs,' analogous to the heart or the visual system or the system of motor coordination and planning. There appears to be no clear demarcation line between physical organs, perceptual and motor systems and organs, perceptual and motor systems and cognitive capacities" (Chomsky 1980, p. 46). Chomsky was firmly convinced that this linguistic organ is innate, because grammatical deep structures are universal. From a neurophilosophical perspective this can only mean that these innate structures are brain structures. This was also Chomsky's opinion. But surprisingly, he also suggested that the complexity of language cannot be explained by natural selection (i.e., evolution theory). "Evolution theory is very informative about many things, but it has little to say, as of now, of questions of this nature (e.g., the evolution of language)" (Chomsky 1988, quote taken from Pinker and Bloom 1990, p. 708; other references given there also). Chomsky shares an aversion to evolutionary explanation for language with rationalist philosophers, such as symbol processing theorist Jerry Fodor. In spite of their naturalistic tendency, both think that evolutionary explanations for rational structures such as language (and for Fodor also thinking) are off the track. That is difficult to understand, but perhaps it can be excused by the fact that it is possible to occupy oneself with the abstract structures of language (which is the job of linguists), without taking into consideration the very physical base on which (at least human) language rests.

The scenery, however, has changed. Authors such as Lenneberg (1977), Liebermann (1984) and Bates, Thai, and Marchman (1989) have attempted explaining language as a biological organ and product of natural selection. Meanwhile, the notion that language is an evolved instinct is even advocated in the Center for Linguistics at MIT in Cambridge. "Evolutionary theory offers clear criteria for when a trait should be attributed to natural selection: complex design for some function, and the absence of alternative processes capable of explaining complexity. Human language meets these criteria: Grammar is a complex mechanism tailored to the transmission of propositional structures through a serial interface" (Pinker and Bloom 1990, p. 707).

Grammatical structures are *realized* by brain structures.

All the points discussed in this book [*The Language Instinct*, H.W.] underscore the *adaptive* complexity of language. The facets are numerous: Syntax, which creates phase structures with its discrete combinatory system, morphology, another combinatory system that forms words, a comprehensive dictionary, a well-furnished vocal tract, phonological rules and structures, language perception, parse algorithms and learning algorithms. *The components are available physically, as structured nerve paths*, which were genetically laid down by numerous interacting and precisely coordinated genetic events. These nerve paths provide us with an extraordinary gift—the capacity to transfer innumerable precisely structured thoughts from one head to another via modulating exhaled breath. Obviously, this gift is an advantage for reproduction. (Pinker 1996, p. 421, emphasis is H.W.'s)

This idea of language supports our theory of adaptive neurosemantics. Naturally, language can only be an instinct when due to evolution, brain structures changed and actually *performed functions*. "The prehistoric brain can only have been rewired if new neural paths had an effect on perception and behavior." (Pinker 1996, p. 408). Admittedly, our knowledge of the genetic underpinnings for the capacity of speech is very modest, but the basic idea is clear. Certain selections of DNA code some proteins, which link particular neurons in the brain to particular networks (provided there are certain environmental conditions), which, in turn, and in junction with the synaptic adaptation in learning processes, serve the purpose of solving a grammatical problem, such as finding an affix or a word. This may be evidenced by the fact that there are hereditary disorders which result in a very specific deficiency in applying grammatical rules (Pinker 1996, p. 374). Theoretically, the main question about understanding language as an instinct is whether the *communication function* of language is actually its proper function (Pinker and Bloom 1990), or whether it developed piggyback on structures with *non-communicative* proper functions (Gould 1987; Piatelli-Palmarini 1989). Advocates of evolutionary theory of language capacity admit the trouble with their thesis. With whom did the first grammar mutant speak? How can grammar develop gradually? How do tiny, gradual changes provide an advantage for survival? It is plausible that certain features of language actually do facilitate survival. A paradigm is the capacity for recursion.

It makes a difference, whether one arrives at a distant region by following a path in front of a big tree, or the path in front of which there is a big tree. It makes a difference if in this region there are animals which one can eat or which may eat you. It makes a difference, whether one finds there fruits that are ripe, or fruits that were ripe, or fruits that will be ripe. It makes a difference, if one arrives there by walking for three days, or whether one arrives and can walk there for three days. (Pinker 1996, p. 428)

On the other hand, evolution theory gives us good reason to assume that there was a change of function, as there was during the development of wings and lungs. But whatever we shall someday discover is not decisive for the theory of proper functions. It is only important that language structures, no matter how they came to be, were selected in the course of continued reproduction because they performed their proper functions.

Now the second problem: In chapter 2 I portrayed connectionistic neurophilosophy as a promising venture for understanding representations. Obviously this idea collides with our evolutionary-linguistic deliberations. Was it not the very idea of connectionism, that neuronal representations do *not* display the properties of language like productivity, systematicity, and inferential coherence? Did I not say that neuronal representations exhibit *no* strong compositional structure, the way that language does? Is not, within the brain, the difference between data structures and rules quite obscure? If language is a tool developed through evolution, then connectionism does need supplementation. Perhaps Fodor and Pylyshyn are right about implementation. Human language has some peculiarities difficult to explain in terms of evolution, but these also enormously increase what it can perform (creativity, nonheredity, discreteness, twofold structure, calculus character; cf. Vollmer 1975, p. 139ff). These very features turn man into a *rational animal* and give him the capacity to develop even artificial languages. Is connectionism on the wrong track?

The question of whether or not the brain is a linguistic machine will someday be answered empirically. Our present reflections rest on the conjecture that the basic principles of neuronal representation are in line with connectionistic notions. So we still need to explain how humans have a capacity to command symbolic language—and make quite good use of it. The clue lies—as in all debate on innate capacities—in an indispensable interweaving of innate structures with experience. Humans can only learn and command symbolic language if they are confronted with it during a critical developmental period. If we view human language skills from a purely internalistic standpoint, be it the mind or the brain, the result will be an inadequate interpretation of mind and brain. An *externalistic* theory such as the TOPF is needed for really grasping the meaning of thought. *Thinking is in the world, not in one's head.* And part of the world, to be precise: Part of the environment of language speaking individuals is language itself. As an external system it is a classical system of symbols.

In my opinion, sophisticated rational intelligible action requires explanation making reference to externalized, symbolic language. My claim ensues from research done by Eckhardt Scheerer (for a similar approach from an entirely different angle see Illich 1988). Scheerer's work *Orality, Literacy, and Cognitive Modeling* defends two interrelated theses:

(a) The "symbolic" level of mental functioning is not a property of the human cognitive system or of the human brain considered in isolation, but can only be understood as a consequence of the historical emergence of written language and other permanent notational system; (b) "Primary" oral language (i.e., language historically antedating the "invention" of writing and ontogenetically the acquisition of written language) and the mental processes underlying it are not symbolic in the sense of the symbol-processing paradigm, but subsymbolic in the sense of the connectionist, or network modeling, approach. (Scheerer 1996, p. 212)

The interesting thing about these conjectures is the claim that the difference between written and oral language has a decisive effect on human thinking. Because we live and think within a culture characterized by writing, to us a connectionistic (neurophilosophical) approach seems inappropriate for explaining symbolic thinking. Scheerer distinguishes between typical ideals of primary orality and typographical literacy.

In line with Ong (1976), "primary orality" is used to denote a linguistic-cultural state and its reflection in the individual person who has made no contact whatever with written language and literate discourse. "Typographic literacy" refers to a state of unrestricted literacy encompassing an entire culture, owing to the universal presence of printed (i.e., standardized) materials and to an educational system in which school attendance is obligatory for everybody. (Scheerer 1996, p. 215)

We are all familiar with literate culture. It is far more difficult to really understand primary orality, because it practically no longer exists and we only have literature on it.[64] From an evolutionary point of view the development of literate culture is very young (the first historically secured and preserved notational systems contain Sumerian economic transactions). Actually primary orality is more relevant for understanding the evolutionary anchors of language. Scheerer discerns four essential properties of primary orality:

1. There is no direct access to phonemes; the smallest unit recognizable as a unit is a syllable.

2. Primarily oral language is coordinating, uses phrases, and is ultimately nonpropositional. Interestingly enough, the evidence that it is nonpropositional is actually neurophilosophical, drawn from studies on patients with language disorders caused by brain damage (patients with aphasia). The speech skill these persons retain reveal older phylogenetic and ontogenetic layers of speech development of vividly nonpropositional nature (see also Brown 1987). This is at least true for so-called global aphasia, which occurs after large parts of the language dominating half of the brain have been destroyed. Using neurological evidence, Scheerer expresses a daring, exciting, yet well founded presumption: Wernicke aphasia, in which mainly language comprehension malfunctions while grammatical speech production remains intact, is a "cultural artifact," resulting from the use of an alphabetic (or at least a phonetic) system of writing. This suggests itself from the pattern of this speech disorder, which is actually a deficiency in discriminating phonemes, and by the fact that Wernicke aphasias have almost never been found in children under the age of seven (some researchers say even under ten). The reason, according to Scheerer, is obvious. In our western culture this is the age when school becomes obligatory and the real literate phase begins.

3. Primarily oral language exhibits natural, situational semantics.

4. Memory in primarily oral languages is reconstructive and interactive; oriented toward meaning in interaction with other speakers or towards meaningful episodes.

Scheerer construes a parallel between the symbol processing approach–literacy on the one side and connectionism–orality on the other. While the first pair is characterized by representations, propositions, an internalistic concept of meaning, and a passive mode of representation, the second pair is marked by holistic representations, a lack of propositions,[65] an externalistic concept of meaning and an active mode of representation. This does not mean that there are two different methods of information processing manifested in two different language variants. Imagine the causal development in reverse. Different language forms (oral and literate) result in different forms of information processing. This illustrates how our thinking, our mental states, are individuated externally. Our mode of thinking depends on the environment we grow up in and with which kind of extraneous, public language we have to deal. This is how Scheerer's theses naturally and apprehensibly combine the debate on an appropriate theory of representation for neuronal states with Millikan's theory.

Scheerer discusses two objections to his theses. The deep theory objection—which is more important for our purposes—states that symbol processing theory does not deal with superficial structures (visible structures of written language), but with deep structures (generative transformation grammar). But Scheerer thinks that even with this, we still lack explanation for how discrete symbols at the deep structure level are created at all! It was not a difficulty, as long as there were no alternatives. But meanwhile there are alternative connectionistic explanations for phenomena, which up until now have only been explained by deep grammar, such as how children acquire language under suboptimal circumstances (*the poverty of stimulus argument*).[66] In the brain, we might add, there is no evidence for discrete symbols that could be atoms of thought. Scheerer's hypotheses help to explain the (cultural) genesis of symbols by beginning with the structures of externalized language. He lists several cultural achievements that could be responsible for it: universal acceptance of Arabic number notation, replacing the abacus with paper and pencil algorithmic arithmetics, widespread use of printed products, and the development of modern musical notation. Presumably, it is not fortuitous that even the earliest philosophical pondering was combined with mathematical reflection. And it is not by chance that Gottfried Wilhelm Leibniz, the first philosopher to equate thinking with formal symbol manipulation, was also the inventor of the first computing device.

What does all this mean for neurosemantics? We can hold fast to connectionistic fundaments. An apparently symbolic character of cognitive activities evolves because external systems of symbols, particularly language, are used by a connectionistic brain. Although the capacity for language is innate, it is less fixed for being symbolic and literate; it originally was more directed toward being oral. We are misled to think otherwise by the ubiquitous usage of symbolic artifacts.

In fact, many cognitive activities cannot be isolated from the symbolic environment in which they take place. Imagine adding two multi-digit numbers in your mind, without using writing utensils. Or, try to solve the following problem without making a sketch. Connect three roads that meet at a crossing in such a way that you can drive from any one onto any other without entering the third—no matter from where you depart nor where you are headed (Dennett 1995). With similar thought experiments, Clark and Chalmers (1997) argue in their paper "The Extended Mind" for an externalistic concept of mind. In principle, they see no difference between a person remembering an address and a forgetful person seeking that address in her personal planer. Naturally, the planner can be separated from the person. But as long as extracorporal assistance is reliable and readily accessible, corporal boundaries are not necessarily essential. The mind is not dictated by the physical boundaries of the brain or the skin, because the way it works already includes outside things and circumstances. This kind of externalism goes beyond developmental history; it relies on close links between cognitive systems and the world necessary for actual cognitive activity. Clark and Chalmers call this *active externalism*.[67] The basic idea of active externalism moves in the same general direction as Kurthen's monistic cophenomenalism (1992) and the theory of dynamical cognitive sciences. Just as the mechanical function of a fish's fin can only be understood within the context of the medium water, so is mental activity of humans comprehensible only within the context (medium) of a cognitive environment. Man navigates through a linguistic environment like the fish in water.

If we reflect, however, on the fact that the meaning of linguistic structures—words, sentences, phrases—can only be explained by recourse to the *history* of their usage, we notice that one of the purposes of language is to remind us of the past. Linguistic meanings can be entirely comprehended only within an extraneous framework that transcends the individual. For starters, the meaning of words and sentences in literate culture does not depend on the meaning an individual speaker may lend them. (Of course, one can attempt to redefine words.) The theory of proper functions explains the intentionality of brain structures on one hand; on the other it explains the meaning of structures exhibited by language constructs. In individuals these two types of meaning crosscut one another. It is this intersecting and entwining that intuitively supports the reproach of circularity directed at the TOPF. Public, symbolic, language—tried and proven in a cultural selection process—is what really makes our thinking intelligible in a strong sense.[68]

2.3.7 Summary   Let me briefly summarize our discussion this far. We aimed to design a theory of teleosemantics suitable for neurosemantics. Unlike Kurthen, we made an effort to sustain guidance by evolution and the historical aspect. That, in turn, evoked the question of how neurosemantics can explain human creativity, for beyond using those historically evolved cognitive patterns, humans are able to generate new semantic content within minute periods. We also came across the question of how the brain relates to language.

I outlined three arguments denying that the evolutionary approach is too limited. The notion that it is inadequate is partly due to a misunderstanding about evolution. Once complex adaptations have taken place, they can be repeatedly applied to new objects. The brain and its cognitive mechanisms are implements—tools for thinking. Besides this, the abstract concept of teleofunction is applicable not only to functions that emerged over phylogenetic periods. In selection type theory teleofunction is appropriate for all devices that evolved through any Darwinian-type selection process. I showed that, presumably, there are selection processes at work in the brain that take place over time spans other than those in terms of phylogenetic time scales. There is quite a bit of empirical evidence that selection processes happen in the course of an individual's development (ontogenesis). If we reduce the time span for observing selection processes to seconds, we can develop complete adaptive neurosemantics. Although their existence has yet to be proven, ultrafast adaptations, following selection type theory rules, are found in contemporary theories on brain function. Finally, the development and existence of external systems of symbols demonstrates very naturally how man belongs to a realm of the intelligible, which always transcends individual reason. For the meaning of public language structures, crucially involved in shaping each personal cognitive system, well exceeds individual experience. And the meaning of language structures can, in turn, be explained using the theory of proper functions. Symbols (and their particular representations) have acquired proper functions in the historical course of being selected, quite independent of individual persons. Symbols hold a treasure of experience related to structures in the world and not to pure thought. In externalistic theory, thinking occurs in the world, and not merely in the head. Thus Oshana's criterion is satisfied, that requests that "the properties constituting autonomy should not be limited to the internal phenomena of the agent" (Oshana 1994, pp. 76f).

In short, with our naturally evolved instrument called the brain, which itself encompasses selective mechanisms, and with assistance from thoroughly tested and trustworthy meaning transporting structures of public language, we, as humans, are in a position to act intelligibly. This also explains how we are in a position to act according to principles and why abstracta play such an important causal part in it. Formulated in language and available in an abundance of physically realized specimens, those structures make up part of our human environment. People come to terms with them, consider them, or ignore them, but ultimately we have no choice: We must deal with them. I feel that the ease with which people can handle literate culture holds one clue to why philosophers think there is a realm of reason causally influencing human action.

Let us now examine how the twofold problem of intelligibility looks under the eyes of adaptive neurosemantics and how neurosemantics contribute a solution.

2.4 Intelligibility and Neurosemantics

2.4.1 Intentional Causation Beliefs and desires are indicative or imperative icons, serving as "blueprints." Human blueprints, that is, intentions, exhibit some peculiarities. Besides certain representational properties they also reveal how thinking and public language are fused. Now, I have not yet set up a theory of human intelligibility or a fully detailed naturalistic successor concept. The phenomenon of consciousness particularly demands closer analysis, instead of essentially speculative notions about ultra fast adaptation. Nevertheless, we want to see how a biologically grounded theory of human intentions would relate to two central controversies about free will.

Let us begin with the discussion about "reasons versus causes," also known as the problem of intentional causation. I have extensively argued the fact that physical brain structures can have intentional content. So the pendulum of action theory apparently swings towards the causalists: Reasons *are* cerebral causes. Or are they? "[H]aving a certain history is not, of course, an attribute that has 'causal powers.' Hence reasons cannot be, as such, causes. More generally, that a thing has a teleofunction is a causally impotent fact about it" (Millikan 1993a, p. 186). This seems to topple our whole set of deliberations. But, ultimately, it is merely the consequence of the teleosemantic approach. Instead of being *identical* with causes, reasons *paraphrase* causes; they provide explanations for the existence of causally effective structures. A neurophilosophical theory of intentional causation must involve the level of representations. But naturalism in Millikan's theory does not imply *identifying* reasons with (causally effective) brain states, it implies rather that mechanisms and brain states that fulfill certain functions can be traced back to a causal history. Acting for reasons means that certain brain structures have representational content that takes on an essential role in the rational explanation of an action (or its justification). Which benefits does the TOPF provide for explaining acting for reasons?

Just as the TOPF characterizes some functions as proper functions, adaptive neurosemantics helps sort out the real reasons for an action from pretentious or merely attributed reasons. We have a "real reason," if causally effective brain structures are related to whatever is the case. That is, they are formulated in speech as a reason, such that those brain structures fulfill their normal function; they correctly represent whatever is the case. "Rationalization" is when they don't. Here is an example: "During a torture session I used electroshocks, because I knew that otherwise my family would be in danger." The person saying this is stating a real reason, only if his brain structures that represent a possible danger for his family actually caused issuing the shocks. But if his brain structures causally effecting the issuance of electroshocks were those having a content of pleasure at administering torture, more or less imperative blueprints, then the reason he stated is a mere rationalization. The fact that brain structures can mean what they mean at all can only be explained teleosemantically, that is, historically. So reasons are not *directly* causally effective. Nevertheless, reasons can be right or wrong; it depends on which brain structures are causally effective.

Taking an intentional stance toward an organism means nothing more than assuming that it functions "normally"—in terms of biological standards. Biological standards are something like "regulative ideas," which—in contrast to a transcendental approach—are not simply presupposed; with factual evidence we can argue that they exist in some systems. Rationality hinges not only on physical or concrete realization, but on the fact that some structure *is supposed* to perform in a certain way and in the best cases actually does. Rationality is a normative concept, just like proper functions are normative entities: "Intentional-attitude explanations of behaviors proceed by subsumption of behaviors under biological norms rather than laws and/or by noting departures from these norms and perhaps causes of these departures" (Millikan 1993a, p. 187). A note is appropriate here. The expression "biological norms" could mislead one to think that acting for reasons refers only to those norms that evolved phylogenetically and are thus genetically anchored. Once again, we are dealing here with the anti-evolutionist misunderstanding discussed earlier. First, this tool called brain can also handle new objects normally, and second, language provides us with meaning-transporting structures that in turn can be represented by neurons and whose meaning likewise can be explained by the theory of proper functions. When these representations are used in a particular way, we can think rationally in the fullest sense of the word.

Let us try to think our way down this middle path between causalists and anti-causalists. If reasons only paraphrase causes, does this not imply epiphenomenalism? In chapter 2, intentional efficacy was conceived of as supervenient causation. As mentioned then, Kim claims we have only the following options: eliminativism, reductionism, or epiphenomenalism—at least if we are unwilling to postulate downward causation. Achim Stephan objected that Kim is only right if we demand of mental efficacy that it be super*duper*venient, which encompasses an explanatory reduction of the relation of supervenience itself. For intentional causation this would mean to explain, via reduction, why an intentional state supervenes on particular physical states and relations. The theory of proper functions provides just this explanatory reduction. A neural state exhibiting intentionality has a wide supervenience base. It supervenes on the brain (*and* most likely also on other corporal states), *and* parts of its adaptive environment, *and* parts of the history of its origin. If we want to explain causal initiation of an action by using reasons, we must make reference to proper functions. If we ignore the past and restrict explanation to momentarily effective causal powers, then we are merely explaining an event with the help of mechanofunctions, but not explaining behavior or actions. If we want to explain why brain states are effective *as* intentional states, we must reduce intentional states to that *broad* supervenience basis mentioned above. The theory of proper functions explains *why* this supervenience relation exists by explaining the production of this state assisted by selection theory. This explanation turns the supervenience relation into a super*duper*venience relation. Intentional causation is thus super*duper*venient causation.

If Kim is right, this means that we must again chose among three options. But instead of ending up with epiphenomenalism, we reach reductive explanation. Why? In biology teleological explanations are merely abbreviated causal explanations. Likewise, intentional explanations (explanations for reasons) are simply abbreviated causal explanations about how a system exhibiting representational and self-representational skills has come to be. We gain the impression that intentional explanations must be more than that, first, because we do not have complete knowledge of the development that led to the action, and second, we—rightly—intuitively do not find it correct to identify an intentional state with a brain state. The reproach of epiphenomenalism is fended off by ultimately achieving a reductionistic solution through explanatory reduction.

2.4.2 The Intelligibility Problem   Earlier on we analyzed the intelligibility problem and discovered two difficulties. On one side, we have the specifically libertarian problem of how an action can be *simultaneously* undetermined and intelligible. Then we have the problem that libertarians and anti-libertarians share. Can intelligible actions be determined by the past without losing their intelligible character? We solved that common difficulty by using the theory of proper functions. Intelligible actions *can* be determined by past events, without losing their intelligible character. According to the TOPF they *must* be determined by the past. This also explains how intelligibility and thus rationality necessarily contain a normative element. This is because meanings themselves are normative.

We still feel uneasy. This might be because our intuitive notions of intelligibility combine the first and second components. And this is right. Even though determined actions can be intelligible, *something* of our intuitive notions has been lost. Ted Honderich describes this discussing the topic of the self-refuting argument:

My confidence in having knowledge depends on my being free to do things, or at least my having been free to do things. There is a connection between confidence and action. [. . .] My confidence in a sentence of this book may depend on my being free to pose certain questions to myself, think of the places where I can find evidence for or against, and so on. [. . .] If determinism is true I'm not free, and if I'm not free I can't engage in real investigations or enquiry (Honderich 1993, p. 78).

Now, it is one thing to contend that determinism threatens our concept of intelligibility and thus knowledge *itself*, and another to claim that it threatens our *faith* in that knowledge. We are dealing here with a psychological reaction, similar to the reaction of a creationist who comes to be convinced one day that the world evolved in a natural way. In chapter 1 we already noted Honderich's reply to the dangers of determinism.

At this point let us proceed to another surprising conclusion of the theory of proper functions. The second part of the intelligibility argument, as outlined in chapter 1, is no longer tenable! To briefly retraverse the argument (the second, presently questionable part, is printed in italics): "A real, intelligible choice ensues from reasons. An indeterministic choice, in contrast, is not determined by reasons. Therefore, indeterministic choices are not intelligible, they are arbitrary, contingent, irrational, not acts, or at least not real choices. *Therefore, intelligibility is not compatible with indeterminism. Intelligibility requires determinism by reasons.*" Determinism by reasons does not exist, according to the TOPF. At least it does not exist if by that we mean that a reason qua its semantic content is causally effective, for only physical structures are causally effectual. From this we can conclude, among other things, that it is not true that intelligibility is incompatible with indeterminism, at least not when we are talking about partial indeterminism. In neurosemantics, intelligible action is the adaptive behavior of an organism in an environment, assisted by cerebral mechanisms representing goals in future scenarios, which are used by the organism in repetitious acts of inference and identification. Indeterministic elements can play an important role in these. In order to flexibly adapt to a changing environment, creative disturbances are perhaps necessary, effecting a system that otherwise functions normally. In other words, indeterminism does not conclusively destroy intelligible action. On the contrary, perhaps the opposite it true; perhaps it fulfills a vital function similar to how random mutations fulfill an important role in adaptation within the process of natural selection. It creates variety.

This is little reward for the libertarian, of course, for normally he advocates an internalistic position on free will. On his view the indeterministic process must take place inside the individual agent—in terms of neurophilosophy this means inside the brain. Three fair objections parry such a theory of partial indeterministic, internalistic intelligibility. The first has already been explained; there is enough evidence that within the brain indeterminism plays no particularly important role. Second, without much ado, the adaptive function of indeterminism can also be performed by deterministic contingency (see Dennett 1981). The influence of stochastic, random processes is sufficient for introducing a disturbance factor into a well-adapted system, in order to generate flexibility and creativity. Indeterminism appears to be compatible with, but not necessary for creative adaptation.[69] Third, even if there are indeterministic processes in the brain that decisively influence intelligible action, we would still want to know whether it holds for self-determined action. We want to know whether indeterministic intelligibility is compatible with agency. The third part of this chapter deals with agency. But first we will take a closer look at two neuroscientific approaches to free will.

2.5   The Will and the Brain

Preceding pages dealt with basic problems of a neurophilosophical theory of intelligibility: how neural states can represent anything at all, how the semantic content of such states can be causally effective, and how these issues contribute to solving the intelligibility problem. Let us now discuss two theories from neuroscience, which make statements about the will and its freedom.

2.5.1   Conscious Volition—Half a Second too Late?   Among other things, our intuitive notion of free will ensues from our daily experience, in which we consciously control and influence our actions, which often consist of bodily movements. A frequent example is raising one's arm. What seems more natural than thinking of willingly raising one's arm— or executing another simple body movement—as a basic specimen of a free act, and then examining just how this is realized in terms of neurobiology. Such research, in fact, does exist. Californian neurobiologist Benjamin Libet conducted experiments and made some exciting findings.[70] Those findings show that presumably consciousness lags up to half a second behind perception and actions. Is free will only an illusion? Let me briefly relate these experiments (see figure 3.2 for a summary) and how they rest on naive notions about intentional causation. Even if libertarian free will is an illusion, Libet's reasons for that are wrong. Let us see why.

In the 1970s, Libet studied the awareness of sensory stimuli. Research was done on subjects who had electrodes implanted in their brains for medical reasons. Those were embedded in the primary somato-sensory cortex. About 0.02 second after applying a simple skin stimulus, an electrical potential, also known as sensory evoked potential (SEP), is noticeable in the *contralateral* cortex. (Both the sensory and the motor tract run crosswise.) SEP can also be registered when the stimulus on the skin is too brief or weak to be noticed consciously. *If* the stimulus does reach consciousness, however, then this happens *directly (approximately 0.02 second) after the skin stimulus occurred.*

Libet stimulated one side of the brain of a subject with very short electrical stimuli directly on the sensory cortex, to which the tactile receptors of the skin project. This type of stimulus causes prickling in the hand

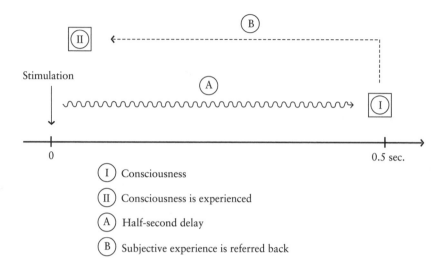

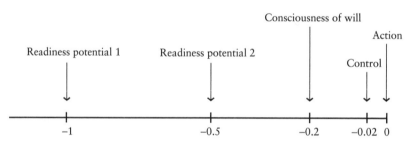

Figure 3.2
Summary of experiments on the delay of consciousness by Libet. Top, from Nørretranders (1994, p. 340); bottom, from Nørretranders (1994, p. 320).

on the opposite side. Pulse sequences of varying lengths were administered. The outcome was surprising: The patients reported prickling only when stimulation lasted longer than 0.5 second.[71] Libet's explanation for this is that it takes a half of a second of cortex activity before an event becomes conscious. It takes this long before *neuronal adequacy* for conscious experience is present. If this hypothesis is generally correct, we need an explanation for cases of normal perception. We experience simple skin stimulation immediately, not with a half-second delay. Why? Libet claims that the brain experiences the stimulation subjectively *as if* it had been aware of it immediately after it happened, although *in reality* it took half a second to become conscious.

This model of *subjective backward referral in time* rests on Libet's very tricky experiment (Libet et al. 1979). It intended to *compare* the moment of subjectively, consciously perceiving a skin stimulus with a direct stimulus of the cortex. The experiment was set up like this. A patient has an electrode in the left somatosensory cortex. Stimulation there generates prickling in the right hand. Next the left hand and the left cortex are stimulated simultaneously. Then the patient is asked in which hand he first felt the irritation. Thus, awareness of the stimulus is captured by indicating one single parameter: left or right. By systematically varying the sequence and the length of time between stimulations, Libet could research the connection between stimulus begin, duration, and awareness.

What happened when first the left hand and then the left cortex (perception in the right hand) were stimulated? If brain stimulation is strong enough, within the first quarter of a second after stimulating the skin, the stimulation can prevent the skin stimulus from being perceived at all—the latter is "masked."[72] This suits Libet's theory well. The skin stimulation does not even get to satisfy the neuronal adequacy for becoming conscious (0.5 second of brain activity). This finding is sufficiently surprising. But very strange indeed is what happened when the cortex was stimulated *prior to* the skin. In this case the test persons reported subjectively experiencing the reverse. They first perceived stimulation on the skin and then in the cortex, provided that the time between both stimulations did not exceed 0.4 second.

To explain these results, Libet suggested that two events take place while registering a skin stimulation. One (the SEP) objectively "marks" the arrival of the stimulus (as mentioned, it can be witnessed at 0.02 second). The other (0.5 second of cortex activity) causes consciousness. Subjective experience of the stimulation is backdated with the help of the objective mark of the SEP, such that one has a subjective impression, *as if* the stimulus had entered consciousness at the time of the SEP. This subjective backward referral for the skin stimulus (see figure 3.2) is a remarkable phenomenon in need of explanation. Libet's theory has been criticized many times.[73] I would like to mention just a few very general points from this complicated debate, which should, at least, provoke caution when evaluating the experiment and its findings.

First, the crucial experiments were undertaken on patients in neuro-surgery who were fully conscious when implanted electrodes in certain places in their brains were stimulated. Today this type of operation is no longer practiced; if it were done, one would have the greatest difficulties getting the experiments approved by an ethics committee. Perhaps this is why Libet's experiments were never repeated. This alone justifies doubting their validity, at least we cannot consider the findings empiri-cally clearly proven. Second, nowhere does Libet say that his experiments contradict traditional physics such that the subjective perception occurs *prior to physical stimulation.* Surprising is merely the *subjective sequence* of perception. Third, the test persons did not report their awareness of stimulation exactly when it occurred. They reported later, usually seconds later, after they had already consciously experienced the stimu-lus. Thus, Libet's experiments cannot be taken as proof that mental events do not fit into the physical world (Popper, and Eccles 1977), nor do they necessitate a new physics of consciousness (Penrose 1991). We must simply take them as empirical phenomena begging for explanation.

Not only does consciousness lag behind perception, even conscious, intended motions occur with delay—at least this is suggested by experi-ments on the readiness potential (RP), a phenomenon discovered by Kornhuber and Deecke. The RP is a slowly developing electric negativ-ity that originates in the brain and can be measured on the skull. It begins up to a second or longer before initiated movements, appears at first on both sides, becomes steep about 500 milliseconds before motion commences, and, at 100 milliseconds before a movement begins, it concentrates over the motor cortex of the moved body part on the contra-lateral side. Since in comparison to other brain activity RP is five to ten times smaller (about 10 microvolts) it is only visibly reproduced, when several movements (at least thirty, usually more) are averaged relative to the commencement of motion. RP is viewed as brain activity correlated with the preparation and initiation of freely willed move-ments. When it begins, its duration and amplitude vary inter-individu-ally and are influenced by many variables such as handedness, strength, complexity of movement, motor learning, attention, and motivation. Many authors locate RP's origin in the so-called "supplementary motor area" (SMA) (Kristeva-Feige 1994). This area belongs to the frontal lobes, on the inside of the hemispheres, and borders the motor cortex from the front.[74]

Libet undertook to research how the "time of conscious intention is related to the onset of cerebral activity (readiness potential)" (Libet et al. 1983). He set up the following test: The test person was instructed, in a relaxed state, to bend his finger whenever he wanted; literally, to let an *urge* to act occur by itself at any time, without planning or concentrating on the act (Libet 1983, p. 625). If this act is repeatedly executed and brain activity measurements averaged, normally negation of the electric potential is exhibited 0.5 to 1 second *prior* to movement commencement. This is startling, compared to our daily experience. In our daily lives there is not a second-long delay between deciding to move and moving! The test persons were also given the task of noting the time and later reporting "the time of appearance of his conscious awareness of 'wanting' to perform a given self-initiated movement. The experience was also described as an 'urge' or 'intention' or 'decision' to move, though subjects usually settled for the words 'wanting' or 'urge'" (Libet et al. 1983, p. 627). For this purpose they kept view of a fast-rotating clock. Using their memory of the position of the clock's indicator, they were later asked to say when they had felt the beginning of the intention.[75] The result was surprising. Test persons registered conscious intention to bend their fingers not until 0.2 second prior to the movement. Readiness potential, in contrast, commenced at 0.5 to 0.7 second prior to movement. In other words, awareness of an intention to act occurs more than 0.3 second after the neural events that initiate that act. Again, here consciousness "delays" the intention to act by about a half second (compared to the commencement of cortex activity). Libet found that this confirmed his earlier findings. Even an intention to act requires 0.5 second of brain activity before we are aware of it.

Libet's experiments were designed to research consciousness. But his findings immediately evoked the query. If we are not aware of our intentions until after the neural machinery for starting the act has already been warmed up, is free will just an illusion?

Libet himself did not draw that conclusion. Consciousness is not entirely impotent. It does not initiate actions, but is does have a veto

(Libet 1985, p. 528), for after all, between commencement of an awareness of an intention and the beginning of action lie 0.2 second (cf. figure
3.2). During this time "consciousness" could prevent the execution of
an initiated action. He concludes: "Processes associated with individual
responsibility and free will would "operate" not to initiate a voluntary
act but to select and control volitional outcomes" (Libet 1985, p. 538).
Thus Libet's theory conspicuously fits into a theory of adaptive neurosemantics. With adaptive neurosemantics, we can explain Libet's findings to mean that various options to act have neuronal representations
and one of them, selected in a process of immediate adaptation, gets
executed. At first glance we could be satisfied. Nothing is more welcome
than confirmation of one's own theory. But we have two reasons for
warning. They hinge on Libet's implicit notion of consciousness and
intentionality.

Consciousness first. As other critics have (see the commentaries in
Libet 1985), Dennett (1991) also finds Libet's theory of consciousness
faulty—a theory that proposes that events become conscious at a particular point in time. In his "theory of multiple drafts" he notes that
within the brain several different information processing procedures run
simultaneously, and there is no clearly defined points where consciousness begins and ends. Spence (1996), in contrast, accepts Libet's theory
of consciousness and concludes that free will is a subjective illusion and
a "free will" is—if anywhere at all—in subconsciousness. At least consciousness cannot be seen as an initiator of acts. But it is misleading to
believe that consciousness alone automatically *guarantees* free will. Conscious states can be just as determined as subconscious states. They must
not be intelligible, and many conscious states are not "our own"—something we can demonstrate with aspects of neurological and psychiatric
disorders. Dennett correctly diagnosed a Cartesian theory of consciousness in Libet's work. Just as Descartes thought that the thinking
substance could causally effect the physical world in almost any (and
ultimately unexplicable) way, Libet's theory contains an implicit notion
that at the very moment in which "consciousness," resulting from neural
processes, "jumps onto the Cartesian stage" (Dennett 1991), it causally
effects those neural processes that otherwise would unavoidably occur.

Besides the issue of consciousness, there is another critical matter ensuing from our previous exposition of neurosemantics. Libet's conclusions rest on a false theory of intentionality and intention. It assumes that a conscious intention (bending one's finger) must be viewed as a causally effective event in the brain, which exists *immediately prior* to the action itself—the way we would expect a proper cause to behave. But is it likely? We can only find an answer using a neurophilosophical theory of intentional causation. Libet's explanations presuppose an enticingly simple, linearly causal (and incorrect) idea of intentional causation. If a cause directly precedes an effect, then a conscious intention must directly precede an act of free will, and the time when this conscious intention occurs can be introspectively determined reliably within the framework of a few hundred milliseconds. And even if there is no directly preceding intention to do something, there must be a directly preceding intention to prevent something (veto rights). But intentions are not direct cerebral causes. We should consider, perhaps, whether Libet's experiments examine the awareness of intentions at all. This is not to say that consciousness plays no part in willed decisions. In Libet's experiments consciousness actually plays a double role, but not the one normally assumed.

According to Millikan, intentions can be viewed as a certain kind of desire. The main proper function of *desires* is to produce conditions in the world that contribute to the satisfaction of those desires. Thus, the hand or finger movement is a (satisfied) desire. The test persons produce the conditions that satisfy their desires, and they do that *prior* to the experiment. What would we reply if asked what the reason was for the movement of the test person's finger? The instructions given prior to the experiment! The test persons were given the instructions to behave, such that in the course of the experiment (precisely, while the clock's indicator rotated once) they should move a hand whenever they wanted. This information was consciously received and generated a conscious goal representation, namely, to execute a (prescribed) movement under certain conditions. Expressed without consciousness-jargon; the test persons must have understood the instructions. The test persons were to execute a movement when they *felt* an urge to do so. I suppose that the test persons certainly (consciously) felt *something*, but *not their intention* to act.

What did they feel? There is experimental data supporting the idea that the test persons felt an internal trigger (like muscle tension in the periphery) to which they selectively guided their attention.[76] The authors of one study conclude that "the general intention to act has been induced by the instruction at the beginning of the experiment. It was the advise to introspectively monitor internal processes which led the subjects to perceive a feeling of 'wanting to move'" (Keller and Heckhausen 1990, p. 360).

If this is true, then a conscious *intention* immediately prior to the movement is of no importance, at most a conscious *feeling* of having passed a threshold. The test persons waited for the start signal with an already fixed intention of moving a finger.

It is not crucial that this interpretation be correct in every detail. The riddle of the half-second delay illustrates that in order to experimentally research desires, intentions, and phenomena of the will, we first need a theory telling us what we are actually looking for and how to interpret our measurements. At any rate, the simple model of causality, derived from folk psychology and used as Libet used it, is inadequate. If the theory of adaptive neurosemantics is correct, then we can assume that within the brain there exist a multitude of neurally realized or non-executed patterns for movement (programs), which get selected in the course of an action. To be intelligible, selection must belong to an overlying scheme of action. In the following I would like to develop an adequate model for the selection of action alternatives that relies neither on Cartesian consciousness, nor on Libet's model of intention.

2.5.2 Frontal Cortex and Intelligibility Imagine that you have invited friends to dinner at the last minute. Since the fridge is empty you must shop on your way home from the office. You quickly make up a shopping list. Time is lacking and you must still drive home and also prepare the meal. You must visit various shops, so you decide upon a sequence. And you must take care not to get distracted by other interesting wares, conversation with the salesperson, or sudden ideas. Normally, performing this task is not a big deal. But it is for patients with lesions of the frontal lobes; they are hopelessly overtaxed. They cannot comply with the demands of this scenario. We plan our actions in advance (anticipation) and choose from various options (selection). When time is limited, it is important that we ignore distractions (suppress response), do not follow up on sudden ideas (control impulses), and stick to our task (concentrate). Finally, we must also remember which shops we have been to and what we have already purchased (working memory). We don't want to serve crackers without cheese!

According to neuropsychological findings, all these functions are attributed to the frontal cortex (Kolb and Wishaw 1996, pp. 305–333). We now need some neuroanatomical information: The frontal cortex comprises three parts: the primary motor cortex, the premotor cortex, and the so-called prefrontal (association) cortex. The primary motor cortex is a thin strip, which on both sides of the head stretches from the middle toward the front up to the temples. It relays motor commands to the muscles via the spinal cord. The premotor region is in front of this strip, it is six times as large and is also concerned with motor functions (Freund 1990). In its medial section sits the supplementary motor area, the SMA, which is presumably the source of the readiness potential.[77] Both areas are closely linked to the biggest part of the frontal cortex, namely the prefrontal cortex. In terms of evolution, it is the youngest part of the human brain. While in cats it makes up only about 3.5% of the cortex surface, in chimpanzees it is about 17%, and in humans it is 29%. That is almost a third of the entire brain surface![78] It is no wonder, then, that the prefrontal cortex is involved in typically human cognitive functions. We roughly distinguish two different sections of the prefrontal cortex. One part lies on the side and top (dorsolateral section) and the other lies below and toward the center (ventromedial section). The ventromedial sections becomes important in our chapter on agency, so we need not discuss it here. The dorsolateral section contains the motor speech center.

Very generally we can say that the function of the frontal cortex is to *organize behavior through time*. While the motor area is concerned with organizing and executing movements, it is the job of the prefrontal cortex to "control" cognitive processes that ensure that suitable movements are selected at the right time for the right place. For intelligible action it is interesting to know *why* a movement occurs. It is reason, which makes a movement understandable, that turns it into an action. Most of our actions are embedded in a larger framework. They are often not spontaneous, but planned. That makes them directly relevant to our topic. Joaquin Fuster, author of a major work on the frontal cortex (Fuster 1989), writes: "What leads to the decision to act, and to act in a certain way? The question is almost inextricable from the argument about free will.... [T]he decision to act, like the formulation of the plan, is the result of the competition between diverse, sometimes conflicting, neural influences converging on prefrontal cortex" (Fuster 1996, p. 51). Patients with larger lesions (damage) of the cortex show a typical clinical syndrome. Their skill of strategic thinking is strongly inhibited, once they have made plans they cannot be swayed to alter them by external stimuli, and they have difficulty adapting their behavior to altered circumstances (Kolb and Wishaw 1996, pp. 305–333). It is as if some ordering instance that controls the coordination and harmonizing of diverse activities were missing. Neuropsychologist Shallice (1988) therefore assigns the frontal cortex the function of *attentive supervision*. Within the hierarchy of cortical systems this has the highest perch above all automatic routine systems. It particularly becomes active when a person is confronted with new situations that cannot be dealt with using habitual behavior routines. It is involved in making plans and selects subroutines appropriate for the situations, while it simultaneously registers and acts on mistakes in executing plans of action.

Now that sounds promising. Aren't these the functions involved in decision-making? Not only lesion studies provide evidence for this. Using functional imaging, it has been proven for normal persons that during willed action a specific activation of the dorsolateral prefrontal cortex occurs (Frith et al. 1991; Hyder et al. 1997; Phelps et al. 1997). In experiments the activation of the brain was measured during movements and while thinking about words. Comparisons were made between passive conditions (moving a touched finger, silently repeating a word) and active, willed, self-generated action (the test person chose one of two movements, or made up a word himself).

In addition, these studies also showed a slight specific activation of the anterior cingulate. That is the foremost part of a cerebral convolution that is shaped like a sickle, situated on the inner surface of the cortex, bordering on both the SMA and the frontal lobes. Many authors consider it as belonging to the frontal cortex. The authors of the work mentioned above only discuss it in passing. But new findings indicate that the anterior cingulate has an important part in "volition." It is involved in many mental functions.[79] Next to its role in selecting action it is an interface between emotion and cognition (see section 3.3.3) and can be viewed as a kind of energy center or driving force. Where there is selective damage, the syndrome of akinetic mutism occurs. Damasio and van Hoesen (1983) describe the case of a woman who had this disorder. Directly after damage, the patient rested in bed with a wide-awake facial expression and apparently reacted not at all to her environment. Closer inspection revealed that she was observing the people in the room. She did not speak voluntarily, nor verbally answer any inquiries. But she did seem to understand the questions, because sometimes she nodded her head. She was able to repeat words and sentences, albeit very slowly. In a nutshell, her reactions to the environment were very limited and rather stereotypical. A month later she had largely recovered. She reported that it had not bothered her not to be able to communicate. Although she was able to follow the conversation, she did not say anything because she "had nothing to say." Her "mind" was "empty." When Francis Crick, discoverer of the DNA double helix and for decades a renowned brain research specialist, read that description, he immediately thought, this woman has lost her will! And so he writes, with naiveness meant to provoke: "I went over for tea one day and announce to Patricia Churchland and Terry Sejnowski that the seat of the Will had been discovered! It is at or near the anterior cingulate" (Crick 1994, p. 268). What did Crick mean? What this woman lacked was obviously any kind of drive, any motivation, to become active. As she herself reported, that was not because she did not understand what was happening around her or because she could not produce any language. It was more that she did not *want* to do or say anything. She did not *make an effort* to do or say anything. A neuroanatomical solution suggests itself. The anterior cingulate lies at the interface between the frontal cortex and motor centers and is part of the limbic system connected with emotions and motivation. Therefore, it is likely that the anterior cingulate plays a part in the behavior of *striving*, which Kane (1996) says is a form of the will (and O'Shaughnessy 1980 calls the *striving will*).

Faced with these findings it is no wonder that some authors try to locate "the will" in the prefrontal cortex or in the anterior cingulate. But let me issue a general warning: When trying to locate things we must be careful not to fall into the homunculi trap and attribute all mental capacities to a little guy (or region) in the brain. While it is true that attributing those functions to the frontal cortex rests on hard neuropsychological facts, the sum of those facts is so great that there is almost nothing that the frontal cortex is *not* supposed to be able to do. Some critics therefore chaff and speak of "frontal lobology" as a new pseudoscience (David 1992). We should, therefore, take pains not to think of the prefrontal cortex as the knowledgeable initiator and top commander of mental planning and decision-making. That would ultimately return us to the regress problem: "Thus, to assign will to any frontal region obviously begs the question of prior command on that region from another structure; the same question can be asked about that other structure, whatever it may be, and then about its precursor, and so on" (Fuster 1995, p. 296). As Fuster emphasizes, it is important to see that the frontal cortex is embedded in a network of actions that he calls the "perception—action—cycle." Sensory information is processed neuronally, which leads to movements, which in turn lead to changes in the environment (internal and external), which again lead to new sensory input, and so on. At the lowest level this cycle is realized as a reflex. Around it and enclosing it there are further cycles—from sensory to motor—with involvement of "control instances" such as the prefrontal cortex. The perception-action-cycle thus consists of several, partially overlapping, bidirectional cycles, with the environment at the bottom. With this idea in the background, an idea which alludes to Viktor von Weizäcker's "Gestaltkreis" (1950), the question of an initiator, an absolute source of actions (first initiation), becomes secondary. We should not conceive of human action as being too linear and not think in terms of stimuli and commands, but rather in terms of intersecting cycles, for which it is arbitrary to determine an absolute point of departure for any act. This is similar to Rheinwald's argumentation (cf. note 74). She insisted that as the matter of ascribing preceding factors becomes less important, the further we move along in a hierarchy of unreal conditional propositions. It would make more sense to speak of modulations of neuronal activity by certain cerebral systems at various levels of organization. It would be the counterpart to Maturana's "perturbation," which comes from without.

But how then does the prefrontal cortex fulfill its selecting function? We get a clue by looking at another deficiency that is evident after damage to the frontal cortex. It concerns the so-called working memory. And, in fact, one of the main functions of the dorsolateral prefrontal cortex is that of a working memory. The prefrontal cortex contains a great quantity of information about objects and can make the representations of those available for planning actions for a while. People with defective working memory depend on hints from the environment to control their behavior. Their behavior is not guided by internalized and active knowledge, but by circumstance. This can be seen in the fact that patients with frontal cortex lesions have difficulty suppressing reactions to external stimuli. In the example given above (shopping for dinner) such patients might suddenly start shopping for shoes or be distracted from their purposes by a conversation.

The prefrontal cortex plays an important role in Changeux and Dehaene's (1989, 1995) theory of mental darwinism. In an approach similar to that of neurosemantics these authors have suggested that we seek the variation-selection process in the brain's cognitive activity in a psychological time screen. They distinguish three kinds of neuronal representations (Changeux and Dahaene 1989, p. 87): (1) percepts, (2) images, concepts, and intentions, and (3) pre-representations. Percepts consist of a correlated activity of neurons that are determined by the outer-world and disintegrate as soon as external stimulation terminates. Images, concepts, and intentions are actualized objects of memory, which result from activating a stable memory trace. (We will recall Edelman's thesis of "remembered present.") Prerepresentations are multiple, spontaneously arising unstable and transient activity patterns that can be selected or eliminated.[80] Prerepresentations that come and go without having meaning could nonetheless acquire meaning when the organism is confronted with new situations. In a new situation the organism might not readily have appropriate representations in store. Selection would occur from an abundance of spontaneously occurring prerepresentations, namely from those that are adequate to the new circumstances and fit existing percepts and concepts. Changeux calls this adaptation process *resonance*. An adaptation process like this also occurs at higher cognitive levels:

> A basic function of the frontal cortex is to capture errors in the unfolding of a motor program. Similarly, intentions might be subjected to internal tests. The validation of a proposition, for example, would then result from a context-dependent compatibility of a chain of mental objects within a given semantic frame with already-stored mental objects. Such tests for compatibility or adequateness might be viewed, from a neural point of view, as analogues of the matching by resonance (or un-matching by dissonance) of percepts with pre-representations. (Changeux and Dehaene 1989, p. 97f)

Changeux and Dehaene have also implemented their theory in a model by designing network models of frontal functions (Changeux and Dehaene 1996).[81] They show that in their model there are rule-coding neurons, whose activity varies randomly and which are then selected in a process in which the matching with memories and external stimuli plays a central role. In their model newly generated rules can be tested in an auto-evaluation process. The authors consider this to be a simple form of thinking.

In summary, planning and making decisions are the result of a selective adaptation process. Representations, or prerepresentations, generated by chance, get selected in an adaptive process (matching, resonance). As in evolution, this could be a random recombination of representations. The meaning of the representations involved is not given by their neuronal form, but by their proper functions. Plans generated in this way are intelligible because they are appropriate for the situation. This happens by matching plans for action with neuronal representations of the situation at hand. The prefrontal cortex fulfills this matching function by providing various representations (working memory). Naturally, linguistically coded representations could therein also be of central importance. Movement does not—as the Libet theory implied—come from nothing; it results from adapting an already available movement pattern in a larger framework. No Cartesian consciousness is necessary for that, no consciousness that performs the whole work of understanding and reason. It is sufficient to have a series of ultra fast adaptation processes which adhere to physiological laws.

Even though all these theories are still fairly hypothetical, it should be obvious by now that the idea of ultrafast adaptation has already been introduced into neurobiological ruminations. Connected with adaptive neurosemantics we can begin to understand how our brains allow us to generate new semantic content in short periods of time. Yet, we still do not have an explanation for what agency can mean from a neurophilosophical perspective.

3 Authenticity in Place of Origination

Synopsis

Every theory of the self or person needs a satisfactory theory of agency. In this chapter we shall look for a neurophilosophical foundation on which we can build a theory of the self. First we shall sketch one kind of incompatibilist theory of agency, namely agent causation, only to dismiss it as inadequate (section 3.1). Then we shall inspect Frankfurt's theory of hierarchical compatibilism (section 3.2). According to this theory the main feature of persons is their capacity to identify with their actions and decisions in a reflective process. Unfortunately, a problem of regress remains. Affective neuroscience, however, does suggests a solution for it (section 3.3). So-called secondary emotions are important for the process of identifying. The incompatibilist concept of agency as the initiation of action can be replaced by the notion of *authenticity*. It is well suited for neurophilosophical theory of cognition because it joins the current states of the brain with the history of the system exhibiting them. It harmonizes with the theses on historicity and externalism of intelligible action that we discussed in section 2. The concept of authenticity illustrates why personal ascription and moral feelings are significant for ethical behavior (section 3.4). Finally, we'll examine whether authenticity is consistent with a compatibilist concept of responsibility.

3.1 Agent Causation

Kant himself clearly expressed the idea of agency. Reason "must see itself as the source of its principles" (Kant 1786/1983, BA 101). "Freedom in cosmological reason" is the capacity for a state to "begin itself." Now, Kant did not propose that there *is* such freedom. But we must postulate it—at least in order to understand ourselves as moral beings. That is the transcendental-philosophical figure of thought. In a similar manner, this idea reoccurs in analytical action theory taking the form of *agent causation*, which, for many libertarians, seems to allow a strong version of free will in our world.[82] This term is sometimes translated into grown as "act causation," "Handlungshausalität"[83] which is unfortunate, because the crucial aspect is precisely that the *agent* (not his action) performs a special kind of causality. It would be correctly translated as "causality of the agent," or, as I shall do in the following, as "agent causation." The notion that a free decision has its origin in the acting person herself is logically independent of the question of whether this decision could have been otherwise, or if it is intelligible: "The theory has to do with [. . .] some thing else, a self or originator. What it comes to is that in each of us there exists an on going entity which is said to originate choices and decisions and hence actions [. . .]" (Honderich 1933, p. 35).

The basic idea of agent causation can perhaps be most easily understood if we relate it to a problem from medieval philosophy.[84] Medieval theists believed that God himself is unchanging. This posed a problem, because all things in nature that cause anything also experience changes in themselves. So how can God be the cause of everything if he himself is unchanging? Philosophers found no real solution. They suggested that we assume there is a special kind of divine causation, so-called *immanent* causation, marked by the fact that while it is effective, the cause itself does not change. To keep them apart, they called nature's causality *event* causation. Roderick Chisholm postulated that agents also have a capacity for *immanent* causation (*agent*, and also *occurent* causation have become common expressions for it). Exaggerating slightly, these theories give humans a divine capacity. The advocates themselves see it this way: "By doing what we do, we cause certain events to happen, and no one and nothing other than ourselves causes us to cause that these events happen . . . if what I have been trying to say is true, then we have a privilege which some would attribute only to God: Each of us, when we really act, is an initial unmoved mover" (Chisholm, quoted from Pothast 1978, p. 82). If an agent acts out of free will, his act is not causally determined by other events, but solely by the agent himself. Is this a solution? Can it explain human action? Notice that the only reason for attributing humans with divine causal powers is to provide them with the capacity to act freely. After introducing this kind of causality it is problematic to claim that we are *explaining* how free human action is possible at all. It is just an ad hoc explanation. An independent reason for postulating this capacity could be that by professing this type of causality we can more easily consider and relate the "commonplace networks of reasons between agents and their actions and facts or events that need explaining" (Rungaldier 1996, p. 144ff). But can we take for granted that our everyday jumble of reasons reflects reality? In light of contemporary knowledge on the common errors in self-attribution, it is highly unlikely that we can.[85] We would be making quite a sacrifice if we were to question the very foundations of natural science out of a denial to revise our everyday notions. Of course, it is justifiable to criticize the concept of causality. Advocates of agent causation do question Hume's regularity theory of causality; the idea captivates us and blinds us for other conceptions of causality (O'Connor 1995b, pp. 182ff). It is true that a reasonable, widely accepted definition for causality is hard to find. In 1913 Russell suggested that we do without it altogether, because science does not at all need it.[86] This advice has never been followed, but more recently critique on causality concepts has again arisen, or it has at least been debated (Heidelberger 1992; Koch 1994), along with the concept of natural laws (Cartwright 1983). This is because the notions of laws of nature, necessity, and causality are interrelated. To this day it has been impossible to define any one of them without using one of the others.[87] But for our purposes we do not need to know which concept of causality is right; we need to know whether it makes sense and is justified to presuppose *two different types of causality.* This debate has been closed inasmuch as even the advocates of agent causation no longer view it as a basically different type of causation! Taylor now thinks that the difference between events and acts lies only in the "difference of contexts, within which they are described—nothing more" (Taylor 1982, p. 226) and Chisholm (1995) envisages agent causation as a subtype of event causation.[88]

Of course, this drains the theory of its suggestiveness. So let us momentarily assume that there is reason to believe that there are two different kinds of causation. Would we still be able to say that agency causation is not an important element of free will? Yes. The main argument for the assumption of agent causation, namely the adequacy of everyday explanations, turns against itself. For the question arises of what the agent in this concept actually is. Our everyday explanations rest on the assumption that the essence of an agent is something at its core, conceived of as a soul or homunculus. Yet advocates of agent causation are particularly careful not to be confused with substance dualists and all the pitfalls of dualism. So just what is the agent in a monistic worldview? According to the theory the definition of agent may not include any properties that could be captured by the categories of event causation, like its body, its history, its natural properties, and so on, because these change while they are causing action. The concept of the agent remains frightfully anemic. But most of all, it contradicts our traditional notions. Furthermore, there is one variant of the intelligibility argument that combats the theory of agent causation. If free decisions are not caused by *anything but* the agent himself, then they are also not caused by reasons. Therefore, they are not intelligible (Kane 1989, p. 226–230; Clarke 1995). It has at least become clear that the only argument for agent causation (adequacy of everyday explanations) is quite fragile. Perhaps the theory well reflects our ideas of origin, of the beginning of a causal chain, and of spontaneity that we impute to our household explanations. But neither the concept of the agent, nor that of intelligible action can be captured in a workaday way with that. In summary, I find that agent causation is not a promising candidate for an adequate theory of agency. So we shall drop it here and turn to compatibilist notions of agency.

3.2   Reflection, Identification, and Responsibility
Compatibilism, you will recall, is the thesis that determinism and free will do not exclude each other. So compatibilists are on the lookout for a concept of agency that does not rest on the idea of agency as initiation.

A weak form of the compatibilist thesis would simply equate the author of an action or decision with the executive instance, as the last member of a causal chain. But this pallid notion is unsatisfactory. For there are many actions and decisions that occur as reflexes or automatically, or that we would rather attribute to the circumstances than to the executive instance. The executive instance should not be merely a *simple* passing station along a causal chain. A compatibilist theory of agency must postulate that the determinants converging in a person are processed in a way that marks the outcome of that processing as an action of that person. In other words, it must be a theory about what makes an executing instance a "self" or "person." Normally, the critics emphasize reason. For example, the sensitivity theories discussed in chapter 1 demand that an action is produced by mechanisms which are sensitive to reasons. But in order to convert action for reasons (intelligibility) into acts of a person (agency), those reasons must not only be relevant to the action, but of a particular kind. So the question is, how can a person make a reason for action her own? An act—using an easily understood everyday intuition also employed in the courts of justice—is attributable to a person, if she has reflected upon it. The capacity for reflection means to weigh reasons for an action against its consequences and competing motives and to relate it to one's own person. Many compatibilists consider this production process to be the central component of any theory of free will: "Processes of free will are personal processes (involvement of the whole structured person) based on motivation conflicts that go through hierarchically ordered recursive loops and to a certain degree consciously represented personality instances" (von Cranach and Foppa 1996, p. 342).

This reflective process is the core of so-called hierarchical theories of free will, which we have previously mentioned several times and which we will now examine more closely. The basic idea was formulated almost simultaneously in the early 1970s by Harry G. Frankfurt and Gerald Dworkin. It has been thoroughly discussed and modified by some authors.[89] Here I will limit our traversal to work of the undoubtedly most prominent representative of this family of theories, namely to Harry Frankfurt, and show how his theory of identification can be considered the compatibilist pendant to agency.

The essential exposition of his volitional theory is found in the essay *Freedom of the Will and the Concept of a Person* (1971).[90] There he differentiates initially between desires of first and second order. The desire to quit work, find a wife, or eat ice cream are first-order desires. If such a desire corresponds to what a person actually does, or—when he is hindered—what he would do, if one would let him do it (if it is an effective or efficient desire), then, and only then, according to Frankfurt, is the first order desire identical to the person's will. The will is thus an effective first-order desire. Second-order desires make reference to first order desires, such as "I wish I did not want to eat ice cream." But this can be desired in two different ways. It can be done rather whimsically, like this: "Oh would it be nice if I didn't want to eat ice cream!" Or, one can desire that this be an *effective* wish, which means that we wish it were our will. Then we have a second order *volition*. Frankfurt explicates freedom of will as follows: "A person's will is free only if he is free to have the will he wants. This means that, with regard to any of his first-order desires, he is free either to make that desire his will or to make some other first-order desire his will instead" (Frankfurt 1988, p. 24). Obviously Frankfurt's concept of free will rests on that of being able to do otherwise. So now we can ask: Do we have free will in the sense propagated by alternativism? Frankfurt does not deal with this issue. So which is his concern? First of all, his explication serves the purpose of characterizing persons as persons. Persons are beings with an interest in coordinating their second-order desires with their effective first order desires (thus: with their will). His example is that of the junkie. He distinguishes three kinds. The compulsive addict doesn't care whether his strong first order desire for narcotics corresponds to his second order desires. He has neither a free nor a bound will and is, in this respect and according to Frankfurt, not a person. (Frankfurt designates him a *wanton*.) The reluctant addict has the first-order desire to consume narcotics, but seriously seeks the second-order desires to live free of drugs. Since he cannot do this, he is not free. Third, we have the willing addict, who—like the unwilling addict—has the first-order desire for narcotics, but also a second-order desire to consume them. His thoughts run like this: It's okay that I'm addicted. I enjoy it." If his drugs would no longer bring him pleasurable effects he would do something to remedy it. In the first-order desire, all three addicts are not free. But Frankfurt says something remarkable about the willing addict: "But when he takes the drug, he takes it freely and of his own free will" (Frankfurt 1988, p. 25). Obviously this is a contradiction. His will is not free, but he takes drugs of his own free will? Has Frankfurt made a mistake, or is he serious? He is serious. What he is trying to do is to define freedom of will analogous to freedom of action. One has freedom of action when one can do what one wants; one has freedom of will when one has a second-order desire to want what one wants. "He takes drugs of his own free will" can be read as "he takes them in accordance with his second order volitions."

Frankfurt has thus developed a modified theory of agency. He explicitly does not adhere to Chisholm's type of agency (Frankfurt 1988, p. 23). But we have good reason to claim that Frankfurt outlines a theory of what it means to act according *to one's own will*. If we slightly modify the above quotation, Frankfurt's statement is reasonable: "The will of an addict is not free, but when he consumes drugs, he does it of his *own* will." Doing something "out of his own will" means that this desire is something belonging to the agent, an expression of himself, it is "real," it is "authentic." When someone does his "own" thing, it seems natural to *attribute* that to him *personally*. As the title of Frankfurt's essay reveals, he links a theory of free will to the concept of person. His aim is to outline a compatibilist theory of freedom of will that gives reasons for responsibility while waiving being able to do otherwise.

But it is not solely agreement among second-order volitions and the will that makes an action to be one's own. More important is how this agreement was reached. A person can very possibly have several second order volitions. How does one gain command? One way would be to have third order volitions. But this ends in regress, as Frankfurt himself acknowledges: "There is no theoretical limit to the length of the series of desires of higher and higher orders, nothing except common sense and, perhaps, a saving fatigue prevents an individual from obsessively refusing to identify himself with any of his desires until he forms a desire of the next higher order" (Frankfurt 1988, p. 21).

How can a person end the series without being arbitrary? "When a person identifies himself *decisively* with one of his first-order desires, this commitment 'resounds' throughout the potentially endless array of higher orders. (Frankfurt 1988, p. 21). But how can a person "decide" to identify herself with something? We understand what Frankfurt means, but does clothing it in words really remedy the regress or merely reformulate the problem? Frankfurt attempts to meet this unavoidable objection in his essay "Identification and Wholeheartedness." He proposes that identification must happen not half-but wholeheartedly. Wholeheartedness, he assures us, is not to be confused with enthusiasm or subjective certainty (Frankfurt 1988, p. 175). But when is identification wholehearted? According to Frankfurt, identification is wholehearted when one has no need of higher-order justifications, when one has the *insight* that no amount of higher order justification will change one's mind. For the sake of illustration, Frankfurt uses the analogy of solving an arithmetic task. When one is finished calculating, one can use various methods and check the solution several times. How does one know when to stop checking? When one has good reasons for believing that there is no other solution and that further checking would not alter the solution. This is the principle of "decisive identification." "[S]uch an identification resounds through an unlimited sequence of possible further reconsiderations of his decision. For a commitment is decisive if and only if it is made without reservation, and making a commitment without reservation means that the person who makes it dies so in the belief that no further accurate inquiry would require him to change his mind. It is therefore pointless to pursue the inquiry any further" (Frankfurt 1988, p. 168). It is the insight that we can waive further justifications that provides a criterion for terminating our checks. Thus, intelligibility is very important for identification. So Frankfurt is a rationalist—as clear as daylight. For it is reason alone that leads us to avoid the threatening regress of higher level volitions.

Frankfurt's approach is appropriate as a model of what it means to make an authentic decision, that is, a decision with which one can identify oneself as a person. Authenticity is not the same as initial causation. But it is important and valuable—an aspect of personality. It is concerned with personal attribution, insofar as it can satisfy some of the intuitions we associate with the third component. But I think that Frankfurt's rationalistic model is entirely wrong. This is because authentic decisions made by humans are not analogous to calculating arithmetic tasks. We need some resources from neurophilosophy in order to set up an empirically plausible model of authenticity, as we shall see shortly.

Some other authors also disagree with Frankfurt's rationalistic theory of identification. Gary Watson criticizes that a hierarchical theory working only with desire hierarchies misses one of the essential points about identification, namely *evaluation*, because "what one desires may not be what one values, and what one most values may not be what one is finally moved to get" (Watson 1982, p. 100). In Watson's opinion, Frankfurt's approach cannot explain to which extent the will of a person is *her own* (Watson 1982, p. 108). That is only possible by making reference to values and values cannot be reduced to desires.[91] So Watson defends a subjectivity variant of evaluation theory.

I believe that Watson is right; values and evaluations are important for the process of identification. It would be desirable to include them in a theory of identification, but why do we need a theory of identification? According to Frankfurt, because it allows us to establish a concept of moral responsibility that can waive being able to do otherwise. Frankfurt thinks that the "principle of alternative possibilities" is wrong, which states that being able to do otherwise is important for responsibility (Frankfurt 1969). This can be demonstrated with the case of the addict. The three types of addicts cannot do other than want their narcotics at the first level. The addict who identifies himself with that desire simultaneously *accepts* the responsibility for it. And that affects his behavior. While the reluctant addict does everything he can to break his addiction, the willingly addicted person will not. The way we morally evaluate this, according to Frankfurt, hinges on identification. Although both kinds of addicts cannot do otherwise, we feel justified to condemn the willing addict for his compulsion, while we do not so strongly disapprove of the reluctant addict. Frankfurt's theory can thus serve as a starting point for a deterministic theory of responsibility.

To summarize, hierarchical compatibilism combines an intuition about agency with the concept of a person. A person brings forth her own acts when she identifies with them, even if she could not do otherwise. I have dubbed this authenticity. The process of identification provides justification for envisioning a person as responsible for her actions, even if she could not have behaved otherwise. Frankfurt's theory has two definite deficiencies. It assumes that the identification process occurs purely rationally, and it neglects the facet of evaluation. As I shall reveal in the following, affective neuroscience provides a solution.

3.3   Affective Neuroscience and Identification

3.3.1   Authentic Decisions and Emotions   The question we want to answer is how a person makes a decision her own. In neurophilosophy, attitudes and beliefs can be understood as sophisticated adaptive brain states, which can be modeled as relaxation states of a neuronal net or as attractors of a multi-dimensioned phase space. A first conclusion from this is that attitudes and beliefs cannot readily be made explicit. In order to know whether a particular action or decision fits into the network of nonexplicit (nonactive) attitudes, it is necessary to compare the plausible decisions with the consequences of one's own attitudes. The way this is realized, it is not always rationally possible, for time is lacking. How can it be achieved? By feelings. The feeling that one has about doing the right thing can take over this role. The intuitive feeling that "something is wrong," a lack of ease while considering a decision, the safe feeling of having made a good decision, the presentiment about going in the right direction; all these play an important part in decision-making processes. My thesis is that decisions do not become authentic purely by exercising reflection and rationally setting one point against another, but by balancing and coordinating them with one's feelings. We shall see why this type of balancing founds authenticity better than a rational reflection process alone.

But first, one objection to this thesis is immediately at hand. Assuming that we could plausibly prove that for most people feelings are central to their decisions, what happens? All the worse for most people! From a normative standpoint, namely, we can claim that things *should* not be this way; the essence of intelligible and moral decisions is that they are guided solely by reason or insight into moral standards or moral codes. Strictly speaking, this means that an act is no longer good if it did not occur for reasons of insight (in the moral law), but for other, subjective reasons. Friedrich Schiller criticized this rational attitude of Kant's with some irony: "Gladly do I serve my friends, but unfortunately that is my bent/And thus it often rankles me, that I am not virtuous" (Schiller, quoted in Höffe 1983, p. 201). An objection such as this would only be significant if it actually were the best to make morally relevant decisions on the grounds of rational insight. Many moral philosophers defend just that opinion, and Frankfurt's rationalistic theory is among them. Yet emotions are a factor in every theory of identification and of morality. Because we are here mainly concerned with the naturalistic aspect of free will, we will only investigate how emotions factor in the process of identification and only brush moral feelings in the conclusion.

The idea that emotions oppose rationality and that they must be overcome and controlled, is dominant not only in moral philosophy. It is also a view widely held within cognitive science. But evidence continues coming in, indicating that this notion—as old and honorable as it may be—is wrong. Psychologists, philosophiers,[92] and also neuroscientists have come to recognize a very close, to a certain extent unseverable connection between cognition and emotions. In the next section I will briefly outline the progress in theories that culminated in this insight and then introduce a model from cognitive neuroscience that demonstrates how certain feelings guide our decisions and why they are serviceable for identification theory.

3.3.2 Emotion and Cognition   The idea that feeling and thinking are two entirely different things is an outcome of dualistic philosophy going back at least to Plato.[93] His idea of the soul imprisoned in the body ends almost directly in separation of intellect and reason, seated in the soul, on one hand, and feelings and emotions, attributed to the body, on the other. Sentiment theories from Descartes to Locke to Hume preserve that tradition. A different tradition begins with Aristotle. In Book II of the Rhetoric, he explains why an emotion contains not merely an element of feeling, but also a factual or value judgment. His idea can also be found in fragments of the Stoics Seneca and Chrysypp, and they surface in a mild version in the work of Saint Thomas Aquinas and Baruch Spinoza, but then remain dormant until late in the twentieth century. The rise of cognitive theories of emotions awakened them once more.[94] In an effort to valorize the cognitive aspect of emotions, some theorists admittedly shot past the mark by claiming that emotions are purely cognitive phenomena. If taken literally, this notion is certainly not correct. But as a rule, most authors emphasize the close connection and inseparable intertwining of both aspects. Luc Ciompi (1982, 1997) argued in his work on affect logics that thinking cannot be conceived of as separated from affects because our acts are determined by a scheme of emotions and thoughts that we cannot evade. In a recently published book, Daniel Goleman (1996) coined the term *emotional intelligence* to express how emotions contribute to intelligent action. Findings from neuroscience are also involved in upgrading emotions; these demonstrate how psychological theses can also be supported or confirmed by an understanding of the neurobiological underpinnings beneath that linkage.

But first some academic remarks on the concepts of cognition and emotion. Cognition is derived from Latin *cognoscere*—to know. In cognitive psychology it includes the functions of perception and recognition, decoding, storing, and remembering, as well as thinking and problem solving, motor control and using language (Strube et al. 1996). There are broader explications claiming that cognition is information processing (Miller, Galanter, and Pribram 1960), or a self-regulating process in living systems (Maturana and Varela 1984). Some psychologists find this definition of cognition quite inflated and would rather reserve it for what we might call "insight" (Dörner 1989). By "emotion" or "affect" we generally mean a temporary agitation with a beginning and an end. We differentiate emotions from mood or temperament, concepts that designate more stable phenomena. Besides being subjectively *experienced*, emotions also effect *behavior* (pain behavior, grief behavior), are visible in expressions (mimic art, gestures, voice) and have a facet of value (they can be characterized as good or bad, advantageous or detrimental). Beyond this, it has been proven that they are founded on *certain physiological processes* in the nervous system.

If we take a look at the progress in emotion theory over the last century we can better understand how neuroscience can bring these diverse components of emotion all together. William James (1884), American philosopher and psychologist, and independently of him Carl Lange (1885), Danish physiologist, stated in theories at the end of the nineteenth century that emotions consist of the perception of bodily changes (see Goller 1992, p. 29f). Somewhat summarized, We don't shake because we are frightened, we are afraid because we are shaking. This notion was criticized by physiologists who pointed out that central, not peripheral physiological processes are crucial for emotions. Today we take this view so widely for granted, that it seems trivial. Naturally, the two theories are not reciprocally exclusive, because—as we know—corporal changes are represented centrally.[95] In spite of the harsh criticism it underwent, the James-Lange theory proved to be astoundingly durable and has been revived in contemporary neurobiology. Papez's (1937) theory is also still interesting, identifying the limbic system as one of the most significant central structures for emotions. It is a structure deep within the brain, old in terms of evolutionary development, and closely coupled with olfaction, emotions, drive, the regulation of autonomous parameters, and memory.[96] Even laymen are acquainted with Paul MacLean's "triune concept of the brain" (1970, 1990), which is based on the limbic system and considers it one of three layers of the brain. Beneath it there lies the evolutionary older reptile brain for reflex behavior, above it is the evolutionary youngest part, the neocortex, which supplies reason. Although something does speak for this theory, it has deeply anchored the notion that the neocortex is the seat of reason while the limbic system is the seat of the emotions and lack of reason. In reality, the matter is more complicated.

In the 1980s a series of emotion theorists picked up ideas from evolution theory.[97] They agree that emotions fulfill some function and have an adaptation value for the organism, or we would not have them. Just as pain indicates an injury to the organism, fear can be positive and adaptive by indicating danger to the organism and motivating an appropriate response. Emotions serve the purpose of allowing an organism to react directly, appropriately and sometimes unavoidably to certain situations. Some basic emotions are innate. While neurobiologists such as Tomkins (1982) and Panksepp (1982) strive to prove this for particular restricted brain structures, Paul Ekman (1982, 1992) took a different route. Based on Darwin's work, *The Expression of Emotions in Humans and Animals* (1872) he has researched the expression and recognition of emotions in mimicry and was able to show that some basic emotions can be transculturally identified. Today this research is considered the best evidence for the fact that basic feelings are universal. These are generally accepted to be the five basic emotions of fear, happiness, sadness, disgust, and anger; others are controversial (surprise, interest); and still others are hot potatoes (excitement, awe, embarrassment).

Tentatively, the most recent class of emotion theories are the so-called cognitive theories of emotion.[98] A forerunner theory was Schachter and Singer's two-factor theory of emotions from the 1960s. These authors postulate that every emotion consists of an unspecific arousal and an additional cognitive evaluation. Although today their theory is considered refuted, the element of evaluation or appraisal has remained the common element of all cognitive theories of emotion. Without getting into details, let us look at the basic idea. The basic assumption of all these theories is that emotion is at least partially defined by appraisal. Appraisal always and inevitably contains cognitive elements because it deals with ranking a certain matter with reference to goals, plans, or functions of an organism. Take sadness as an example. We can try to understand sorrow as an entirely subjective feeling. We can study the underlying physiological brain activity during an episode of sadness. We can further analyze the typical facial expressions and behavior of a sad person. But we cannot understand what sadness is, according to the cognitive emotion theorist, if we do not also understand sadness as a state that is a reaction to the loss of a loved one or the failure to reach a goal. By being sorrowful, we *know* this kind of loss or failure. We realize that this kind of knowing is a part of sadness because news of the opposite—that the loss did not happen—normally ends the sorrow abruptly.

This does not mean that subjective experience and appraisal cannot dissociate. In some psychopathological processes they actually do. Nevertheless, a period of sadness that continues although the person learns that there is no reason for it is incomplete. It is a subjective feeling *like* sorrow, but not real sorrow. A real feeling is defined by *all* of the components; if they are not present, the feeling is not real. We would intuitively hesitate to attribute real pain to a person who claims to suffer from extreme pain but does not exhibit a trace of pain behavior.

Several theorists have drafted models of this appraisal process. They vary in the number and differentiae of the steps of appraisal, at the level in a hierarchy at which an evaluation takes place, and when precisely it happens. We need not concern ourselves with these details (see Power and Dalgleish 1996). At this point I would only like to point out that an evaluative component does not contradict evolutionary biological and neurobiological theories, they are actually well compatible. For sophisticated organisms such as humans, higher emotions, such as those concerned with social behavior, can be well explained by cognitive emotion theories. Some examples are altruistic or ethical feelings.[99]

In the 1980s emotion psychology witnessed the Lazarus-Zajonc debate, a famed quarrel about the priority of emotions over cognition (cf. Goller 1992, p. 178). Although they are intertwined, one of the two elements was thought to be effective first, for example when perceiving an emotionally relevant stimulus. While Lazarus contended that cognitive processing precedes emotional processing, Zajonc cleverly argued that every perception is already emotionally tainted. Leventhal and Scherer (1987) criticized that quarrel as a sterile semantic controversy about the meaning of words. Their claim is that it is meaningless to search for a definite answer to the question of just *what* exactly an emotion or a cognition is. Both terms refer to complex patterns of behavior that change during the lifetime of an organism; they are products of a changing processing system made up of several components. While it is true that these words demarcate two separate realms in everyday experience as well as in research (see my explication above), their underlying mechanisms and elements of information processing are not specific to those realms.[100] Instead of searching for specific conceptual demarcations, we should study which contribution certain processing components make to emotional experience and behavior.

In their own emotion theory, Leventhal and Scherer tackle this from a psychological viewpoint. But meanwhile there exists a wealth of neuroscientific findings on neurobiological mechanisms of emotions.[101] These deal with the "humoral" side (findings on transmitters and hormones), as well as the "neurocomputational" side (knowledge of the structures, circuits, and the interaction between certain networks and the relay stations of the brain). It would take a whole book to describe these. So here we will very selectively take a look at the most recent findings in the neurophysiology of patients with brain damage, which I find directly demonstrate the relevance that neurobiological knowledge has for the theory of authenticity.

3.3.3 Feeling, Thinking, and Deciding: The Embodied Mind Psychological and neurobiological research on emotions concentrated mainly on basic emotions: fear, sadness, anger, disgust, happiness. Meanwhile, we know the neuroanatomical bases of these emotions. One special member of the limbic system, the amygdala (almond), a little, round, bunch of cells deep within the brain, plays an important role in them. LeDoux (1994, 1996), using the example of fear, demonstrated that there is a kind of emotional memory that helps organisms to direct their emotions prior to making use of their higher, but clearly slower cognitive functions. He proved that there are two different neuroanatomical ways of processing information from emotional stimuli. One way leads directly from the sense organs to the amygdala. Input information about an emotionally laden stimulus—say, a snake—is ready prior to rational processing in the cortex. We feel frightened before we know why. The fact that we judge faces as being nice or not, before we even know them, may also occur along these lines. Normally, information processing takes place when two pathways interact. Their reciprocal influence is shaped by the complexity of the input stimuli and what the organism has already learned. Processing is not strictly parallel, but interactive, and the higher cognitive strategies rely on and also change the lower ones. Hebb and Thompson postulated as early as 1968 that the more highly developed the intellectual capacity of a species is, the more complex its emotions become.

The traditional Bayesian model is still the predominate model for rational decision making. It is particularly favored by economists as it assumes that a person thinks over possible alternatives, sorts out the advantages and disadvantages, rationally determines the best decision, and then decides accordingly (Sugden 1991; Joyce 1995). But normally people do not follow this pattern. Studies on patients with brain damage provide evidence that feelings are not only *helpful* in decision-making, they are *irreplaceable*, and when feelings are left out of decision processes, the outcomes turn out to be "poor" decisions. Feelings, premonitions, and appraisals have a guiding and stabilizing function that saves us from becoming victims of outside circumstances, as the high level of flexibility in our cognitive skills would actually allow. So-called secondary emotions are the basis of the neuronal self. Emotions are important for making decisions authentic. Studies on patients with brain damage show that the ventromedial frontal lobes function as a mediator between reason and emotions and they are involved in making decisions under real conditions. This theses is particularly advocated by a work group lead by neurologist Antonio Damasio[102] and has basically been confirmed by other researchers (Rolls et al. 1994; Hornak et al. 1996; Elliott et al. 1997). The following exposition mainly regards the Damasio group findings.

It is not surprising that damage to the limbic system influences the realm of emotions. A patient called SM, for example, whose amygdala has been destroyed, no longer has any feeling of fear. At a "rational" level she knows what fear is, but she exhibits no fear reactions in dangerous situations, a behavior that naturally can be very harmful. For a patient named Elliott the emotional disturbance was more complicated and is more significant for our purposes. Elliott's ventromedial frontal lobes (the part of the cortex lying toward the middle and below) was destroyed on both sides by a tumor.[103] Elliott recovered well from the operation and initially appeared to have no essential cognitive losses. His IQ of 140 remained stable, his store of knowledge was available, he could answer questions appropriately, and he had no complaints. But his daily life changed dramatically. Previously a reliable accountant and loving family member, Elliott converted into an irresponsible, disorderly, and unsociable person. Since his intelligence had not suffered, first conjectures were that he had a psychiatric, not a neurological problem. That was an error.

As described in section 2.5.2, patients with lesions in the dorsolateral frontal lobes exhibit specific losses in cognition. But neuropsychological tests done on Elliott to check these functions exhibited no deficits. His disorder, which transformed his social life, communication, and moral choices made it appear as if he had lost social competence or insight. A series of tests were set up to examine skills for imagining appropriate reactions to social situations, for spontaneously weighing the outcomes of certain reactions, for thinking up ways to achieve social goals, for predicting social situations and for making higher level moral judgments. Yet even in those areas Elliott displayed an astonishingly almost normal performance. Why, in real life, was he so changed and restricted, such that we would be likely to say that his disorder was an "acquired socio-pathic disorder?" Damasio's answer is that there is a difference between knowing about decisions and actually making decisions in real life.[104] After Damasio and his coresearchers had ruled out all purely cognitive deficits, they proposed that the disturbance in decision making might have something to do with a lack of feelings. In contrast to the patient SM, Elliot was able to feel fear in certain situations. The disturbance was in the emotional background music of daily life. He had emotional anemia. Elliott was passionless and uninvolved, and he himself did not suffer from those deficits or the consequences of his actions. Together with his colleague Bechara, Damasio drafted a test meant to simulate near-to-life decisions (Bechara et al. 1994). Using that, it was possible to check their theses on emotionally disturbed decision making.

The test consisted of a card game. Four stacks of cards and an initial budget of $2,000 play money is placed in front of the test person. He is instructed to pick up cards and win as much money as possible and lose as little as possible. Each time he turns a card over, he receives a reward ($100 for stacks A and B, $50 for stacks C and D). Some cards, however, bring punishment. These are distributed such that they come up frequently in stacks A and B and rarely in stacks C and D. The distribution of punishment cards is not predictable and even normal test persons were not able to exactly calculate their "accounts." The test person is also not told how many cards must be taken before the game terminates. (It will be 100.)

On the average, it pays to play stacks C and D, the "good" stacks, even though the reward per card is lower, and to avoid the "bad" stacks. Normal people do just that, after having gathered some experience with the stacks. Patients with damage in other parts of the brain also do so. But Elliott and some patients with damage in the ventromedial area of the frontal cortex (VM patients) prefer to play the "bad" stacks, which promises immediate high rewards. What control experiments and qualitative observation show is that this is not due to sensitivity to rewards or insensitivity toward punishment; it is a general lack of concern for the future that guides their decisions.

Another experiment (Bechara et al. 1997) revealed an even more exciting outcome, for in this case the state of the body—as James had supposed—was involved in the process. Measurements of the electric skin conductance on normal persons exhibited no skin response during the first repetitions of the experiment. A change in the skin conductance response (SCR) is a classic sign indicating that the vegetative nervous system controlled by the body is reacting. But after about the tenth repetition, the skin of normal people began to respond directly before their choice to take a card from the bad stacks. At this stage, normal people began to avoid the bad stacks. After about 50 repetitions they reported an intuitive feeling that "something was wrong" with some of the stacks. After about 80 repetitions they knew rationally which stacks were bad and why. In other words, before they *knew* why they selected certain stacks, they made their decisions "intuitively," they had a feeling about which ones were wrong. That feeling could be registered physiologically, namely as SCR. VM patients on the other hand exhibited neither discomfort nor a skin response, neither at the beginning nor the end of the game, although in other circumstances they did exhibit high rates of skin response. In the case of the card game their bodies did not tell them what to do.

Particularly interesting was their behavior at the end of the game, *after* they understood which stacks were good or bad, which was the case for 70% of the normal persons and 50% of the VM patients. Although the VM patients rationally knew exactly and could explain which stacks were good and which were bad, their knowledge did not effect their behavior. They continued to prefer the bad stacks. On the other hand, the normal persons who did not rationally check what was going on right up to the end of the game continued "listening" to their body signals and avoided the bad piles. It looks as though the body not only helps during intuitive decisions, but also when rational insights must be turned into deeds.

The theory Damasio established based on these findings is called the *theory of somatic markers* (Damasio 1995). We need to briefly survey his theory of emotions (Damasio 1994, pp. 178–226), which belongs to the class of evaluative emotion theories. Similar to those, Damasio distinguishes emotions from the subjective feelings associated with them. A feeling, according to his theses, "depends on the juxtaposition of an image of the body proper to an image of something else, such as the visual image of a face or the auditory image of a melody" (Damasio 1994, p. 201). Damasio also differentiates between primary and secondary emotions. Primary emotions are *innate* and are controlled by the limbic system. Secondary emotions exploit the same "brain machinery," but they have been *learned*. They are associated with individual experience. In the brain there exists a constantly active and unstable representation of the state of the body, marked by feelings. This picture exists parallel to cognitive activities and is closely involved with them. When a person experiences certain situations, these are automatically accompanied by felt bodily representations, which include a value mark. Value marking says something about what is good or bad for a person in that situation. Value marks express more than can be rationally comprehended because the body reacts to the entirety of a situation and thus also to secondary features of it and reacts to things that are—let us dare to say it—subconscious. The associations of the "somatic" marker are stored in memory along with complicated stimuli, scenes, and situations.

In a situation that demands a decision the following happens. While weighing diverse alternatives for action we not only make plans and think up arguments, we also imagine the possible outcomes of possible decisions, that is, we imagine future scenarios. Expressed somewhat more technically, we mentally simulate counterfactual situations. The prefrontal cortex generates these scenarios of future events (see section 2.5.2). Simultaneously the amygdala and hypothalamus (hormone control center) also effect one's body, particularly the visceral functions (heart, intestines, blood pressure, etc.). The body reacts as it has done in similar past situations and, via feedback loops, it reports its state back to the brain. A feeling for future situations that arises in this way is usually a fairly reliable sign for decisions—similar to the way in which a pain is a feeling that without much thought or rationalization—tells us whether our present situation is okay or whether we must change something. VM patients are unable to make evaluations using their feelings because the relevant region in their brains is damaged, namely the region that coordinates the integration of body state representations and imagined scenarios, that is, the ventromedial section of the frontal cortex. Loss of that function severs the physiological link between the prefrontal cortex, the limbic system, and body-state representations. That their bodies no longer react as in healthy persons is evidenced by a lack of electric skin response. This is a neurobiological explanation for a disorder in cognitive procedure brought about by interrupting emotional mechanisms. Since a decision cannot be supported by the feeling that it is the right decision, many of the decisions these patients make are useless and not in their own interests. So, not only is insight crucial, but also whether a decision falls into line with one's emotional values!

Damasio's guess is that once it has been established, the juxtaposition of cognitive contents and somatic markers can also take place without participation of the body, (Damasio 1994, pp. 213ff). The frontal cortex sections, which are closely connected to the limbic system and generate ideas of counterfactual situations, could also directly influence body representations via "as-if loops." But an as-if loop is second choice. The real body generates intricate changes more adequate to reality than the prefrontal cortex could ever simulate them, particularly regarding the humoral realm. The body, or better, the representation of it which the brain constantly holds *online*, is also a factor in "pure thinking" happening in the brain.

Another important aspect of Damasio's theory is that decisions are coupled with the neural basis of the self through the body-base of secondary emotions. According to Damasio, the unity of self constitutes itself based on the central nervous system's representations of the body. Three brain systems are involved. First is the brain stem and the hypothalamus, which coordinate and represent the vegetative and biochemical (hormone) regulation of the body. Second is the secondary and tertiary somato-sensory cortex, particularly belonging of the right half of the brain, which represents our muscles, tendons, and skin and their potential movements. Third is the insula, crucial for visceral feelings—feeling the inner organs of the body.[105]

This thesis is supported by the clinical syndrome of anosognosia (Kolb and Wishaw 1996, p. 273ff; Damasio 1994, pp. 98–107). Anosognosia is the failure to recognize that one is ill. After a normal stroke, which effects only the primary somato-sensory cortex, patients know that they are paralyzed. For anosognosia this is different. Objectively, patients are paralyzed, but they deny it. One can try to convince them that they are paralyzed and they might believe it for a short while, but then they forget it. Even if they do recognize the fact that they are paralyzed, it does not seem to impress them. It is interesting that this kind of anosognosia occurs after damage in the right hemisphere in those regions which Damasio says hold the foundations for our self's body image. It is as if these patients had forgotten that a part of their body belongs to them, as soon as they no longer are attentive to that part. This indicates the role for somatic markers: They are amplifiers for the continued activity of working memory and attention.

There is a conspicuous and even empirically supported objection to Damasio's theory. It claims that in evaluating our bodies we are fairly unreliable, as interoception research has shown (Vaitl 1995). Yet Damasio's theory does not require that secondary emotions be conscious feelings about what is happening in the body. What we become aware of is their evaluating aspect.

But does this reply immunize the theory from empirical arguments? Not at all. Damasio's hypotheses are indeed speculative, yet empirically testable. His statements, which can be falsified, are about which brain members must be active during decision making, namely just those brain parts that generate the basis for the body self image. We can empirically examine whether his thesis is right or wrong. In an extremely interesting study using functional methods on normal persons (PET), Elliott, Frith, and Dolan (1997) were able to show that the ventromedial frontal lobes were active during planning and decision tasks, if emotional feedback occurred. The more difficult it is to control the task, the stronger the activity, that is, the more the decision hinges on intuitive evaluations. In some areas Damasio's original assumptions have already been falsified. Initially he had assumed that patients with ventromedial damage were especially restricted in making social decisions. Experiments with the Wason selection test have, meanwhile, proven this incorrect (Adolphs et al. 1995). Not in the social realm, but in the realm of what one is *familiar* with is where those persons make the worst decisions. Another way of testing Damasio's theses is to examine patients with antisocial personality disorders not due to brain damage (Walter 1996d). The symptoms are similar, although patients with VM lesions generally exhibit less criminal energy. This alone does not guarantee that the underlying neurobiological mechanisms are the same, but it is a plausible assumption. Research has been done on cases of antisocial personality disorders—formally called "psychopathy"—using electric skin response tests (Hare and Quinn 1971) and EEG studies on evoked potentials (Forth and Hare 1989). Neurophysiological studies showed "ventral frontal deficits in psychopaths" (Lapierre, Braun, and Hodgins 1995). And using new methods in functional imaging it could soon become possible to study exactly those structures that Damasio suggests are involved in the genesis of sociopathic behavior. There is actually already one study being done on the role of the amygdala in the emotions of patients with social phobia which will be extended to patients with antisocial personality disorder (Schneider et al. 1999). Here lies an advantage of neurophilosophical strategy. Further developments are not left to thought experiments alone, but rest on feedback with empirical science.

Meanwhile, there is direct empirical evidence that interruption in the circuits described above proceeds with a disturbance in the feeling of agency. One pathological symptom discussed in this regard is the *alien hand syndrome* (Goldberg and Bloom 1990; Gasquoine 1993). It occurs after damage in the anterior cingulate and neighboring areas. A person with this disorder makes movements with his left hand, for example, but does not feel *responsible* for that action. Usually this involves rather simple and stereotype motions. It can happen that the hand grasps for a nearby object "by itself," as it were. In some cases the patient cannot let go of the object with his sick hand and must pry it out using his healthy hand. In another case a patient could not willingly open his hand, but he was able to do so by giving his hand a command. He said out loud, "Let go!" At the level of conscious experience we would say that the movement did not happen willingly. But what we are essentially saying is that the owner of the hand is no longer the *agent* of the movement. One patient described by Spence (1996) reported that his hand "has a will of its own." In agreement with Damasio's theory these phenomena can be explained by noting that the connection has been severed that normally exists between the regions controlling the movement of the hand and the other parts of the neural body-self.

Psychiatry provides a wealth of disturbances in volition and agency that certainly will be a major source for future empirically supported theories of autonomy. The development of neuroimaging opens a new era of explanation for some well known phenomena. An appropriate portrayal of these sources would require a book by itself. But I would like to mention a few findings relevant to our topic. For depression as well as for a subclass of schizophrenia, it has been shown that there is reduced activity in the left dorsolateral frontal lobes (Andreasen 1997). This finding is not considered specific for the illness, but specific for the symptom, because both disorders exhibit a "hypovolitional" syndrome, which means drive reduction and impeded initiative, that is combined with flat affects in some schizophrenics (the syndrome of psychomotor poverty; Liddle 1987). This fits the dorsolateral prefrontal cortex function for "willed action." Another important subclass of schizophrenic patients, who clinically are said to have disorganization syndrome, exhibited reduced activity in the right ventromedial frontal cortex and hyperactivity in the cingulate anterior on the right (Liddle et al. 1992; Liddle 1994). The authors propose that these patients exhibit an abnormality in the ventromedial cortex that causes a tendency for inappropriate behavior.

Another important illness, obsessive compulsive disorder (OCD), exhibits just the opposite. In this case functional neuroimaging has shown that the ventromedial cortex (and the subcortical motor regions connected to it) exhibit increased activity (Baxter 1992; Breiter et al. 1996). Patients suffering from OCD must do certain things or must think certain thoughts, although they claim that they do not want to and often desperately try to fight it. Baxter's hypothesis (Baxter 1992, see also Kischka et al. 1997) is that this occurs because a "worry input" entered through the frontal lobes is fed into the subcortical basal ganglia via the ventromedial cortex. The ganglia's (probably primarily) reduced filter function reduces the impeding effect of another structure (the thalamus) on the ventromedial cortex, so that a positive feedback loop occurs, whose activity then spreads to other brain regions. The reason patients with compulsory disorders do not feel that they themselves produce their thoughts and actions has an explanation. In my view, the circuit has become autonomous and uncoupled from the representation of the body-self.

One of the most interesting phenomena for the feeling of agency is, perhaps, the so-called "I-disorder" (Ichstörungen).[106] Typically, it is exhibited by schizophrenics. The patient feels that his own psychic procedures no longer belong to himself; he experiences them as being produced outside of himself. Patients are under the impression that their thoughts can spread to other people, that their thoughts are taken away from them, or that foreign ideas get put into their minds. It is also sometimes thought of as a disorder of "belonging to oneself" (or "me-ness" as Metzinger puts it). It includes more experiences of alien control. Patients have the feeling that they can control things that they really cannot control ("I control the movements of the sun!"), or that they are influenced by things which do not really influence them ("An electronic remote control is controlling me!"). What could cause these types of phenomena? Obviously, they are phenomenologically connected to the concept of agency. Philosophically interested psychiatrists discuss these phenomena in connection with Frankfurt's compatibilistic theory of agency (Stephen and Graham 1994). We can speculate that "Ichstörungen" have something to do with irregularity in those brain sections dealing with agency, that is, in the ventromedial cortex, including the anterior cingulate or the body representations in the right hemisphere. There are, in fact, some empirical findings that indicate this. In a recent, and—for this field of work—methodically very tidy study, Spence et al. (1997) used positron emission tomography to investigate the brain activity of schizophrenic patients suffering from passivity phenomena (one form of "Ichstörungen") during a willed motor task. Symptom-specific activity was discovered when the data were compared with brain activity of normal persons and with that of schizophrenic patients *not* suffering from passivity phenomena. Which brain regions were involved? As expected, activity was in the motor, premotor, and parietal regions. The seven patients with self-disorders, five of which experienced passivity phenomena *during* the experiment (exclaiming: "I feel like a machine" or "I feel guided by a female spirit who has entered me"), in addition also exhibited symptom-specific activity. This activity was found in exactly those areas previously discussed, namely, in the right inferior parietal cortex and the anterior cingulate. Both regions are central for the representation of a body-self during willed actions, but, activity in those regions was increased and not reduced. This is not necessarily inconsistent with the hypothesis of the neural base of a self-body image. Instead of thinking along the lines of reduced or increased brain activity in particular brain regions, we should perhaps speak of regulation disorders in cerebral circuits. Over-activity, for example, could be an attempt to compensate for a functional disconnection to another station in the circuit.

In summary, the traditional notion that feelings get in the way of reflective and responsible decision-making is not true. Emotions actually constitute a foundation for our subjective values. We cannot do without them when making authentic and prudent decisions having implications for our own futures. Central body-representation joins the emotional basis of decisions with the physical basis of the self, by implicitly containing the past history of the individual. This neurophilosophical thesis about the components of the agency of willed actions is based on empirical findings, thereby changing the phenomenon of agency from a philosophically obscure thesis to an empirically researchable topic.

3.4   Authenticity and Its Implications

3.4.1   Personal Ascription   What do all these considerations have to do with Frankfurt's theory? I am not criticizing Frankfurt's reflective model itself, because reflection is also an important part of natural autonomy. I do resist the rationalistic solution to the regress problem in identification, because of the analogy to arithmetical calculation. Instead, I postulate a central role for mechanisms, which rely very heavily on emotional valuations. When we look at practical decisions that we make everyday, it is obvious that among them there is hardly one we could make as if we were solving a math problem. It is too time consuming. Many decisions must be made so quickly that it is impossible to consider all relevant factors. And most decisions are made with a certain degree of uncertainty. The relevant data is not always available to enable us to make prudent and adequate decisions; the outcomes of decisions are not always foreseeable. This is particularly true for important decisions in life, like changing one's occupation, marrying, or moving one's household. These decisions need time to mature, before one makes up his mind. So here the network in the brain needs a longer period before it can relax at an energy minimum. In cases like these it is not the pro and con reasons that have changed, but rather, how they have been weighted. Suddenly, we just know the wrong or right thing to do. This requires a repeated reflection process that just keeps on entering our reasons into emotional loops, until a point is reached at which we just feel what is right. The emotional decision produces a subjective feeling of certainty, which, in turn, prevents us from starting to deliberate all over again. And finally, making responsible decisions is something that must be *learned*. We are not born with it and it requires practice, by making concrete decisions and shouldering the consequences, that is, by *accepting* responsibility. To make a correct decision would then be something like recognizing a pattern in the mesh of various factors. And neuronal networks are particularly good at recognizing patterns. But pattern recognition only works when the network has been trained with a wide selection of samples; when it has gone through similar situations and thereby gained specific, in the case of human brains presumably individual, weightings for the connections. Experience and life's wisdom become indispensable advisors and are effective through our feelings.

My answer to the regress problem can thus be stated: Regress of ever higher leveled volitions is terminated when a person emotionally identifies with her self-representations. The emotional balance of our decisions depends on the body-self, but it can also occur in higher-level models of the self (cf. Metzinger 1993). Somatic markers, for instance, connect decisions with autobiographical key experiences, and linguistically represented models of the self, as well as narrative models of the self can be included in the identification process. Nonetheless, all models of the self are founded on our neuronal body-self. It is, so to say, the matrix upon which the cognitive content of one's self is written.[107] Decisions made in this way are not just any decisions. They are authentic, because they were made using pattern recognition processes that take place based on the neuronal body-self and are thereby connected to the individual history of the person and all her deeply anchored emotions.

A neurophilosophical theory of authenticity can help us to understand when it is that we consider decisions and actions to be *personal*, that is, when we justifiably attribute them to the active person. If a person makes a decision in line with what she has previously experienced, done, or decided up until this time, then we do feel justified in saying that this decision was a decision of that person, it is *hers*. For what does a person consist of, if not the totality of her dispositions and experiences, which presents itself as a whole in every new moment? Frankfurt correctly titled his basic work "Freedom of will and the concept of a person." We would certainly have a strange idea of what it means to be a person if we would not attribute a decision to a person, when that decision (ideally) is fully in line with what that person thinks, feels, and has done in her life so far. In fact, the neurophilosophical theory of authenticity well satifies two classical criteria for discerning the identity of persons: physical (bodily) criteria and psychological criteria (continuity and connectedness of mental states).[108]

Of course, this does not mean that our emotions can always help us to arrive at clear decisions. It can happen, and it certainly does, that somatic markers do not indicate a clear route. Many decisions that people make are just not authentic, they are the result of pressures, like time, or random factors, and so on. But I did not claim that human decisions are always authentic. I was interested in the question of what it means that one's decisions are *one's own*, and how a theory of authenticity can help us to understand that.

3.4.2 Moral Sentiments   Personal ascription and feelings also play an important role in moral decisions. Opposed to the traditional concept of responsibility as influencing future behavior, we can see that in everyday situations we mean more by responsibility than just the addressee of measures for change. In particular, the fact that we also attribute misbehavior to other persons does not seem to be captured by the traditional concept. An argument proposed by Sabini and Silver (1987) is of interest in this context. They suggest that our evaluations of other people depend on the fact that they are emotionally susceptible in a way that cannot be controlled. While rational arguments and reasons are easy to manipulate and can be used to deceive others, our sentiments are difficult to control. Therefore, they reveal something about the person and her character. Based on those sentiments, say Sabini and Silver, our judgments of people, are more of an aesthetic than an ethical nature. Although an ethical judgment justifies condemning and punishing a person, aesthetic judgments do not justify those kind of consequences. But they might justify that we avoid a certain person, that we warn friends about her, and that we hope our children will not become like her.

I think that emotions are more important for a theory of moral behavior than Sabini and Silver will admit. For just as daily decisions based solely on rational deliberations are often not prudent and often detrimental, moral behavior without sentiments is also hard to imagine. As Strawson (1962) correctly noted, moral values exhibit an analogy to reactive personal feelings. If someone malevolently and purposefully injures me, I do resent it. That is a natural psychological reaction, independent of any ruminations on determinism. A moral value is similar to this kind of personal reaction. Moral disapproval is analogous to taking offense, one feels offended in place of that other person who was insulted, or whose rights were violated. Strawson considers the practice of giving moral praise or showing disapproval not as purely a means for controlling another's behavior, but as an expression of our nature as persons. Just as moral values, reactive personal attitudes (praise, blame, love, and so on) belong in a network of quasi transcendental conditions of human communion, which we cannot simply dispose of. It is unfortunate, that "talk of moral sentiments has gone out of fashion" (Strawson 1962, p. 231). I take this as a plea for a new evaluation of theories about moral sentiments, as advocated by Hume. The poor reputation of these kinds of theories is, in my opinion, the result of placing feelings at a subjective opposite pole to rational thinking. Meanwhile, we have seen how misleading this notion is.

The theory of somatic markers can explain various kinds of decisions in which reason alone does not lead us toward clear decisions, situations in which after rationally evaluating all our reasons we still do not know what we should do. These are precisely the choice situations for which the libertarian demands free will (van Inwagen 1989, pp. 233ff): Situations in which our reasons for alternative strategies are equally important, situations in which there is a conflict among obligations and penchants (long term interests and short term desires), and situations in which we must decide from among incompatible values. All these decisions contain an irrational element that determines our action preferences. These are based on feelings about what is right to do in a given situation. Our choice is not derived from behavioral principles based on highly moral basic principles, it is derived from our experience in solving moral conflicts. Sentiments cannot replace rationality or reflection, but they can assist in reaching a decision. The example with the VM patients has shown how rationality without emotional attachments can lead to detrimental and irresponsible behavior.

The economist Frank (1992) had similar ideas, although seen from an entirely different perspective. He argues against the model of subjectively expected utility. That model can hardly explain the kind of altruistic behavior people exhibit in situations in which, according to the model, it would be rational not to be cooperative. Why do people often not cheat, although they can be certain that no one will notice it? Why do we want justice to win, even when bygone injustice will not be amended by that? Why do people say the truth, even though it brings them tremendous disadvantages? In general; why do people *want* to act morally, even when, according to the model of personal utility, there are no rational reasons for doing so? Frank's reply is that their moral sentiments have determined this behavior. According to the model an honest person is someone who values trustworthiness *for itself*. He is not interested in the fact that he could have material gains by changing his attitude. Exactly because he does have this attitude, he can be trusted in situations in which his behavior cannot be controlled. Someone who has scruples about cheating will do it less often, whether he wants to have those scruples or not. Feelings are thus better for fixing morals, because it is difficult to influence them willingly and normally they are hard to hide. So they make our attitudes readily visible to others. Frank argues that emotion attachments are therefore the basis for mutual trust, predictability, and assessment. This does not mean that reflection and rationality are useless. Purely rational considerations might also lead us to the conclusion that it is wrong to cheat. But who do we trust more, someone who abhors cheating or someone who does not cheat because it has disadvantages?

There is another argument for the indispensability of moral feelings (P. S. Churchland 1995). It appeals to the fact that moral behavior must be learned. Aristotle himself pointed out that there is a relationship between habits and self-control. Whether we learn to deal with the world, to delay small gains in favor of long term success, to find appropriate forms of expression for anger and sympathy, or to show courage depends on whether we acquire appropriate decision-making habits. Expressed in the jargon of dynamical system theory, we must model the terrain of the neuronal phase space such that the appropriate behavioral trajectories are deeply engraved. We learn moral concepts like "just" and "unjust," "good" and "bad" when, as children, we are confronted with prototype samples, and because of our capacity for pattern recognition, we can also apply these concepts to new situations. It seems to be necessary for learning moral concepts that the basic circuits for emotions are intact. Prototypical situations in which there are unmoral acts provoke uncomfortable feelings of fright, concern, or sympathy. While simple situations can be ordered without the help of evaluative feelings, more complex scenarios require more than just applying rules to situations. We acquire moral education not just in practical life. Tales and stories also play an important role, accounts in which imagination and empathy, the ability to put oneself in the other's shoes, are prerequisites for understanding the point of the story properly (Johnson 1993). In other words, moral learning requires the simulation of counterfactual situations with emotional adjustment. Moral decision-making is a *practical* skill. It is less like mathematical calculation, and more like exercising an occupation. Six years of studying medicine by the books does not make a good physician, just as purely rational considerations do not make us morally reasonable people. Textbook knowledge and moral principles are helpful, but are of little use without practical experience. In this sense, moral feelings are probably indispensable indicators in moral conflict situations. They do not replace reflection, but we must have them, if they are to help us achieve morally established behavior.

These thoughts show why a realistic theory of natural autonomy is important for moral issues. If we want our fellow humans to act morally, we must also take their neuronal "design" into consideration. Moral philosophy that neglects moral psychology may, perhaps, be valuable for philosophical conventions, but not for practical living (see also Flanagan 1991).

3.5   Natural Autonomy and Responsibility

We now approach the completion of my exposition. I have analyzed all three components of the concept of free will and tried to find out how they are compatible with what we know about the brain. The result is disillusioning. For free will, as it is traditionally conceived, things look pretty sober. The notions that under identical circumstances we could do other than we actually do, that we simultaneously act for understandable reasons, and that we ourselves are the source of our actions, are, taken together, an illusion. The point can be argued not only philosophically, but also neurophilosophically. Indeterminism, for all we know, plays no role in brain mechanisms. Reason is not an instance floating about our brain, but a capacity due to certain brain mechanisms, involvement with the environment, and the development of public language. Self-determined behavior is not a result of rational considerations, instead we learn to make clever and socially responsible decisions with the aid of our emotions. When we possess all these skills, we have natural autonomy. What implications does this have for the concept of responsibility?

There is no "ultimate responsibility" of the kind postulated by libertarians. In a deterministic universe, no one can be absolutely responsible for the kind of person he or she is. The fact that there are also undetermined events in our world does not change that. Because no one, in any sense of the word, is responsible for undetermined events. Ultimate responsibility is a libertarian illusion. But, as I have repeatedly emphasized, we cannot conclude that the concept of responsibility is meaningless or that all moral order breaks down. We must, however, revise the concept of responsibility. In this work I have dealt with free will as a challenge to natural philosophy, not as an ethical issue. But any revision of the concept of responsibility is also always a challenge to ethics, because the revised concept might not be compatible with moral theory.[109] I have not tackled the task of redefining the concept. But I would like to convey an idea of the kind of concept of responsibility that would be possible based on a theory of natural autonomy.

We are responsible when our actions ensue for reasons that are our own. It is necessary that we have a capacity to reflect and evaluate. But it is also necessary that we have some leeway, a certain degree of flexibility, and freedom, so that we consequently do not always behave according to a given scheme (a weak form of being able to do otherwise). Thinking is flexible and adaptive due to the mechanisms that have brought it forth. Through language we are in a position to also neuronally represent our norms and principles and include them in our reflections. And it is furthermore crucial to our moral behavior, whether or not we identify with our actions and decisions. Being emotionally fixed sometimes restricts dangerous cognitive flexibility and enables reliable social interaction. It is also a mechanism that makes our actions and decisions authentic and is thereby a basis for the personal attribution of decisions.

There is a second compatibilistic answer to the question of why we should hold others responsible. That is because doing so is the best strategy for encouraging them to behave morally. I suspect that this is one of the best reasons we can find. Of course, it is open to empirical criticism. Experience shows that the boundaries are not easily discovered for when the attribution of responsibility has desirable effects. The art of upbringing, for instance, lies in giving children just the right amount of responsibility that they can learn to accept, but not so much that they become overtaxed. In a mild form, this is also true for people with geriatric obstinacy, for the mentally ill who do not possess certain capacities, for healthy insecure persons, and for people in many other situations. Whether attributing responsibility is always the best strategy for producing moral behavior would need to be proven for each individual case. But there is no time for that. We don't know enough; defining boundaries is difficult and to a degree arbitrary; feeble-mindedness can be precisely diagnosed only in clear cases. Whatever reasons we accept as excuses, I suspect, depends on the question of being able to do otherwise in similar circumstances. Research on the phenomena of weak will and impulse control would be relevant for that issue. But granting responsibility is not solely a means for controlling behavior. It includes a theory of what it means to take a person seriously. When we acknowledge that other people have natural autonomy, we grant them the right to found their decisions and actions on their *own* convictions and values. Desiring to be treated this way also implies a willingness to accept the sanctions justified by a concept of natural autonomy.

4   Conclusion

Synopsis

Free will, in the libertarian sense of the word, does not exist. We can do justice to many libertarian intuitions, however, with a neurophilosophical concept of autonomy that includes mild forms of all three components. New is the emphasis on the fact that being able to do otherwise is nonlinear. The insight is that human action and volition can be understood by a theory in which there is no room for rationality dualism, but which does make reference to the past, a theory that also acknowledges that secondary emotions are indispensable for authentic and socially responsible actions. The illusions involved in the libertarian variety of free will are presumably as intractable as optical illusions. But now we can explain what the evidence in its favor actually implies. What remains is a kind of autonomy, that, loyal to a naturalistic approach, I call *natural autonomy*.

In chapter 1 we discussed, rearranged, and analyzed the challenge of free will as it is dealt with in contemporary analytical philosophy of mind. We saw that it is not one isolated, but a series of several interwoven perplexities. I proposed that each of the most important philosophical theories on free will contains at least one of three components: *the ability to do otherwise, the condition of being understandable (intelligibility),* and *the postulate of agency.* These components were demonstrated using Kant's theory of freedom. They are best understood as fundamental intuitions about the human free will used for general orientation by all theorists. Various theories can be set up by combining the three components in varying degrees.

Many studies on free will emphasize our capacity to do otherwise, which is the issue of whether or not and how behavioral alternatives are open to us. The debate pivots on whether determinism and freedom to do otherwise are compatible (compatibilism) or not (incompatibilism). Acknowledging its significance, we took a closer look at determinism. We were particularly interested in whether contemporary physics is deterministic. It is probably not. Two surprising outcomes resulted from that analysis. First, contrary to traditional notions, Newton's physics and the theories of particles in specific relativity theory are not necessarily deterministic. Second, at the quantum level, quantum mechanics is a deterministic theory. The indeterminism of quantum theory manifests itself at the transition from the quantum level to the classical level of physics.

In contrast to other work in this field, we also gave the other components of free will their due. This was necessary for more than one reason. First, several arguments in the debate on alternativism usually implicitly refer to those components. It is questionable whether the components are compatible at all. Second, the nature of intelligibility is a problem for deterministic and indeterministic theories alike. Third, the component of agency is more pressing for issues concerning responsibility and personal ascription than is generally acknowledged.

After clarifying concepts, I asked whether there is free will in the sense meant by libertarianism. We understand libertarianism to be the thesis that there exists a form of free will that simultaneously satisfies all three components in their strong interpretations. We apposed, discussed, and evaluated the most important relevant arguments. The consequence argument and the intelligibility argument are central for our outcome. There is no free will in the libertarian sense, because it is compatible with neither determinism nor indeterminism. The notion of noncausally determined rationality was important for the self-refutation argument. We outlined the logic of arguments from moral philosophy and demonstrated formally why the idea that there is no such thing as responsibility does not necessarily follow from the nonexistence of libertarian free will.

As incompatibilists, libertarians nevertheless continue to believe that indeterminism, which they find indispensable, must be compatible with the other components. Compatibilist theories can be understood as combining mild versions of one or more of the three components. However, if we dilute the components enough, then the existential claim becomes trivially true. But we do not want to answer the question of the nature of free will purely by definition. We want to test whether and how we can soften those components, so that they can be realized in our world.

This requires that we include empirical findings. The task of a naturalistic theory of free will consists, among other things, of testing which components must be weakened in which way for empirical reasons, and which unnecessary censures we can avoid.

In chapter 2 I introduced the approach of neurophilosophy. We understand it as a bridge discipline between neurosciences and philosophy. There are two ways of doing it. For one, neurophilosophy *utilizes* neuroscientific findings for solving philosophical problems, or at least for making them easier to apprehend. That is the approach taken here. On the other hand, neurophilosophy is concerned with philosophical issues that arise within neuroscience itself. After first introducing the historical precursors to neurophilosophy, explaining the mind-body problem, and reductionism, we took a closer look at two neurophilosophical theories: Maturana's neurobiological constructivism and the Churchlands' eliminative materialism. Both forfeit plausibility for the sake of radicalness. They do, however, contribute new impulses to neurophilosophy. Constructivism gives us ideas on biological self-organization and eliminative materialism is linked to connectionism (the theory of neuronal nets). We discussed connectionism and its central problem of compositionality somewhat extensively, because it is so important for neurophilosophy.

Finally, after some systematic reflections, I outlined a program of *Minimal Neurophilosophy*. Minimal neurophilosophy is based on the conviction that mental states rest on (are realized by) brain processes and that therefore, by studying brain processes we can learn something about mental states and free will. This minimal strategy was motivated by two findings. First, metaphysical background assumptions are so drastically different for various neurophilosophies that those variants deny each other's advantages—an unfavorable circumstance for gaining knowledge at all. Second, it is not clear at all whether one and the same physical relation can be assumed to be valid for all mental states. There is the serious option that different mental states exhibit different kinds of relations to physical states (thesis of differential metaphysics). I propose that we choose the relation of supervenience of mental states on physical states as an appropriate point of departure for a neurophilosophy of the free will. We introduced and discussed that concept, as well as the concept of emergence. We also traversed the problem of mental causation and explained what it means to hold mental causation for supervenient causation. We acknowledged the problem of explanatorily reducing the supervenience of mental states to physical states. Finally, we outlined the notion of naturalism that underlies neurophilosophy.

In chapter 3 we used neurophilosophy to analyze all three components. The purpose of this analysis was to find out how much of the strong interpretations of those components we must skim off in order to formulate a neurophilosophically plausible theory of autonomy. To get there, I had to sketch a neurophilosophical theory of the mental, because without such a theory it is impossible to say anything about the specific features of mental processes that are pertinent to free will. Let me, once again, attempt to coherently explain the outcome of that analysis.

We need indeterminism for a strong interpretation of being able to do otherwise. Going by contemporary physics, it should be of a quantum-physical nature. An examination of the oldest (Pascual Jordan) and the most recent (Roger Penrose and Stuart Hameroff) theories of this kind shows that there is no convincing evidence that quantum mechanical events play any crucial role in brain processes (and therefore not for mental processes); there are, in fact, good neurophilosophical arguments to the contrary. A milder form of being able to do otherwise under *almost* identical circumstances, on the other hand, is empirically plausible. This is supported by nonlinear, chaotic systems dynamics of the brain. The advantage that chaotic brain processes bring for a theory of autonomy is that it does not succumb to the intelligibility argument as easily as those theories relying on absolute chance as found in quantum mechanics. This is because certain chaotic ordering states can serve as a physical basis for behavior-guiding neuronal representations, in spite of their sensitivity.

If deterministic chaos should, in fact, turn out to be a ubiquitous phenomenon within the nervous system, that would explain why we can make different choices in similar situations. It would explain why even in comparable situations we do not always take the same path, explain how we keep natural alternatives open and why our thinking is so flexible. It would also explain why the subjective impression of being able to do otherwise seems so irrefutable. Often enough, we do experience a feeling that in comparable situations we would act differently, although we cannot always explain it rationally. Not only can chaotic processes help explain quasi indeterministic capacities to act otherwise and flexibility; under certain conditions they also produce stable and predictable behavior. Part of our predictable behavior is presumably within the realm of intermittence—in a realm of order in the midst of chaos.

Intelligibility (the term I chose to mean "understandable actions due to reasons") is the most difficult, and traditionally, the least discussed component of free will. It is closely connected to the problem of intentional causation, that is, the question of how reasons can be causally effective. For the dualist, mankind belongs to a second, intelligible world. This creates the problem of how that world can be causally effective within the first, and natural, world. In connection with the concept of consciousness, the second component is often taken as evidence for the notion that free decisions are not predetermined by past events, but made with the assistance of reason. On the other hand, indeterminism is hardly compatible with a notion of intelligible behavior. So, without introducing rationality dualism, it is difficult to theoretically apprehend intelligibility. The only alternative is to design a naturalistic theory of intelligibility. This is achieved by first adopting a naturalistic theory of meaning. The neurophilosophical thesis runs like this. Neuronal states gain their semantic content, their meaning, from being embedded in nature. I outlined this kind of theory as *adaptive neurosemantics*. It rests on the notion of teleosemantics. Teleosemantics traces semantic content back to the concept of proper function, and this, in turn, back to an evolutionary, or evolution-analogous process. The meaningfulness of physical structures (organs, kinds of behavior, natural signs, structures of knowledge) is not only compatible to being determined by past events; it actually depends on it. I thoroughly explained, and rejected, criticism directed at the notion of proper function.

In order to do justice to human flexibility and adaptation capacities, the theory requires some supplement. We examined whether and how selection processes in time spans shorter than phylogenic ones play a role. Based on this idea, I sketched the framework of *adaptive neurosemantics*. We showed that different theories of brain function contain ultrafast selection processes as central elements of cognitive mechanisms.

Neuronal states, however, do not contain meaning by themselves, just due to their structure. Not only its history, but also the fact that an organism is embedded in its environment is an absolutely essential factor for a neurosemantic theory of meaning (active externalism). It follows that intentional states supervene not only on brain states, but on brain states plus portions of their history and the environment relative to the system. Since neurosemantics explains why that is the case, we have thus achieved an explanatory reduction of the supervenience relation. Expressed in philosophical jargon. Intentional causation is superdupervenient causation.

I have further shown how language and thinking mutually affect each other via their physical manifestations (written language and the brain) in a way that enables rational intelligibility. Just as we can only understand a fish's capacity to swim by understanding the medium—water—in which it swims, we can understand the intelligibility of human behavior through its embeddedness in the medium of public language.

Finally, we made an amazing discovery. Chance plays an important role in adaptive neurosemantics, as a generator of variability. This, however, does not provide an argument that absolute chance plays a constitutive role. First, quasi chance can also generate the required variability. Second, arguments against the factual importance of absolute chance (indeterminism) in the brain remain untouched by this. And third, randomly generated variability is not self-caused.

In conclusion, I analyzed and evaluated some neurophilosophical hypotheses from empirical scientists on free will. Libet's well-discussed experiments on readiness potential are based not only on an inadequate theory of consciousness, but also on a naive, workaday notion of mental causation. They have little to say on free will. Other scientists try to correlate the free will with certain parts of the brain, like the prefrontal cortex or the anterior cingulate. Some of those hypotheses actually do suit a theory of natural autonomy, but on the whole, we must view attempts to localize the free will skeptically. They need to be woven into a comprehensive theory of human action and decisions. A central role in that could be taken on by a neurophilosophically plausible theory of agency.

For the component called agency, I discussed the most important theories of incompatibilism and compatibilism. We reject the incompatibilistic theory of *agent causation* that views agency as origination through the agent alone. *Hierarchical compatibilism* centers around the concept of *identification*. That is the process through which a person makes her volitions *her own*. This, according to neurophilosophical arguments, does not in fact—as the theory assumes—happen purely rationally, but rather, it is the result of essentially *emotional* mechanisms. An emotional break-off mechanism solves the regress problem of traditional identification theories. There are concrete neurobiological hypotheses about this mechanism. The dorsolateral section of the frontal cortex is important in simulating future counterfactual situations. The ventromedial section admits mental sample actions into the evaluation circuit. This circuit joins emotional centers, the body, and its neuronal representation. Changes in the body's state and the secondary emotions associated with that contain a subjective, experience-dependent evaluation aspect. Emotionally fixed points thus prevent purely rational reflection from ending in a regress. We can describe the process of emotional identification as a cognitively nontransparent, but economical and efficient test for whether actions are consistent with one's own past. It thus fulfills the function of a self-compatibility-test. I suggest to call this kind of agency *authenticity*. Presumably, the neuronal body-image is a necessary basis of a self-model, in which, during the course of a lifetime, other, more sophisticated cognitive models of the self become integrated.

Based on this kind of a theory of authenticity we can justify personally attributing actions and decisions. Namely, when a person not only rationally reflects her actions and their consequences, but also takes possession of them as a person with a particular history and experience. This idea is compatible with the notion that a person's history is due to events from the distant past. We should not characterize persons based on their capacity to originate actions, but on the capacity to combine their current state and their history to make a coherent whole. Secondary emotions in the form of moral sentiments could play an important part in morally relevant decisions.

I want to summarize the idea of natural autonomy in one sentence. We possess natural autonomy when under very similar circumstances we could also do other than we actually do (because of the chaotic nature of our brain). This choice is understandable (intelligible—it is determined by past events, by immediate adaptation processes in the brain, and partially by our linguistically formed environment), and it is authentic (when through reflection loops with emotional adjustments we can identify with that action). This kind of autonomy suits a compatibilistic concept of responsibility and supplements it in some areas.

Some features of natural autonomy are easily recognizable; they have repeatedly played an important role in the course of our discussion: the feedback principle, externalism and history. Let us, once again, emphasize this. Feedback is important in all three components. Chaos, for instance, arises in mathematics when simple, nonlinear equations contain terms that are repeatedly multiplied with themselves. This means that the result on one calculation enters the result of the next calculation in a nonlinear way. The brain physically realizes this principle. It exhibits an extremely high degree of positive and negative feedback. While discussing intelligibility I mentioned several neuronal models relevant for ultra fast adaptations: Edelman's *reentrant loops*, Mumford's *Ping Pong System*, and Changeux and Dehaene's *mental Darwinism*. Crucial to all these models is that a subsystem's neural activity serves as input for another subsystem, after which the altered activity is reentered into the system. According to the hypothesis of evolutionary theory of knowledge, reflection is sample action in mental space. Using these models, we can now make this hypothesis more precise. Reflection is the simulation of counterfactual situations tested in several feedback loops. The fact that neuronal states can simulate situations, that is, that they can *mean* something, is explained by neurosemantics. Rational thinking is distinguished by the fact that the representations used in the simulation process are explicit (Millikan's expression). To put it colloquially; they are conscious. In a catchword, we know what we do. In explicit reflection (feedback between the prefrontal cortex and the other brain areas), mentally simulated scenarios of decision situations are not only tested for logical consistency and compatibility with internal and external standards.

Above all, they are made self-compatible, which brings us now to the third component. Repeated reentry into the body-loop and the as-if-loop makes decisions authentic. That does not mean that we begin new causal chains of events with such decisions. It means merely that they are made consistent with ourselves, as the persons we have historically come to be.

Another element of particular importance for a neurophilosophical theory of autonomy is that of externalism. Neuronal processes are not purely internal or structurally determined processes in the way that the theory of autopoiesis assumes. This became obvious in the thesis of dynamical cognitive science, in which the idea that cognitive mechanisms are tightly linked to the environment plays an important role. The more reliable the invariances of an environment are, the more a cognitive system can afford to be flexible and fluid. Adaptive neurosemantics is also externalistic. Having meanings depends on using meaningful structures for specific purposes, as well as on interaction with the system in which a thing is embedded. In the same way, active externalism says that the way a brain currently behaves depends on external matters. Even the evaluation loop providing authenticity is connected to actions and the experience that results therefrom.

The history factor became most obvious for the theory of adaptive neurosemantics. In this case, meaningfulness is traced back to the history of the origin of a structure in a process analogous to evolution. But even the chaotic way a brain functions, exhibits an historical aspect. Since the behavior of chaotic systems cannot always be predicted, in the end they can only be controlled by learning to regulate the control parameters in such a way that the behavior they produce is appropriate. A well-adapted chaotic system can only acquire fine-tuning through learning processes, which, in turn, also help to explain current behavior. And the same holds for the concept of authenticity. We need the backgrounds or our individual biographies in order to acquire more and more authenticity. Taken together, control, meaning, and authenticity are properties that must unfold, such that an individual possesses them *as* an individual, and not just as a representative member of his species.

Natural autonomy, let it be said once more, is even possible in an entirely determined world. Nonetheless, an indeterministic world somehow is more appealing. The thought, that our futures are not already fixed has something comforting about it, even though we cannot precisely describe what that is. This also seems to be true when freedom is not within reach. Even absolute chance can be a valuable ally. As externalism and the history factor demonstrate, indeterministic events need not be located in the brain in order to decisively influence our mental states. That doesn't support a libertarian theory of free will. But if it is a fear of a deterministically fixed block world that drives us into the arms of libertarian illusions, the ideas worked out here may help us to accept a more realistic theory of natural autonomy.

Notes

Preface

1. Odo Marquard holds this opinion: The only office left for philosophy is that of explaining its own incompetence. Formerly, philosophy was an all-encompassing science. In the course of history it lost competence to individual sciences (Marquard 1981: 23–28).

Chapter 1

1. See Kane 1996, p. 13, and Dennett 1981, pp. 286f.

2. A Libertarian (Latin *liber*, free) is the philosophical term for someone who believes in a strong version of the freedom of will.

3. Prauss 1983 and Allison 1990 discuss Kant's philosophy of freedom; see also Funke 1990, Schroeter 1993, Stekeler-Weithofer 1990 and essays in Part IV of Schönrich + Kato 1996.

4. This moral law, also known as "categorical imperative" reads in its simplest wording: "Act according to a maxim which can also make itself a universal law" (Kant 1786/1983: BA 81; alternative formulations can be found at BA 52, BA 67/68, BA 82).

5. An overview of the relevant discourse up until about 1978 is given in Pothast 1978, 1980. A recommended introduction on the subject is in Patzig 1994 or Honderich 1995. A good survey of the more recent discussion can be found in Fischer 1994 and Kane 1996.

6. Seebass considers freedom, volition, and agency the three ultimate components. His book *Wollen*, however, is an intricate language analysis for volition, which I will not pursue further here.

7. A comprehensive analysis of volition can be found in O'Shaughnessy 1980; Seebass 1992 discusses volition in detail. See also Kane 1996, and section 3.1. in this chapter.

8. This kind of argument is also known as the defiant argument, cf. Steinvorth 1995, pp. 413–415.

9. As we shall see later, however, some—particularly political—philosophers do define the freedom of will in this weak sense as a freedom from foreign coercion.

10. Austin claims that determinism is at best a "term for nothing distinct" (cited in Pothast, 1978, p. 195), Gerent (1993: 41) considers a detailed discussion on determinism unnecessary and Strawson (1989) declares that the issue of determinism is unimportant for the question of the freedom of will. I do not share this opinion. But I do agree with these authors that by discussing determinism we cannot exhaustively meet the challenge of the freedom of will.

11. For the history of the concept of determinism, see Frey 1971, therein also the reference to Snell.

12. Predeterminedness differs from determinedness in that *someone* fixes the course taken.

13. Luther thought that our moral decisions are determined, but our daily decisions (whole wheat cereal roll or croissant) on the contrary are free.

14. Kant 1789/1983, B 473; Ayers 1968; Anscombe 1981, p. 141; von Wright 1974, p. 21; Taylor 1974, p. 115; van Inwagen 1986, p. 3; Watson 1992a; Pothast 1980, p. 42; Seebass 1993, p. 1; Gerent 1993, p. 42.

15. There are basically two different strategies for handling these concepts. The normal strategy, which we intend to adhere to here for the most part, is to go along with the definition of these terms as they occur in current physics, the recognized fundamental science. The other strategy considers the acceptance of these concepts responsible for the problem of free will. Some philosophers go so far as to assume that everyday psychological usage of these terms is more fundamental than that of physics, for example, the concept of causation. This will become apparent in our discussion of mental causation.

16. Using this we can distinguish between various types of determinism. Edwards (1967) distinguishes between ethical, logical, theological, physical, and finally psychological determinism; Pothast (1980) counts seven variations of determinism.

17. In Laplace, P. S., *A philosophical essay on probabilities,* quoted in Gerent 1993, p. 3.

18. An informative exposition can be found in Buschlinger 1993, p. 98–110.

19. The distinction between historic and futuristic determinism can be found in Earman 1986, p. 13; the distinction between postdictive and predictive determinism can be found in Koch 1994, p. 100.

20. To be precise, relativistic *field* theories *are* deterministic; they are even the best example of deterministic theory in physics. Relativistic *particle* theories are not deterministic, if tachyons exist and the Minkowski space-time cone is pervious.

21. For example, when we assume the existence of a Cauchy surface for the class of all physically possible worlds (Earman, 1986, p. 183).

22. See Penrose 1991, pp. 322–338.

23. We cannot, however, save determinism in the micro-world without giving up something else. We *can* formulate a deterministic interpretation of quantum mechanics; but to do so we must sacrifice so-called locality. A vivid explanation of theses connections is given in Koch 1991.

24. According to Double, Chisholm, Taylor, von Inwagen, Campbell, and Kant are non-valerian libertarians, while Dennett, Kane, and he himself are valerians.

25. At most, this argument cannot be applied to the very first selection of a *daimon*. But then there is the question of how the soul came to exist at all. If it has been created by God, then it is not free either (see Horn 1996, p. 117).

26. For a detailed discussion on the highly faceted concept of will in the history of philosophy and psychology please refer to the specialized books and essays such as O'Schaugnessy 1980; Dihle 1985; Heckhausen, Gollwitzer, and Weiner 1987; Seebass 1992; and von Cranach and Foppa 1996.

27. The general difference of these traditions is that the first held intentionality to be a phenomenon of consciousness (Husserl, Heidegger, Sartre, Merleau-Ponty), and the second placed more emphasis on the mutual aspects the term has with language (Russell, Chisholm, Sellars, Quine). A survey can be found in Bechtel 1988a, pp. 40–78; see also Searle 1983.

28. Quote taken from Dennett, 1984, p. 21. Dr. Bramhall, Bishop of London-derry was a Libertarian and opponent to Thomas Hobbes.

29. If we knew more about consciousness we could define intelligibility as follows: A person acts intelligibly when he is capable of being conscious of future circumstances (conscious of alternatives and their consequences), is conscious of the decision-making situation itself (reflective consciousness), and consciously realizes one alternative action for particular reasons.

30. Representatives of causal action views, for example, Carl G. Hemp, Alvin Goldman, Paul Churchland, Robert Audi, and, in a wider sense, Donald David-son. While the first group attempts to explain human action similarly to phenomena in natural science with deductive-nomological methods, Davidson's theory of anomal monism refutes strict laws for actions.

31. This view developed from Wittgenstein's late philosophy and from the debate on explanation in the social sciences.

32. Cf. Röska-Hardy 1995, pp. 267f. Representatives of an anticausal view of action are Elizabeth Anscombe, Abraham I. Melden, Anthony Kenny, George Henrik v. Wright, and Charles Taylor, among others.

33. This conclusion is nothing other than the basic structure of the theodicy problem. Streminger (1992) deals with it in detail.

34. Compare the Roman legal maxim: *Ultra posse nemo obligatur* (Do not ask more of someone than he is capable of doing). The original version (Celsus in

Corpus iuris civilis) exhibits even greater proximity to the issue discussed here: *Impossibilum nulla obligata est* (We are not obligated to do the impossible). Cf. Bartels and Huber 1981, p. 58, who find a similar thought as early as Herodot.

35. The philosopher of law Schünemann demonstrates that free will is not a prerequisite for all areas in German law. Civil law gets along without it. Public law is a more difficult case and German penal law is not thinkable without assuming free will (Schünemann 1997).

36. Court ruling of the Federal Court of Justice from March 18, 1952 (quote taken from Schreiber (1994, p. 5)), which deals with the issue from a psychiatric viewpoint. A survey of the relevant debate in the philosophy of law can be found in Pothast 1980, and particularly in Dreher 1987, which includes a detailed description of various positions with their representatives.

37. See Wilson 1979. For authors in the philosophy of law consult Pothast 1980 and Dreher 1987.

38. Not to confuse retaliation with atonement nor with revenge. Atonement is an evil accepted voluntarily by the wrongdoer, revenge is an individual need. Retaliation can be considered an instrument of reconciliation between society and the wrongdoer. The principle of retaliation fulfills functions that cannot be achieved by pure negative prevention. For example, it satisfies a population's feeling of justice. This function is also sometimes called positive general prevention. And finally, it gives us an idea of the principle of proper proportion of deed and punishment. See Ebert 1988 for a comprehensive debate on these topics. A survey of newer literature in English can be found in Ellis 1995.

39. Foremost we should mention Dennett here, who allots an entire chapter to the concept of control and self-control (Dennett 1984). Fischer subtitles his book *The Metaphysics of Free Will: An Essay on Control.* He distinguishes between absolute regulative control and *guidance control.* The later is compatible with determinism and would render responsibility possible. (Fischer 1994, pp. 160–189).

40. Similar to Wilson 1979, who organizes the consequences of determinism into four categories: Human self-concepts; responsibility, praise, rebuke, and excuse; interpersonal attitudes; and social institutions. A marked difference is Honderich's emphasis on the concept of knowledge, which we will return to when discussing the argument for self-contradiction.

41. A large portion of the American attitude toward life is based on this illusion. When Frank Sinatra appeared before the audience in Madison Square Garden on October 13th, 1974, to begin his much-quoted song *My Way,* he announced: "Ladies and Gentlemen, now I'm going to sing the *national anthem,* but—*you need not rise.*"

42. How often we really do act freely is quite controversial. See Albritton 1985/6, who claims that we always do, and Van Inwagen 1989, who claims that we very rarely do. Treatments of this claim can be found in Fischer and Ravizza 1992, with a reply in Van Inwagen 1994.

43. Strawson (1986, p. 5) distinguishes seven variants of compatibilism; see also O'Leary-Hawthorne and Pettit 1996, who discuss different compatibilistic strategies.

44. As I discovered after finishing this manuscript, in his newest book Double suggests that we recognize two further theories other than classic compatibilism and incompatibilism: theories that view free will as compatible with neither determinism nor indeterminism (*no-free-will-either-way-theory*), and theories that hold free will to be compatible with both determinism and indeterminism (*free-will-either-way-theory*) (see Double 1996, p. 101). The treatment for compatibility claims developed independently of Double in 6.2 in the end turns out to be a *no-free-will-either-way* argument.

45. Steinvorth 1995, pp. 413–415.

46. Perhaps our conviction that we possess free will is analogous to such a sensory illusion, which cannot be deceived by experience. Even if we *know* that we have no free will, we can hardly do otherwise than to *feel free* (see Searle 1986, chap. 6). This could be due to our emotionally familiar distinction between active doing and passive suffering.

47. Well-known and commonly used intuition pumps for the problem of free will are, for example, the drug addict (Frankfurt 1971), the physiologist who influences our volitions by pressing buttons (Taylor 1974, p. 50), the ruthless neuro-surgeon who manipulates us (Fischer 1982, p. 26), the hypnotist (Slote 1980, p. 137), the man from Mars who influences us by remote control (van Inwagen 1986, p. 109), and the cosmic child whose playthings we are (Lem 1980). Dennett (1984) discusses such thought experiments critically. See also Double 1991, pp. 31–62 and Buschlinger 1993.

48. Dennett (1984) thinks that it is the fear that is called forth by such thought experiments that is the real problem of the freedom of will.

49. The question of just what exactly an argument is, is particularly difficult for determinists to answer. Compare the discussion about the self-contradiction argument.

50. No confusion here. The traditional claim is that Christianity assumes free will and Islam is fatalist and thus determinist. But this generalization is incorrect. Christian Calvinism preaches predestination for salvation or damnation. God decides which fraction a person belongs to and *it is not within our power* to influence this. Orthodox Islam preaches determinism that correctly results from the concept of Allah as an absolute, omnipotent ruler and explains the fatalist attitude of many Moslems. But Moslem Kadarites, an unorthodox minority, deny this and teach the freedom of will (cf. von Glasenapp 1992, p. 326). Mediating theologians like al-Ash'ari tried to settle the difference by advocating the omnipotence of Allah and the freedom of man simultaneously—a feat that every theology student is similarly confronted with in the form of the theodicy problem.

51. The consequence argument has been supported by many authors: Ginet 1978; Wiggins 1973; van Inwagen 1975, 1986; and Fischer 1983, 1994. An

extensive bibliography for the consequence argument can be found in Fischer 1994, p. 219, footnote 10, and Kane 1989, p. 220, footnote 4.

52. Fischer (1994: 8) indexes N relative to a person and time.

53. Fischer clothes this statement in principles. The principle of the fixed past and the principle of fixed laws of nature. Van Inwagen and Fischer view things slightly differently. In contrast to van Inwagen, Fischer thinks that the principle of the fixed past and the principle of fixed laws of nature are sufficient for constructing an argument against compatibilism and that the transfer principle is not needed at all. He actually believes that these principles can be stated such that a "basal" version of the argument for incompatibilism results (cf. Fischer 1994: chap. 5). But these details are of little interest here.

54. Cf. Slote 1982; Hill 1992; Dennett 1986, pp. 111ff; Schnädelbach 1987, pp. 117ff; and Gerent 1993, pp. 217–223.

55. It was already known to Hobbes, Hume, and Schopenhauer (cf. Kane 1996, p. 229, footnote 1). Van Inwagen (1986, p. 16) calls it the *Mind* argument, because it has been dealt with so often in the philosophical quarterly with the same name (cf. Hobart 1934; Nowell-Smith 1948, 1954; and Smart 1961). It is a compatibilist's argument, but is discussed here because of the internal connection to the consequence argument.

56. This is an example of Double's so-called *free-will-neither-way theory* (see Double 1996, p. 101).

57. Naturally, libertarians try anyway to show how an indeterminist freedom of will could be intelligible. We will discuss these attempts later on.

58. Popper and Eccles 1977 offer substance-dualist arguments. Such arguments are also implicit in most Christian-oriented philosophical debates on free will. Immanuel Kant advocates reason dualism.

59. This important principle of scientific theory goes back to William of Ockham (approx. 1280–1347). It states that we should not accept pluralities without coercion. In other words, if we can explain something with one entity (one cause, one substance, one principle, etc.), then we should not add an additional different cause, substance, or principle to our explanation without having a *compelling* reason for doing so.

60. This argument has been brought forth by many philosophers, as we have seen earlier, even by Kant. The most important advocates in the twentieth century were Heinrich Rickert, Taylor, J. R. Lucas, Norman Malcolm, Chomsky, Alisdair MacIntyre, Snyder, Boyle/Grisez/Tollefsen, Popper/Eccles and Denyer (see Pothast 1980, pp. 258ff; Honderich 1990b, pp. 360ff, and Honderich 1995, pp. 112–116. Two variants of this type of argumentation, which emphasizes our epistemological limits, use Newcomb's Paradox (Schlesinger 1974) and Goedel's axioms for nonprovability (Lucas 1970) to prove the freedom of will (cf. Honderich 1990b).

61. The naturalistic fallacy is more well-known. It is the conclusion from purely descriptive statements to deontological or normative statements. The deonto-

logical fallacy is thus a reversed naturalistic fallacy. With the help of modern logic, Stuhlmann-Laiesz (1983) has demonstrated that both cases are actually invalid conclusions.

62. Double calls his theory *anarchistic* subjectivism, in order to contrast it with *universal* subjectivism, as in evolutionary ethics, for example, which claims the existence of subjective, but nonetheless shared moral properties.

63. Williams 1976/1984; Nagel 1976/1984; and Patzig 1994.

64. Patzig (1994) says that this argument expresses our lack of knowledge about the degree to which an action is an expression of the agent's character. Also see Richards 1986.

65. See Schlick 1930/1978; Hobart 1934; Nowell-Smith 1954; Smart 1961; Dennett 1986; Tugendhat 1987; and Nathan 1992.

66. See Davidson 1970a; Gerent 1993: 27–30; Charlton 1998; and Mele 1995: part I.

67. Problematic is the issue of just what exactly an inner force is.

68. Moore 1912/1970. Austin 1961 argues against Moore and for a categorial analysis of the ability to do otherwise. See Frankfurt 1988 for a conditional analysis of the second level. Watson 1982 offers a conditional analysis that includes values (cf. the argument of objective morals). See also Wolf 1980, 1990.

69. See Bergson 1888/1989; Planck 1936/1978; Hampshire and Hart 1958; McKay 1967/1978.

70. Many authors on epistemic indeterminism, however, do think that fundamental nonpredictability does imply indeterminism and thus makes determinism impossible. Thus McKay refers to corresponding theses in Popper 1950. However, this conclusion is false (see section 1 of chapter 2).

71. In his essay "Lösen die Naturwissenschaften das Leib-Seele-Problem?" (Can Natural Science Solve the Mind-Body Problem?) Tetens does not claim to argue against determinism or for free will; he is concerned solely with the empirical impossibility of behavior prognosis using measurements of brain states in general. See also Tetens 1994.

72. The regress argument can also be found in works of classic authors such as Hobbes, Locke, Hume, and Leibniz (see Seebass 1993, footnote 29). In analytical philosophy see Nowell-Smith 1954, pp. 286f; Kenny 1975, pp. 147f; Strawson 1986, pp. 28f; Shatz 1986, pp. 462–468.

73. Rosemarie Rheinwald (1990) gives a quite interesting retort to the regress argument. She concedes that the conditional solution leads to a hierarchy of continually higher-level, unreal conditional axioms. The higher we advance in this hierarchy, the less we *know* the determinant factors. They become increasingly less significant. Particularly in the case of apologetic reasons for behavior, they play an increasingly smaller part. Therefore, says Rheinwald, we can say that we are "freer" the longer the chain becomes between the action or choice in question and the determinant factors. Rheinwald sets up *epistemic* (Which

determinant factors are recognizable?) and *normative* (Up to which level do we expect and demand conditional freedom?) criteria with which we can evaluate whether an action is "free." Although this retort describes the actual usage of the word "free" fairly well, the decisive question for incompatibilists, namely whether we could have acted otherwise under identical circumstances, remains unanswered. A criticism is offered by Grewe 1994.

74. These forms of dualism are not as distinctly separable as this classification may make it seem. We could also add value theories. I will not consider property dualism with respect to phenomenal consciousness (Chalmers 1996a, 1996b), because in its present form it makes no contribution to a theory of the freedom of will.

75. See Taylor 1974; Chisholm 1978; Clarke 1993; and O'Connor 1995b.

76. Lucas 1993 claims that voluntary action must be uncaused; Ginet 1990 and McCall 1994 say that it must be either uncaused or indeterministic.

77. Kane 1985, 1988; Nozick 1981; and Clarke 1993 argue for this, and in a weaker version so does McCall 1994.

78. An affirmative answer is given by Eells 1991, a negative answer by Rosenberg 1992.

79. Nestor of these identification theories is Harry G. Frankfurt. See the collection of his essays up until 1987 in Frankfurt 1988 and 1992. Criticism of these approaches can be found in Shatz 1986.

80. See Watson 1987 and Scanlon 1988. Double 1991 sets up a theory like this only to show that it does not work.

81. See Fischer and Ravizza 1994 and Christman 1991, as well as his critic, Mele 1992.

82. Shatz (1988), who coined the term *valuational compatibilism* distinguishes value theories using another dimension, depending on whether values and valuations play a role in producing voluntary actions or whether responsiveness to values is decisive.

83. Our action is only free when it is founded on insight in moral law, so that "a free will and a will that follows moral laws become one and the same." (Kant 1786/1983, BA 98).

84. However, Wolf understands "being able to do otherwise" only as psychological indeterminism, which in turn is compatible with absolute determinism. Criticism on this position can be found in Watson 1992b and Shatz 1988, pp. 170f.

85. Valuation compatibilists of one type or the other are numerous. David Shatz mentions, among others, Paul Benson, Lawrence Davis, Daniel Dennett, Herbert Fingarette, John M. Fischer, Bernard Geert and Timothy Duggan, Jonathan Glover, Patricia Greenspan, Michael Levin, Alisdair MacIntyre, Wright Neely, and Robert Nozick. See Shatz 1988, p. 194, footnote 9.

Chapter 2

1. Once we start looking we even find concepts such as neuro-didactics (Preiss and Forster 1994) and neuro-theology (Ashbrook 1984). It probably won't be long until we have neurosociology or neuropolitics!

2. For the following, see particularly Oeser and Seitelberger 1988, pp. 1–49; Vogeley 1995, pp. 38–55; Popper in Popper and Eccles 1987, pp. 188–258; Doty 1965; Florey and Breidbach 1993; and Breidbach 1997.

3. In Phaedo (96–98) he also tells how Socrates—contemplating Anaxagoras' teachings—explains the difference between (physical) causes and (rational) reasons. We will return to this difference in chapter 3. Socrates asks what the cause is of his sitting in the dungeon. He refuses to think that the direct cause is the state of his bones and tendons. He sees the "real cause" in the decision of the Athenians who condemned him and in his decision to undergo that punishment.

4. The notion of a cooling aggregate in the brain is not as naïve as we might suppose. It is actually the case that deep within the brain a network of vessels, the so-called *sinus cavernosus* has this function (see Baker 1980).

5. The Persian doctor Avicenna (980–1037 A.D.) is supposed to have conjectured that there is an appendix between the first and the other two ventricles, which acts as a vent and when closed prevents sense perceptions and ideas from being processed by the brain or stored in memory.

6. See Hans-Peter Schütt *Rediscovering the Father of Philosophy (Die Wieder-entdeckung des Vaters der Philosophie)*, 1996. A reconstruction of Descartes' arguments for dualism can be found in Beckermann 1986.

7. The draft was first published posthumously. The first three sections (the fourth on resistance was never completed) had been jotted down in two notebooks and found among the papers of Freud's acquaintance and pen-friend Wilhelm Fleiss, after his death. See Sulloway 1982 for a description and discussion of the draft's content.

8. One might complain that this is already an inappropriate constraint on the mind-body problem. It is certainly a restriction, but not without reasons. It also does not exclude our widening the inquiry, if for example we should discover that the body or meta-individual things are absolutely necessary for theoretically understanding mental states.

9. For summaries of the mind-body problem in German, see Brüntrup 1996, Wiesendanger 1987, Metzinger 1985, Bunge 1984; and anthologies Bieri 1993, Warner and Szubka 1994, and Metzinger 1995.

10. Classic twentieth-century advocates are Popper and Eccles 1987, in German literature Seifert 1989. For watered-down dualism cf. Swinburne 1997. Recent years have seen dualism's resurgence: cf. Carrier and Mittelstraß 1989; Part V in Warner and Szubka 1994; Smythies and Beloff 1989; and Foster 1991.

11. C-fibers are nerve filaments (thin nerve threads without marrow sheaths) that conduct the activation of pain receptors in the periphery to the central nervous system.

12. Leibniz gives us two versions of the principle of indiscernibility. The onto-logical version says: "In nature there are never two beings, one of which is exactly like the other and for which it would not be possible to find an inner difference or a difference based on an inner difference" (Monadology § 9, Philosophical Writings VI, 608). The logical version states: "Identical are those [terms], for which one can be inserted for the other while retaining truth [i.e. truth values]" (*Specimen calculi universalis*, Philosophical Writings VII, 219). Mixing both ver-sions in a sentence about identity can be treacherous because the validity of logical identity can only be predicated when well-defined realms of objects ordered in individual entities can be assumed (quoted from Lorenz 1984, pp. 189f).

13. In his analysis of modal predicates Kripke (1972) opines that identity pred-icates can never be contingent; they must be necessarily true or false.

14. That mental events are not subject to strict laws follows from ideas about the holism of the mental, the indeterminacy of translation when attributing psy-chological properties, and the normative assumption of rationality (cf. Wiesen-danger 1987, pp. 211–235).

15. For a brief but good exposition of the problem cf. Stöcker 1992.

16. Bridge laws must not necessarily join laws together, they can also merely regularly connect concepts of two theories.

17. This is approximately what Kim means by *local* reductionism (cf. the species specific identity theory by Lewis 1989, p. 50). When we only have correlations for individual events (the token identity theorist's position), we can also speak of point-to-point reduction (cf. Stephan 1999).

18. There is Von Foerster and Von Glasfeld's radical constructivism, the theory of science constructivism in the Erlanger School, Piaget's constructivism, con-structive naturalism by Owen Flanagan, and much more.

19. We can name further sources. Constructivists make reference to findings in psychology, particularly Piaget's developmental psychology. But we should not be mislead by the attribute "constructivistic." Not every constructivism works as a fundament for *radical* constructivism. Piaget's theories, for example, are also used especially by *realistic* knowledge theorists.

20. All works are in German. *Über das Konstruieren von Wirklichkeiten*, von Foerster 1975; *Die erfundene Wirklichkeit*, Watzlawick 1975; *Die Kontrolle von Wahrnehmung und die Konstruktion der Realität*, Richards and von Glaserfeld 1984.

21. A survey of the spectrum of radical constructivism can be found in Schmidt 1987.

22. Young, by the way, also considers himself a neurophilosopher, as the title of his book reveals: J. Z. Young *Philosophy and the Brain*, 1989.

23. Maturana 1985, p. 17. For an up-to-date depiction of the neurophilosophy of color vision, see Zeki 1993. An exposition on the philosophical aspects of color vision can be found in the extraordinary monographs by Hardin 1988 and Thompson 1994.

24. According to Maturana, "structure" is the entirety of all relations among the parts of a system, which themselves are independent. "Organization" is the entirety of relations that define a system as a unit, without reference to the (material) peculiarity of the parts. The structure therefore can only be understood by observing the system, the organization only by considering its *function* with reference to the milieu (Maturana 1985, pp. 240f, 314f).

25. This thesis of state determination would let us suppose that Maturana must be a strict determinist. Surprisingly, he believes in free will, but his opinions on the issue are quite diffuse (Maturana 1985, pp. 269ff).

26. Actually this should be the consensual realm of the third order. But for unknown reasons Maturana does not continue numeration here.

27. This depiction only covers the part of the theory important for cognitive issues. Maturana draws extensive political and social conclusions from the relativity of knowledge. He thinks, for example, that his theory fortifies the individual and that dictatorships can be prevented by making theories subject-dependent (since dictatorships basically rest on an absolute claim to truth) and further, that if we would take his theory seriously, we could instate comprehensive liberty and democracy in the social world. (Taken from a lecture held at the NeuroWorlds Conference in Düsseldorf, 1994).

28. Another option would be a transcendental position along Kantian lines. Some constructivist's statements actually do sound rather like transcendental philosophy. But at work they always claim more than a standpoint in transcendental philosophy would allow.

29. Gerhard Roth (1994) tries to disperse this conflict by distinguishing between an "actual" (german: *wirklichen*) and a "real" (german: *realem*) brain. The *actual* brain is the brain as we construe it; the *real* brain is the one that is independent of our constructs. This distinction only conceals the difficulties of radical constructivism, instead of mastering them. As Roth correctly observes, one's evaluation of radical constructivism depends in the end on which epistemological position one advances. On those terms and in my opinion hypothetical realism still looks best.

30. The following exposition was taken from Mainzer 1995; Spitzer 1996, 1997 (in German); and Bechtel and Abrahamsen 1991, as well as Churchland and Sejnowski 1992.

31. In 1949 Canadian psychologist Hebb postulated a mechanism for altering synaptic transmission dependent on experience. Known as the "Hebb Rule," it states that the more often a connection is used, the stronger it becomes. In 1973 a mechanism of this type was first discovered in the brain, the long term potential (LTP). Initially this was described as being located in the hippocampus, but has been proved to be in the cortex. LTP occurs in glutamatergic synapses and

is transmitted via NMDA receptors. There is also proof of inhibitory connections among the output neurons in the biological brain that are realized there by gabaergic inter-neurons (cf. Spitzer 1997, pp. 23f).

32. It is characterized by error feedback to several layers within the network. In biological brains there is no equivalent for this algorithm, however. As a result, the significance that this algorithm has for connectionism furnishes evidence for doubt about whether some connectionist notions are applicable to neurobiology.

33. There are also critics among neurobiologists who point out that connectionistic networks are extremely different from real neural nets in the brain in many ways. Neurons are built differently; the brain is organized topologically; it has various forms of transmission; it knows no back propagation algorithm; and and so on. This is certainly correct. But first, some neuronal network models are being developed in a direction that strives to accommodate other properties of neurons as well, and second, this fact is irrelevant for the essential disagreement between symbol processing theorists and connectionists, which will be demonstrated in the following.

34. The discussion of rules is closely associated with the development of modern linguistics and thus with the work of Noam Chomsky. Chomsky supports the notion that there is a kind of innate language organ in the brain. Since language can generate an unlimited number of well-formed sentences, which obey a limited and relatively small number of grammatical rules, perhaps merely these construction rules are innate. This presumption is obviously contrary to the principle of connectionism that states that rules exist at best implicitly in the nets (cf. Pinker and Prince 1988; Clark 1991, pp. 161–176; Bechtel and Abrahamsen 1991, pp. 210–254).

35. The central texts of Smolensky on one side and of Fodor and Pylyshyn on the other, as well as additional replies and a summarized exposition can be found in MacDonald and MacDonald 1995, pp. 1–290; see also Chalmers 1993; van Gelder 1990, 1993. Summaries of the discussion are also given in Clark 1991, pp. 143–160; and Bechtel and Abrahamsen 1991, pp. 210–254.

36. These are the so-called tensor product representations. They are simply products of activity vectors. With parametric procedures it is possible to portray classic parse trees on superposition and tensor product vectors (for technical details see Smolensky in MacDonald and MacDonald 1995, chapters 4 and 6).

37. I understand neuroscience here very widely. It includes not only scientific neuro-disciplines, but also clinical subjects such as neurology and psychiatry.

38. Vollmer 1985, pp. 217–267, particularly pp. 236ff gives a definition of a "virtuoso" circle.

39. The controversial expression "metaphysics," disputed in meaning and usage, is used here more or less to denote "ontology." It serves as a name for that abstract part of philosophy concerned with what really exists and how what exists is distinguished from other things and how that is possible (see Hamlyn 1995, p. 556).

40. At least in analytic philosophy of mind. There are a few exceptions, such as Lyons (1980) and de Sousa (1987).

41. A possible objection to the thesis of differential metaphysics is that it is ridiculous to speak of one system of metaphysics that accommodates contradictory assumptions about mental states. Either it is simply wrong, or there must be superior unified metaphysics. This type of objection is motivated by the idea of the unity of science. Without pressing this issue, we can reply. Admittedly, there could be a consistent superior metaphysics, perhaps there *must* be one. But this does not alter the fact that in such a superior metaphysics mental states presumably do not appear as a unified class. It is an empirical question—independent of the normative idea of unified science. Here is a useful example from another discipline. Physicians used to speak generally of the illness dropsy. But it turned out that very different pathological processes are subsumed under this heading (kidney disease, heart insufficiency, etc.), which only belong to the same category when analysis is very superficial. Another possible objection to differential metaphysics is that we are not really talking about metaphysics, but about ontology. There is nothing wrong with talking about "differential ontology." But this does not alter the thesis at hand. It is not the name, but the topic that matters. Let it also be said that in the philosophy of mind the line between metaphysics and ontology is notoriously ambiguous.

42. This is also the reason why I have not adopted an attractive alternative formulation suggested in conversation by Thomas Metzinger, namely, "For every mental process there is one true biological description." In order to not exclude externalistic explanations for mental processes we must either provide a very wide concept of neurobiology or use the term "(partial) description," which does not seem particularly appropriate. If identity theory were true for all mental states, we could no doubt use this alternative suggestion.

43. You may wonder why I so stubbornly try to keep neurophilosophy open for dualists. My aim is to lure dualists to be open for the insights and findings of neuroscience in order to see why their dualistic theory is superfluous.

44. Mental states cannot be identical with neural states because they are functional and thus can be manifested in a variety of ways.

45. See Kim 1994 for a brief and well arranged synopsis. The *idea* of supervenience was introduced by Moore (1912); the term was first used by Hare (1952). Davidson (1970b) was the first to apply it to the mind-body problem. The main philosopher of supervenience is Jaegwon Kim (1993).

46. Physical properties are mass, charge, position in space and time, field properties and the exercise of the four basic powers, etc. It does not matter whether contemporary physics is complete or correct. The concept of supervenience is also applicable to future physics.

47. This is said under the assumption that facts belonging to a particular class can be characterized by clearly determining the properties of the objects in question.

48. In German a distinction is made between *physisch* and *physikalisch*. (In English both meanings are expressed by the word *physical*. In philosophy, physical (here: *physikalisch*) properties are a subclass of physical (here: *physisch*) properties, "physical" in this second usage meaning "natural, found in nature" (Duden, *Foreign Terms Dictionary*). [Translator's note: Physical properties are a subclass of natural properties.] Nonphysical properties are then such things as logical and abstract properties—and even mental properties (although that *is* questionable). Commonplace usage of "physical" denotes "bodily."

49. We can ask an analogous question for the case of phenomenal consciousness: Couldn't a physical theory of conscious organisms be true without there being any particular organism actually exhibiting consciousness? This idea has been dubbed the "Tibetan Prayer Wheel" (Bieri 1992), in Anglo-American literature it is also known as the "Zombie Argument."

50. Normally this type of reflection employs the concept of "possible worlds" (cf. Lewis 1986), as we shall see in the following. A possible world is a world that is different from ours in possible respects: like a world in which tigers have no stripes or in which there is no Coca-Cola, or in which persons do not exist. Talking of possible worlds is a way of expressing modal intuitions, which means thinking about what is or is not possible. In a first approximation we can imagine a possible world to be a universe parallel to ours, in which the same natural laws hold as in ours, but in which many marginal conditions and random developments are different.

51. The third kind of supervenience is *global* supervenience. It quantifies only over possible worlds and not over individuals. Strong supervenience implies weak as well as global supervenience. In contrast, global supervenience, formally does not imply both other varieties, but together with some plausible metaphysical assumptions it does include strong supervenience. Although global supervenience is of interest to some philosophers for the very reason that it does not imply type-type relations between mental and physical states (cf. Kim 1994, p. 580), it is negligible for our concerns because to date it has been of minor significance in the discussion on the mind-body problem.

52. To be more exact, we have here two non-empty families of properties that are closed under normal Boolean operations (complementation, conjunction, and disjunction) (cf. Stephan 1999).

53. Following Peter Bieri, who formulated this trilemma in 1981 in the introduction to his reader titled *Analytische Philosphie des Geistes* (*Analytic Philosophy of Mind*), distinguishing two varieties (from the standpoints of substance dualism and substance monism, respectively; see the second edition, Bieri 1993, pp. 5, 9). His exposition of the problem is still directive; I have chosen Brüntrup's version because it deals particularly with supervenience and emergence.

54. Another way of denying that this trilemma is a serious problem is to question the prevalent concept of causality entirely. I won't pursue this option now. See Quante 1993 for a discussion on the difficulty of mental causation.

55. In order to deny premise (2), Brüntrup himself—in good company with Dummett, Goodman, Rorty, and Putnam—favors semantic antirealism. Starkly abbreviated we can think of semantic antirealism as the thesis that not every statement about our world is unambiguously true or false independent of the way is which we recognize its truth conditions (Tennant 1995). In other words, antirealism adheres to an epistemic concept of truth. Since my work is founded on a correspondence theory of truth, I find this solution unattractive.

56. I have chosen linear causation of individual causes for simplicity. But the same scheme can be used to understand causal networks and backwards-directed causality.

57. This portrayal is taken from Merricks 1995; all quotations are from Kim 1993.

58. The whole argument can be formulated either in events ontology or in an ontology of properties and relations.

59. See Stephan's excellent comprehensive monograph (1999) and papers in Beckermann, Flohr, and Kim 1992. A synopsis and introduction are given in Hoyningen-Heune 1994 and Stephan and Beckermann 1994.

60. The discussion of emergence within the context of evolution theory, such as in Lloyd C. Morgan's book *Emergent Evolution* from 1923, is part of the second phase of the usage of this concept (cf. Hoyningen-Huene 1994, pp. 166–168; Stephan 1999, part I).

61. A brief exposition of the other variations: By adding the dimension of time (thesis of originality) to weak emergence we get weak diachronic emergence. Similarly, strong diachronic emergence is synchronic emergence plus the originality thesis. So-called structure emergentism is structural nonpredictiveness added to weak diachronic emergence. This kind is interesting, inasmuch as it could be possible to foretell systemic properties without it being possible to foretell the structure of the system in question (Stephan's example is that of deterministic chaos theory).

62. Stephan (1999, pp. 32–44) distinguishes two kinds of irreducibility: the irreducibility of a system's behavior and the irreducibility of a property that cannot be analyzed in terms of behavior. The latter refers to qualia and phenomenal consciousness.

63. Hoyningen-Heune (1994, pp. 172–175) distinguishes four causes of unpredictability: It can result from (a) missing or incomplete microdetermination, (b) purely probabilistic microdetermination (quantum phenomena), (c) a property's not being deducible as defined above, or (d) a lack of information about tiny but decisive degrees of haziness (deterministic chaos).

64. Meanwhile Kim also finds mereological supervenience to be the most interesting way of understanding the relation between physical and mental states (Kim 1994, p. 582).

65. See Stephan 1999 and Hoyningen-Heune 1994, pp. 175–179, as well as the relevant papers in Beckermann, Kim, and Flohr 1992.

66. See Sperry 1980, 1986. Sperry gained renown through his neuropsychological studies on split-brain patients (cf. Springer and Deutsch 1995). For medical reasons (such as treating epilepsy) the two halves of the brain were disconnected by severing the *corpus callosum*. Such patients exhibit a kind of doubled consciousness, a phenomenon that—long before the theory of blindsight—aroused philosophical interest and incited the first boom in neurophilosophy.

67. For a key to naturalism see Vollmer 1992b; Wagner and Wagner 1993; French, Vehling, and Wettstein 1994; and Keil 1993b.

68. For Ruse naturalism does not automatically lead to materialism or atheism. This is worthy of debate.

Chapter 3

1. At least if there are no hidden parameters that would make quantum physics deterministic.

2. Compton 1935; Munn 1962; Margenau 1967; Thorp 1980; Jonas 1981; Kane 1985, 1996; Beck and Eccles 1992; and Harkavay 1995. See also the entries in Consciousness Research Abstracts of Tuscon II, *Journal of Consciousness Studies* 1996, pp. 57–58.

3. Eccles tried to exploit quantum theory for interactionistic dualism (Eccles 1990, see also Beck and Eccles 1992). He claims that the probability of emptying a vesicle (a small sac containing transmitter fluid) at a synapse (the locus of contact between nerve cells for the purpose of signal transmission) is statistically so minute that it is equal to the slight probability of random oscillation in a quantum field; therefore, one might unknowingly "violate" the law of conservation of energy. Because there are innumerable synapses, this micro-influence could have a macro-effect. The mind would be analogous to a quantum probability field. This "explanation," it would seem, uses only an analogy (and an inadequate one at that) and does not in the least circumvent the problem that interaction faces in terms of violating the law of the conservation of energy.

4. It was primarily conceived as a theory of consciousness. The mingling of intentionality and consciousness is a delicate matter, for which I will express some speculative thoughts in the section on intelligibility. Perhaps free decisions must also always be conscious ones. But a solution to this difficulty is not prerequisite for neurophilosophically investigating whether P and H's theory has any chance of being successful.

5. The following critique was laid out by Grush and Churchland 1995. Further sources are the discussion in the electronic forum of the periodical *Psyche* (*http://www.znet.co.uk/imprint*) and papers in Hameroff, Kaszniak, and Sott 1996.

6. It is an amusing observation for the theory of science that Kant, in his arguments contra Soemmering, used an "argument of unordered water."

7. See Churchland 1981a, 1981b; Dennett 1994, pp. 203–215; and Spence 1996.

8. Introductions to chaos theory are Crutchfield et al. 1987, Gleick 1988, and Briggs and Peat 1990. A good survey from a lexicographic standpoint is given in Ravn 1995, a good synopsis in Küppers 1996; for a scientific description see Thomas and Leiber 1994.

9. In his original work Lorenz wrote of a seagull flapping its wings, but later changed it to the butterfly. Apparently he thought that for human imagination a bird's wing, compared to a butterfly's wing, was not small enough to be impressive. Would knowledge of chaos theory have spread quicker if he had thought of a fly's leg shivering?

10. Presently we distinguish between three types of mathematically conceptualized chaos: (1) statistic chaos (Brown's molecular movement, undesirable noise in electronic circuits, etc.), (2) Hamilton's chaos (for example Poincaré's the three body problem), and (3) dissipative chaos (turbulent currents) (cf. Thomas and Leiber 1994).

11. A fractal structure is characterized by constant similarity with itself in any proportions. A classic example is the coast of England. It exhibits a similar structure, whether viewed from a satellite, an airplane, a hill, the beach, or under a magnifying glass. Benoit Mandelbrot (1977) is the founder of fractal geometry.

12. Verhulst discovered this equation in 1845; it is modified by standardizing the size of the population with *relative* values.

13. The best synopsis on chaos within the nervous system is found in Elbert et al. 1994; see also Babloyantz and Lourenço 1994; Kelso 1995. An adequate introduction is given in Basar and Roth 1996.

14. Self-organization is the creation of structures through reciprocal effects of unstructured elements, without intervention from outside of the system. A survey of self-organization theories is offered in Paslack 1991, and Krohn and Küppers 1992.

15. Other examples of synergetics are chemical clocks (chemical mixtures that change color according to certain patterns and rhythms), structure generation in mucus fungi, and the development of patterns in liquids heated from one side (a.k.a. the Bénard problem); see Haken 1983.

16. Haken suggests, for example, that we view the workplace atmosphere or folk characteristics as ordering factors that have causal influence on employees or people in general, a standpoint that met with justifiable criticism.

17. Kruse et al. also discuss the relevance of synergetics for psychotherapeutic intervention.

18. A comprehensive survey in German is given by Jaeger 1996; see also Pasemann 1996. Volumes with quantitative models are Port and van Gelder 1995; models for developmental psycho-biology are given in Thelen and Smith 1994. Philosophical implications are portrayed in an ambitious article titled *"What might cognition be, if not computation?"* by van Gelder 1995. A critique of the approach is in Eliasmith 1996.

19. Kanitschneider 1993 also fights the case against mystifying chaos.

20. Waller 1988 and 1993 demarcates his theory against those of Frankfurt 1988 and Wolf (1980, 1990), who claim that reason serves the purpose of helping man to do what is true, right, and good (Wolf 1990). His intuition seems more than plausible, because approaches that interpret autonomy as "going the right way" (and Kant is among them) lead to paradox consequences. One would only be acting autonomously if one were doing the "right" thing. There would be no autonomous "wrong" actions. See also the last part of chapter 1.

21. If it should turn out that our brain possesses a kind of amplifier mechanism for noncausal micro events, then we would be absolutely free. Under identical constraints and initial conditions a person could do otherwise, albeit randomly. But I do not want to presuppose that.

22. Joyce 1995 surveys modern developments in this field; Hampton 1994 and Sugden 1991 discuss empirical problems of this model.

23. The idea of synchronized chaos is simple, yet ingenious. When two almost identical systems *of the appropriate kind* are started by the same input signals, both produce the same—unpredictable—output signal. The difficulty of this simple idea is to *design* systems of the appropriate kind (see Ditto and Pecora 1993, pp. 48–51).

24. An artificial system (a robot) rigidly programmed to adhere to a categorical imperative would hardly exist for long without the extremely careful protection of others. But if it were possible to program the categorical imperative into a device (robot) in such a way that that rule it is not exercised obstinately, always, and without exception, but pragmatically and cleverly, then I think we would have difficulty not viewing that robot as a morally thinking thing.

25. From a neurophilosophical perspective, a maxim is solely a very general notion that guides behavior, instantiated in the form of neuronal representations.

26. Up to this point we have avoided the term "free," but here we must use it. Following normal language usage it is inevitable. This may serve as evidence for how the notion of chaos at least partially satisfies our intuitions.

27. Stadler and his coworkers have presented a model of psychotic frenzy based on the idea of the balancing act. The diversion is too lengthy for our purposes, but the model can be found in Stadler, Kruze, and Carmsin 1996, pp. 339–351.

28. Double has objected that a decision-making process P can only explain a choice A as *rational* when, providing P, the likelihood of P choosing A is greater than that of not selecting A (Double 1988, 1991, pp. 203–204). In contrast, Kane holds that a decision can also be dual when this is not the case (Kane 1988, p. 445; 1996, pp. 174–178). In the most recent version of his theory, Kane (1996) has responded to this criticism by supplementing his thesis of *dual* rationality to become a thesis of *plural* rationality (1996, pp. 135ff.) This improvement is not tangential to his assumption that reasons are determinant causes (even though are not unambiguously determinant).

29. Searle 1990, 1992, claims the opposite.

30. Naturally this is merely a sketch for the sake of illustration, because cows with and without udders were never in competition for survival. Evolutionary explanations require that even slight changes issue functional changes that bring advantages in terms of selection. This presupposes a change of function or a combined succession of functions (see the following text).

31. Ernst Mayr (1991, pp. 51–86, slightly altered edition of an essay from 1974) calls such explanations *teleonomous*, in order to demarcate them from the term "teleological," which is historically somewhat tainted. But his usage has not become customary.

32. Her fundamental work is *Language, thought and other biological categories* (Millikan 1984). Further publications differentiate, explicate, advocate, and deliberate with competing standpoints. Later essays are compiled in Millikan 1993a. See also Millikan 1993b, 1998.

33. Further independent teleosemantic theories of intentionality have been suggested by Papineau 1987, 1993 and Dretske 1988; see also early work by Fodor 1984, who later gave up the teleosemantic approach. Millikan's theory of meaning was probably not widely received until recent years because it is quite complicated and difficult to access. Suitable introductions and summaries are given in Cummins 1989, pp. 147–163, Lyons 1992, and Kurthen 1992.

34. Meaning rationalism is the notion that the meaning of speech units or thoughts can be grasped by a rational person a priori, prior to any empirical experience. Millikan claims that a rational person cannot recognize a priori whether an actual thought is the same as or different from another one, whether it is unambiguous or whether it has meaning at all. This claim is only plausible when phenomenal consciousness is theoretically isolated from intentional consciousness. Millikan would not object to the claim that we have phenomenal experience due to the fact of our internal structure. What she denies is that we know the meaning of our thoughts *solely* because we have phenomenal experience.

35. The concept of proper function, associated with von Wright's etiological theory of functions, is well discussed independently of the problem of intentionality in the theory of the science of biology. See Bigelow and Pargetter 1987; Griffiths 1993; Kitcher 1993; Amundson and Lauder 1994; and Allen and Bekoff 1995. Neander 1991a, 1991b also developed an etiological theory of biological functions independently of Millikan.

36. See Millikan 1984, pp. 31–49. Beyond the subgroups mentioned she also introduces stabilizing, standardizing, historically proximate, distal, disjunctive, conjunctive, serial, and focused proper functions.

37. Bee dances consist of certain figurations with defined elements. By dancing it, one bee shows others where she has found nectar relative to the location of their hive. [Translator's note: To prevent confusing a B with a bee (particularly when reading aloud), I have changed Millikan's symbol from B to N (nectar) for this example.]

38. For a dispositional theory of function see Bigelow and Pargetter 1987.

39. Dr. Pangloss in Voltaire's *Candide*—a satire on Leibniz' notion that we live in the "best of all possible worlds ... for since everything was created for a purpose, it necessarily serves the best purpose. Notice, please, that noses were made to hold up spectacles, therefore we have eyeglasses. Feet were obviously made for footwear, hence we have shoes." (Voltaire in *Candide*, quoted from the German version Grewendorf 1995, p. 155).

40. Griffiths (1995) argues analogously for understanding adaptation as a several-phased process.

41. The basic idea of this thought experiment is derived from Putnam's (1975) twin earth notion; cf. also Burge 1979.

42. Being *supposed to* perform some function does not imply that some intelligent being has planned it.

43. A third type of function can be isolated from mechano- and teleofunctions, as analyzed by Cummins. To ascribe a function to an item means to ascribe a capacity to that item which fulfills a role in the analyses of the capacity of the system to which that item belongs (Cummins 1975, p. 765). An example is the function of a cog wheel in a gear or the function of an enzyme for digestion. Since this concerns the function of a *part* of a system (Greek: *meros*: part), I call this kind of function a *mereofunction*. Thus we have three different subtypes of functions: (1) mechanofunctions—everything an item can do or for which it can be used; (2) mereofunctions—the role which a particular item performs within a system for that system; and (3) teleofunctions—whatever an item was naturally selected for or for which it was produced. These kinds of functions can coincide, but they must not necessarily do so. In biological systems a mereofunction is also simultaneously a proper function. For an attempt to develop a concept of functions which encompasses teleo- *and* mereofunctions see Kitcher 1993 and Griffiths 1993; for the preference within biology for the concept of mereofunction see Amundson and Lauder 1994.

44. Of course, this example has been cleverly construed. Normally a change of function happens over a long time period and is accompanied by some structural changes. But since function changes are possible without structural changes, Colin Allen and Mark Bekoff suggest that we differentiate between function and design. A feature M can only have an effect X as a natural design, if M is a function of T and there is evidence of structural changes of M in M's phylogeny , which have given T an advantage in selection (Allen and Bekoff 1995, p. 619).

45. Frege (1892) distinguished between the German "Sinn" (literal: sense) of an expression and its "Bedeutung" (literal: meaning). For Frege "Bedeutung" is the denoted thing (to what the name refers to), and "Sinn" is something given. The planet Venus, for example, is called the morning star, but also the evening star. Both expressions *mean* the same, because they refer to the same planet. Frege applied this distinction to sentences and predicates. Although the details differ, Carnap made a similar distinction between extension (corresponding roughly to Fregean "Bedeutung") and intension (corresponding roughly to Fregean "Sinn").

This is why Fregean "Sinn," i.e., Fregean sense and the intension of an expression are often considered one and the same. However, today we use "reference" where Frege used "Bedeutung" and "meaning" or "sense" where Frege used "Sinn." It is easy to get lost in terminology! Here is a table for ordering this jumble.

"morning star"	Frege	Literal translation	Contemporary common usage	Carnap
the real planet Venus	"Bedeutung"	meaning	reference denotation	extension
the star seen in the morning	"Sinn"	sense	meaning sense	intension

Millikans's theory of meaning is intended to divide the amalgam of meaning + intension (Millikan 1984, p. 127) into two distinct sectors, namely the Fregean sense on one side and intension on the other.

46. Millikan adopts the term "icon" from Charles Pierce, since it is not overly commonplace and does not stimulate unintended associations.

47. Millikan (1993b) calls more simple forms (mimicry phenomena, biological clockworks, the design of the inner ear) *tacit suppositions*. Representations go beyond them and fulfill *additional* conditions, which we will discuss next.

48. Millikan defends her theory against objections of the type Putnam-Kripke-Wittgenstein, that is, against "metaphysical realism" in Millikan 1993a, chapters 10 and 11.

49. The icon rules are not to be confused with covariance, that is, the demand that the circumstances specified in the icon rules always exist when the icon exists. This only means that one of the normal conditions of the proper function of intentional icons is that these circumstances do indeed exist.

50. This does not imply a language of thought with a structure similar to that of public language. It is the task of future applied neurosemantics to discover the actual relationship of public language and inner representations.

51. If we think of thoughts or inner cerebral states as intentional icons, then the producer and the user can be in one and the same organism. This means that there must be a mechanism in the brain that *produces* the icons and another mechanism in the same brain that *uses* those icons. The trouble with this is that intention (internal usage within a system) and Fregean sense (the correspondence of a device to being supposed to do something) are not always easy to separate.

52. The act of identification holds a central position in Millikan's theory (see Millikan 1984, pp. 239–256).

53. If an intentional icon actually corresponds to a thing to which it is supposed to correspond, then this concrete circumstance is its "real value." [Translator's note: "What an intentional icon is 'of' I will call its 'real value.'" Millikan 1984,

p. 101.] A real value is not the same thing as a referent. The real value of a warning screech is a present danger, the referent—in contrast—is something particular: a concrete, individual predator. Contrary to the referent, the real value can have indefinite meaning; it could be meant for a type of things.

54. This proximity to logic is not haphazard. Although Millikan emphasizes that human thinking differs from formal logic, she does try to anchor laws of logic in her theory of knowledge. The law of the freedom of contradiction, for example, is not only a law of logic, but also an epistemological criteria we use in conceptual thinking. It helps us to distinguish empty from valid, correct from incorrect ideas (see Millikan 1984, chapter 18).

55. Besides acts of identification, inference mechanisms, subject-predicate structure, and the possibility of negation, Millikan adds three more features of *human* representations, which distinguish them from intentional icons in the animal world. Human representations include self-representing elements; they can be stored, and their indicative aspects can be isolated from their imperative aspects (Millikan 1993a, pp. 97–101).

56. For beliefs these normal conditions correspond to truth conditions, see Papineau (1993, chapter 3.8f). In order to meet the objection that desires can be satisfied by false beliefs, Papineau defines truth conditions as conditions that *guarantee* the satisfaction of a desire: "The truth condition of every belief is the condition which guarantees that actions brought forth by these beliefs fulfill the biological purpose of satisfying the desire" (Papineau 1993, p. 80; see also Papineau 1987, pp. 61f).

57. In outlining his theory, Kurthen also—as I myself do—borrows some notions from Millikan, Maturana, and connectionism. But he also includes reflections by Wittgenstein, Heidegger, and the hermeneutic cognitive sciences (cf. Kurthen 1994).

58. The philosopher Dretske (1988) designed a teleosemantic theory propagating ideas similar to those of Millikan, but with the difference that he considers the vital functions to be those that develop in the course of individual learning. In other words, he examines not only the phylogenetic, but also the ontogenetic time span.

59. There are more selection theories not mentioned by Darden and Cain, which are important to mention because this demonstrates that not all selection theories have been successful. There was the selection theory of organs by the developmental biologist Wilhelm Roux (1881), the bacteria selection theory by the biologist August Weismann (1895), an early selection theory for the production of antibodies by the physician Paul Ehrlich (1897), and the selection theory for neuronal connections by E. L. Thorndike (1908) (see Amundson 1989, pp. 414f).

60. See Young 1964; Dawkins 1971; Changeux and Danchin 1976; Changeux 1983; Johnson and Karmiloff-Smith 1990; Edelman 1978, 1989, 1992, 1992; Moreno et al. 1997; Calvin 1987, 1996; Changeux and Dahaene 1989, 1995; and Sporns and Tonini 1994.

61. Richard Dawkins (1976) introduced the term "mem." A mem is a kind of cultural gene: an idea, a concept, a word, that—once it has been put into the world—is reproduced and spreads throughout a population (see also Dennett 1991, pp. 263–298 and Dennett 1995).

62. It is interesting and certainly not fortuitous that Edelman was an immunologist before turning to brain research. He received a Nobel prize for his work in that field.

63. A neurobiological theory of development emphasizing the parceling process can be found in Ebbeson 1980.

64. Thus we only have information about it from indirect sources, particularly reconstruction and interpretation by ethnological, anthropological studies. Existing preliterate societies today are almost all "contaminated" by contact with literate cultures and their interpretations. Scheerer's other sources include findings about the invention and effects of notational systems of symbols in advanced ancient cultures, studies on oral poetry in Yugoslavia, earliest written reports like the Beowulf Saga, the Odyssey, and the Bible, language experiments with chimpanzees, and the study of analphabets, children, and patients with speech disorders.

65. Scheerer employs the paradigm of negation to demonstrate the nonpropositional character of primarily oral languages. The standard function of negation in oral cultures presupposes certain conditions, such as that the hearer believes the negated matter. Certain kinds of negation, like those that refer to an unlimited object, never occur in oral cultures, although they are grammatically possible. In other words, negation is generative only to a limited extent!

66. Seidenberg (1997) argues that the development of connectionism shows that much scorned statistic-probabilistic explanations for language acquisition perform better than originally anticipated. Connectionistic networks are very useful for multiple constraint satisfaction. This capacity explains how individual bits of information contribute in a nonlinear manner to a network's quick convergence to a correct interpretation of an incomplete stimulus. A child must not identify rules of grammar, it must *use* language. Emphasis on performance (in contrast to the emphasis on competence made in traditional theories) draws language acquisition closer to *skilled processing*. Prince and Smolensky (1997) use a theory of harmonic functions to explain how networks generate grammatical performance by simply *ranking* constraints. This approach is attractive because it explains why children are able to understand grammatically very differentiated utterances, although they themselves still make mistakes. It also relates what all languages have in common (universal constraints) and what makes them different (their rankings).

67. It differs from arguments for passive externalism as brought forth by Putnam (1975) and Burge (1979) in thought experiments about twin earth. If *I* think that water (H_2O on earth) is wet and my *twin* thinks that water (XYZ on his planet) is wet, then the circumstances that exist for difference of meaning in both of our

statements are *distal* and *historical*; they lie at the other end of a long causal chain.

68. However, not only language makes thinking intelligible. Having interaction with other persons (social externalism) and being embedded in social institutions and standards (community externalism) contribute as well. If autonomy requires intelligibility in this broad sense, then it must refer to culture as a whole. A similar idea, although it serves a quite different purpose, is proposed by Quante (1997), who examines the concept of personal autonomy in Hegel's philosophy of law.

69. In biology, stochastic contingency is also the most important element. It is presumably less a matter of mutations, which we intuitively are most likely to classify as consequences of indeterministic processes (such as ionizing rays), but more stochastic recombinations of chromosome sets from both parents, which constitute the main source of diversity so important for selection theory.

70. See Libet et al. 1979, 1983 as two trend-setting original pieces of work and Libet and commentators 1985, Libet 1993 for summaries and a discussion.

71. At this point we must note that the time required for perception depends on how strong the impulses are.

72. How the cortex stimulus masks the skin stimulus remains to be explained.

73. See Churchland 1981a, 1981b, and Libet 1981; commentaries in Libet 1985 and Dennett 1994.

74. The SMA is attributed with the central role in programming and timing voluntary, particularly double-sided movements (Goldberg 1985; Freund 1990; Kandel, Schwartz, and Jessel 1996, pp. 541–562). Particularly fascinating is the fact that SMA is not only active when movements are actually executed, but also when they are merely imagined, as measurements of brain circulation have shown. No wonder that dualists attribute the SMA the role of a "liaison brain" between mind and brain (Eccles 1982).

75. This is a variation on Wundt's "compilation clock," with a quickly rotating point used as an indicator, on which five traditional seconds correspond to 0.2 seconds.

76. The authors conducted three experiments. Experiment 2 repeated Libet's experiment. In experiment 1 readiness potential prior to small, subconscious movements was registered, while the test persons were distracted by an addition task. In Experiment 3 the test persons were instructed to introspectively pay attention to their arms. If a spontaneous movement occurred, they were asked what they had felt prior to that movement. All three experiments demonstrated BP approximately 500 milliseconds prior to the movement. Differences were only in amplitude (presumably caused by differences in strength) and potential distribution over the head (the potentials of conscious movements were characteristically up front and toward the middle).

77. The lateral sections of the premotor cortex are particularly relevant for movements triggered by external stimuli, while the medial sections (including

SMA) are concerned with internally generated (not directly initiated by external stimuli) movements (Passingham 1993).

78. Newest research questions the exceptional status of humans. The differences in size of the frontal cortex are not noteworthy within the family of primates (H. Damasio 1996, p. 12).

79. The best survey is in Devinsky et al. 1995. See also Joseph 1996.

80. Changeux and Dahaene sometimes call the prefrontal cortex the *generator of diversity* (which incidentally forms the acronym *god*). But it is unclear whether it performs that task, or whether diversity occurs spontaneously.

81. These are models of two widely used neuropsychological tests that are held to be specifically for frontal functions; the *delayed response test* and the *Wisconsin card sorting test*.

82. See Thalberg 1967; Taylor 1974; Chisholm 1978; resuscitated by Clarke 1993; O'Connoer 1995b; see also van Inwagen 1986.

83. Translator's note. This clarification deals with using the German expression *"Handlungskausalität"* to mean agent causation, which, according to the author, should be translated as *"Kausalität des Handelnden,"* or better; *"Akteurskausalität."*

84. See van Inwagen 1986, pp. 135ff.

85. See Nisbett and Roos 1980; Cook and Levin 1990.

86. On Russell see Keil 1996. A discussion of diverse causality concepts can be found in Brüntrup 1994, pp. 195–228 and Koch 1994.

87. Some science theorists rationally reconstruct causality as nomologicalness (being law-like). Hempel views causality as nothing more than a special case of deductive-nomological explanation. Stegmüller defines the cause of an event *E* the "totality of all antecedent conditions of an adequate explanation for *E*" (cf. Keil 1996, pp. 527f). Vollmer (1994) gives a good synopsis of the difficulties in defining laws of nature. None of the features suggested (synthetic all-propositions held to be true and formulated as conditional propositions, support for counterfactual conditional propositions, naturally necessary validity) is sufficient for a satisfactory explication of the concept of laws of nature. The notions of necessity and constraints, especially, lack explication without recourse to the concept of laws of nature. Vollmer suggests that we tentatively define laws of nature as "regularities in the behavior of real systems."

88. According to Clarke, Chisholm turns away from his own theory of agent causation as early as 1986, in a contribution to Radu J. Bogdan (ed.): *Roderick M. Chisholm*. Reidel 1986.

89. See a collection of papers in Frankfurt 1988, 1992, and the collection of essays by Dworkin 1988. Essays by other authors can be found in Christman 1989; Fischer 1986; and Fischer and Ravizza 1993. Fischer 1986, and Shatz 1986 discuss hierarchic compatibilist theories. Seebass (1992) uncovers the historical roots of these theories in Aristotle and Locke.

90. This and other essays are in Frankfurt's collection published in 1988.

91. Meanwhile, Watson thinks that even reference to values cannot explain all the acts we call free. A case in point are "perverse" situations, in which a person consciously does something clearly contrary to her own system of values (Watson 1987, p. 150).

92. Analytical philosophy, however, hardly takes notice of any philosophy of emotions. In this field, the important works of the past two decades are Lyons 1980 and de Sousa 1987. In contrast, phenomenology has more consistently dealt with emotions (see Fink-Eitel and Lohmann 1993).

93. A history of the philosophical treatment of emotions can be found in Power and Dalgleish 1996, pp. 17–64.

94. Oatley and Johnson-Laird's work *Towards a Cognitive Theory of Emotions* is a milestone. It was also the first essay contributed to the periodical *Cognition and Emotion*, published since 1987. An up-to-date and extensive report on cognitive emotion theories and their importance for understanding psychic disorders is available in Power and Dalgleish 1996. Goller 1992 provides an excellent survey of emotion theories. A more general introduction is given in Rost 1990, an unusual and artful book.

95. Neurobiological research always strove to locate emotions. The Cannon-Bard theory wanted to seat them in the thalamus (Cannon 1927). Papez (1937) located emotions in the limbic system, an idea later picked up by MacLean (1970, 1990). Among the centralist theories is Lindsley's activation theory (Lindsley 1951), which attributed a pivotal role to the ascending reticular activation system (ARAS). A whole school of contemporary emotion-EEG research is based on that work (see Davidson 1993 for a survey). Laterality research has also worked on emotions (for an introduction see Springer and Deutsch 1995, pp. 201–211). The initial hypothesis is that emotions are mainly processed or registered in the right hemisphere. But a series of neurophysiological studies and medical evidence for patients with epilepsy and brain damage provides a more differentiated picture (cf. Davidson 1993; Haaland 1992; Borod 1992). The left hemisphere seems to be specialized in positive emotions, such as happiness, while negative emotions are lateralized to the right. But further research using EEG data questions this hemisphere specialization (Machleidt, Gutjahr, and Mügge 1989).

96. Actually it is not a *single* structure, but a number of interconnected structures and systems that form a circuit, the so-called Papez circle. It normally includes the hippocampus, the septum, the gyrus cingulus anterior, the amygdala, mammila bodies, and sometimes also the hypothalamus. But what exactly belongs to the limbic system and whether in light of more exact findings this term is meaningful at all is quite controversial (see survey work by Kötter and Meyer 1992). The one part of the limbic system that has gained the most attention in recent years is the amygdala, the almond (cf. Aggleton 1992; LeDoux 1996).

97. To mention the most important of them: Plutchik 1980, Tomkins 1982, Panksepp 1982, and Nesse 1989.

98. The classics are Schachter and Singer 1962; Lazarus 1982; Leventhal and Scherer 1987; and Oatley and Johnson-Laird 1987. For a new version that incorporates clinical experience see Power and Dalgleish (1996). It also contains a useful survey of more cognitive theories of emotion (Power and Dalgleish 1998, pp. 65–114); also see Goller 1992, pp. 149–198.

99. See Nesse 1989; Oakley 1992.

100. From this explication, one might be tempted to conclude that one realm is emotion-specific and not characteristic for cognition, namely that of subjective experience and feeling. But that is also incorrect. The fact that cognitive processes, such as the perception of a red blotch, also have an element of subjectively felt experience is the basis of the entire philosophical qualia industry!

101. See Springer and Deutsch 1995; Machleidt 1989; Davidson 1993; Scherer 1993; LeDoux 1994, 1996; Damasio 1994; Gazzaniga 1995; chapter 7; and Ciompi 1997.

102. Saver and Damasio 1991; Nahm et al. 1993; Bechara et al. 1994, 1995, 1997; and Adolphs et al. 1995. A summarized exposition is given in Damasio 1994. For an essay on the meaning of these theories for the problem of the free will see Walter 1996d, 1997a.

103. Viewed in terms of neuroanatomy, the ventromedial section is everything that is not in the dorsolateral part of the frontal lobes. It comprises the orbitofrontal sections and the rostral section of the anterior cingulate. Damage to this section is very rare without the neighboring area also being damaged. The deficiency usually is the result of a state after a nonmalignant tumor has been operatively removed from this area, or after a stroke in the supply area of the anterior communicating brain artery.

104. Compare: The will is not an instance of theoretical, but of *practical* reason (Kant).

105. Edelman also proposes a neuronal self that provides value direction. He thinks, however, that it is in the subcortical systems, which regulate the homeostasis of the body and are mostly innate (see Edelman 1992, p. 120).

106. Philosophers may find it interesting that the classification as "I-disorder" is only common in German psychiatric discourse, where it is called "Ich-Störung." Anglo-American literature calls this phenomena "delusion of alien control" or "passivity phenomena." This may be due to Kant's influence and the associated idea of a transcendental self.

107. The idea that our body and its central nervous system representations are the foundation for our mental model of the self has increasingly gained attention in philosophical considerations. Cf. Johnson 1987 and the contributions in Bermudez, Marcel, and Eilan 1995.

108. A third criteria is the so-called simple criteria as suggested by Richard Swinburne. Persons are simple, immaterial, and irreducible entities. This corresponds to notions of substance dualism and agency causation. There have been

attempts to combine all three criteria (Wiggens 1993). For a discussion of these criteria see Brüntrup and Gillitzer 1997.

109. I suspect that the notion of "ultimate responsibility" and the attempt to find (impossible) ultimate reasons for ethical principles practically always go hand in hand. Here is a typical example: "Ethics, if it is supposed to be a sufficient reason for morals, must take recourse to something absolute and ultimately valid, that guarantees its normative claim. In the principle of morality, ethics says this absolute thing is freedom, a freedom that has no reason beyond itself, a freedom that is its own reason" (Pieper 1985, p. 35).

References

Adler, M. (1958). *The idea of freedom: A dialectical examination of the conceptions of freedom*. Garden City, NY.

Adolphs, R., Tranel, D., Bechara, A., Damasio, H., and Damasio, A. R. (1995). Neuropsychological approaches to reasoning and decision-making. In: Damasio et al. (1995), pp. 157–180.

Aggleton, J. P. (1992) (Ed.). *The amygdala: Neurobiological aspects of emotion, memory, and mental dysfunction*. New York.

Albritton, R. (1985/1986). Freedom of will and freedom of action. *Proceedings and Addresses of the American Philosophical Association*, 59, pp. 239–251.

Allen, C., and Bekoff, M. (1995). Biological function, adaptation and natural design. *Philosophy of Science*, 62, pp. 609–622.

Allison, H. (1990). *Kant's theory of freedom*. Cambridge, MA: MIT Press.

Amundson, R. (1989). The trials and tribulations of selectionist explanations. In: Hahlweg, K., and Hooker, C.A. (Eds.), *Issues in evolutionary epistemology*. Albany: State University Press of New York, pp. 413–432.

Amundson, R., and Lauder, G. V. (1994). Function without purpose: The uses of causal role function in evolutionary biology. *Biology and Philosophy*, 9, pp. 443–469.

Andreasen, N. C. (1997). Linking mind and brain in the study of mental illnesses: A project for scientific psychopathology. *Science*, 275, pp. 1586–1593.

Anscombe, G. E. M. (1981). Causality and determinism. In: Anscombe, G.E.M., *Collected papers*, Vol. 2, Oxford: Basil Blackwell.

Ashbrook, J. B. (1984). Neurotheology: The working brain and the work of theology. *Zygon*, 19, pp. 331–350.

Audi, R. (1986). Acting for reasons. *Philosophical Review*, 95, pp. 511–546.

Austin, J. L. (1961). Ifs and Cans. *Philosophical Papers*. London.

Ayala, F. J. (1974). Introduction. In: Ayala, F. J., and Dobzhansky T. (Eds.), *Studies in the philosophy of biology*. Berkeley.

Ayer, A. J. (1954). Freedom and Necessity. In: Ayer, A. J., *Philosophical Essays*, London.

Ayers, M. R. (1968). *The refutation of determinism*. London: Methuen.

Babloyantz, A., and Lourenço, C. (1994). Computation with chaos: A paradigm for cortical activity. *Proceedings of the National Academy of Sciences*, 91, pp. 9027–9031.

Baker, L. R. (1993). Metaphysics and mental causation. In: Heil, and Mele (1993), pp. 75–95.

Baker, L. R. (1995). *Explaining attitudes*. Cambridge: Cambridge University Press.

Baker, M. A. (1980). Ein Kühlsystem im Gehirn von Säugetieren [A cooling system in the brains of mammals.] In: *Gehirn und Nervensystem*. Weinheim: Spektrum, pp. 178–185.

Barkow, J. H., Cosmides, L., and Tooby, J. (1992). *The adapted mind*. Oxford: Oxford University Press.

Bartels, K., and Huber, L. (1981). *Veni, vidi, vici*, fifth edition. Zürich: Artemis.

Basar, E., and Roth, G. (1996). Ordnung aus dem Chaos. Kooperative Gehirnprozessen bei kognitiven Leistungen [Order from Chaos. Cooperative brain processes in cognitive performance]. In: Küppers, G. (Ed.), *Chaos und Ordnung*. Stuttgart: Reclam, pp. 290–322.

Bates, E., Thal, D., and Marchman, V. (1989). Symbols and syntax: A Darwinian approach to language development. In: Krasnegor, N., Rumbaugh, D., Studdert-Kennedy, M., and Schiefelbusch, R. (Eds.), *The biological foundations of language development*. Oxford: Oxford University Press.

Baxter, L. E., Schwartz, J. M., Bergman, K. S., et al. (1992). Caudate glucose metabolism rate changes with both drug and behavior therapy for obsessive compulsive disorder. *Archives of General Psychiatry*, 49, pp. 687–689.

Baxter, L. E. J., Schwartz, J. M., Guze, B. H., Bergman, K. S., and Szuba, M. P. (1990). Neuroimaging in obsessive-compulsive disorder: Seeking the mediating neuroanatomy. In: Jenike, M.A., Bear, L., and Minichiello, W. E. (Eds.), *Obsessive-compulsive disorders: Theory and management*. St. Louis, MO: Mosby Yearbook, pp. 167–188.

Bayertz, K. (1993). *Evolution und Ethik* [Evolution and Ethics]. Stuttgart: Reclam.

Bechara, A., Damasio, A. R., Damasio, H., and Anderson, S. W. (1994). Insensitivity to future consequences following damage to the human prefrontal cortex. *Cognition*, 50, pp. 7–15.

Bechara, A., Damasio, H., Tranel, D., and Damasio, A. (1997). Deciding advantageously before knowing the advantageous strategy. *Science*, 275, pp. 1293–1294.

Bechara, A., Tranel, D., Damasio, H., Adolphs, R., Rockland, Ch., and Damasio, A. R. (1997). Double dissociation of conditioning and declarative knowledge relative to the amygdala and hippocampus in humans. *Science*, 269, pp. 1115–1118.

Bechtel, W. (1988a). *Philosophy of mind*. Hillsdale, NJ: Lawrence Erlbaum.

Bechtel, W. (1998b). *Philosophy of science*. Hillsdale, NJ: Lawrence Erlbaum.

Bechtel, W. (1993). *Discovering complexity: Decomposition and localization as strategies in scientific research*. Princeton: Princeton University Press.

Bechtel, W., and Abrahamsen, A. (1991). *Connectionism and the mind*. Oxford: Basil Blackwell.

Beck, R., and Eccles, J. C. (1992). Quantum aspects of consciousness and the role of consciousness. *Proceedings of the National Academy of Science*, 89, pp. 11357–11361.

Beckermann, A. (1986). *Descartes' metaphysischer Beweis für den Dualismus* [Descartes' metaphysical proof of dualism]. Munich: Alber.

Beckermann, A. (1996). Eigenschaftsphysikalismus. [Property physicalism]. *Zeitschrift für philosophische Forschung*, 50, pp. 3–25.

Beckermann, A., Flohr, H., and Kim, J. (1992) (Eds.). *Emergence or reduction?* Berlin, New York: Springer.

Bergson, H. (1888/1989). *Zeit und Freiheit* [Time and Freedom]. Frankfurt: Athenäum.

Bermudez, J. L., Marcel, A., and Eilan, N. (1995) (Eds.). *The body and the self*. Cambridge, MA: MIT Press.

Bickle, J. (1992). Mental anomaly and the new mind-brain reductionism. *Philosophy of Science*, 59, pp. 217–230.

Bickle, J. (1995). Psychoneural reduction of the genuinely cognitive: Some accomplished facts. *Philosophical Psychology*, 8, pp. 265–285.

Biedermann, E. (1991). Bemerkungen zur Willensfreiheit [Remarks on the Freedom of Will]. *Zeitschrift für philosophische Forschung*, 45, pp. 585–595.

Bieri, P. (1992). Was mach Bewusstsein zu einem Rätsel? [Why is Consciousness a Puzzle?], *Spektrum der Wissenschaft*, Oct. 1992, pp. 48–56.

Bieri, P. (1993) (Ed.). *Analytische Philosophie des Geistes* [Analytical Philosophy of Mind]. Second revised edition, Bodenheim: Athenäum.

Bigelow, J., and Pargetter, R. (1987). Functions. *Journal of Philosophy*, 84, pp. 181–198.

Birnbacher, D. (1993). Freiheit durch Selbsterkenntnis. Spinoza—Schopenhauer—Freud. [Freedom through knowing oneself. Spinoza-Schopenhauer-Freud]. *Schopenhauer-Jahrbuch*, 74, pp. 87–102.

Birnbacher, D. (1995). *Tun und Unterlassen*. [Action and Omission] Stuttgart: Reclam.

Block, N. (1980). Troubles with functionalism. In: Block, N. (Ed.), Readings in the philosophy of psychology. 2 Vols., Cambridge, MA: Harvard University Press, pp. 268–305.

Block, N. (1980) (Ed.). *Readings in the philosophy of psychology*, Vol. 1, Cambridge, MA: Harvard University Press.

Borod, J. C. (1992). Interhemispheric and intrahemispheric control of emotion: A focus on unilateral brain damage. *Journal of Consulting and Clinical Psychology*, 60, pp. 339–348.

Boyle, J. M., Grisez, G., and Tollefsen, O. (1976). *Free choice: A self-referential argument*. London.

Breidbach, O. (1997). *Die Materialisierung des Ichs* [Materializing the Self]. Frankfurt: Suhrkamp.

Breiter, H. C., Rauch, S. I., Kwong, K. K., et al. (1996). Functional magnetic resonance imaging of symptom provocation in obsessive compulsive disorder. *Archives of General Psychiatry*, 53, pp. 595–606.

Briggs, J., and Peat, D. F. (1990). *Die Entdeckung des Chaos*. [Discovering Chaos]. Munich, Vienna: Hanser.

Brown, J. (1987). *The life of the mind*. Hillsdale, NJ: Erlbaum.

Brown, J. (1991). *Self and process: Brain states and the conscious present*. Berlin, New York: Springer.

Brüntrup, G. (1994). *Mentale Verursachung* [Mental Causation]. Stuttgart: Kohlhammer.

Brüntrup, G. (1996). *Das Leib-Seele-Problem* [The Mind-Body Problem]. Stuttgart: Kohlhammer.

Brüntrup, G., and Gillitzer, B. (1997). Der Streit um die Person. [The quarrel over persons]. *Information Philosophie*, 4, pp. 18–27.

Bunge, M. (1977). Emergence and the mind. *Neuroscience*, 2, pp. 501–509.

Bunge, M. (1984). *Das Leib-Seele-Problem* [The mind-body problem]. Tübingen: Mohr.

Bünning, E. (1935). Sind die Organismen mikrophysicalische Systeme? Entgegnung a P. Jordan. [Are organisms micro-physical systems? Reply to P. Jordan]. *Erkenntnis*, 5, pp. 337–347.

Bünning, E. (1943). Quantenmechanik und biologie [Quantum mechanics and biology]. *Naturwissenschaften*, 31, pp. 194–197.

Burge, T. (1979). Individualism and the mental. *Midwest Studies in Psychology*, 4, pp. 73–122.

Buschlinger, W. (1993). *Denkkapriolen* [Caprioles of thought]. Würzburg: Könighausen und Neumann.

Busemeyer, J. R., and Townsend, J. T. (1993). Decision field theory: A Dynamic-cognitive approach to decision making in an uncertain environment. *Psychological Review*, 100, pp. 432–459.

Buss, E. M. (1995). Evolutionary psychology: A new paradigm for psychological science. *Psychological Inquiry*, 6, pp. 1–30.

Buss, S. (1994). Autonomy reconsidered. *Midwest Studies in Philosophy*, 14, pp. 95–121.

Calvin, W. H. (1987). The brain as a Darwin machine. *Nature*, 330, pp. 33–34.

Calvin, W. H. (1989). *The cerebral symphony*. New York: Bantam.

Calvin, W. H. (1995). Cortical columns, modules, and Hebbian cell assemblies. In: Arbib, M.A. (Ed.), *Handbook of brain theory and neural networks*. Cambridge, MA: MIT Press, pp. 269–272.

Calvin, W. H. (1996). *The cerebral code*. Cambridge, MA: MIT Press.

Campbell, D. T. (1974). Evolutionary epistemology. In: Schilpp, P. A. (Ed.), *The philosophy of Karl Popper*. La Salle: Open Court, pp. 413–463.

Cannon, W. B. (1927). The James-Lange theory of emotions: A critical examination and an alternative theory. *American Journal of Psychology*, 39, pp. 106–124.

Carrier, M., and Mittelstrass, J. (1989). *Geist, Gehirn, Verhalten*. [Mind, brain, behavior]. Berlin: de Gruyter.

Cartwright, N. (1983). *How the laws of physics lie*. Oxford, New York.

Chalmers, D. (1993). Connectionism and compositionality: Why Fodor and Pylyshyn were wrong. *Philosophical Psychology*, 6, pp. 305–319.

Chalmers, D. (1996a). *The conscious mind*. Oxford: Oxford University Press.

Chalmers, D. (1996b). Das Rätsel bewussten Erlebens [The puzzle of conscious experience]. *Spektrum der Wissenschaft*, Feb., pp. 40–47.

Changeux, J.-P. (1983). *L'homme neuronal* [Neuronal Man]. Paris: Librairie Arthème Fayard.

Changeux, J.-P., and Dahaene, S. (1989). Neuronal models of cognitive functions. *Cognition*, 33, pp. 63–109.

Changeux, J.-P., and Dahaene, S. (1996). Neuronal models of cognitive functions associated with the prefrontal cortex. In: Damasio, A.R., Damasio, H., and Christen, Y. (Eds.), *Neurobiology of Decision-making*. New York: Springer, pp. 125–144.

Changeux, J. P., and Danchin, A. (1976). Selective stabilization of developing synapses as a mechanism for the specification of neuronal networks. *Nature*, 264, pp. 705–711.

Charlton, W. (1988). *Weakness of the will*. Oxford: Blackwell.

Chisholm, R. (1978). Human freedom and the self. Lindsey lecture at the University of Kansas. German translation in: Pothast (Ed.), *Seminar: Freies Handelin und Determinismus*. Frankfurt: Suhrkamp, pp. 71–87.

Chisholm. R. (1995). Agents, causes, and events. In: O'Connor, T. (Ed.), *Agents, causes, events*. Oxford: Oxford University Press, pp. 95–100.

Chomsky, N. (1980). *Rules and representations*. Oxford: Blackwell.

Christman, J. (1989). *The inner citadel*. Oxford: Oxford University Press.

Christman, J. (1991). Autonomy and personal history. *Canadian Journal of Philosophy*, 21, pp. 1–24.

Churchland, P. M. (1984). *Matter and consciousness*. Cambridge, MA: MIT Press.

Churchland, P. M. (1989). *A neurocomputational perspective*. Cambridge, MA: MIT Press.

Churchland, P. M. (1995). *The engine of reason, the seat of the soul*. Cambridge, MA: MIT Press.

Churchland, P. S. (1981a). On the alleged backward referral of experiences and its relevance to the mind-body problem. *Philosophy of Science*, 48, pp. 165–181.

Churchland, P. S. (1981b). The timing of sensations: Reply to Libet. *Philosophy of Science*, 48, pp. 492–497.

Churchland, P. S. (1986). *Neurophilosophy*. Cambridge, MA: MIT Press.

Churchland, P. S. (1991). Our brains, our selves: Reflections on neuroethical questions. In: Roy, D., Wynne, B. W., and Old, R. W. (Eds.), *Bioscience and society*. West Sussex: Wiley & Sons, pp. 77–96.

Churchland, P. S. (1995a). Can neurobiology teach us anything about consciousness? Presidential address to the American Philosophical Association, Pacific Division. *Proceedings and Addresses to the American Philosophical Association*. Lancaster, P.A.: Lancaster Press, 67(4), pp. 23–40. Also in: Morowitz, H.J. (Ed.) (1995), The Mind, the brain and complex adaptive systems. *Proceedings*. Vol. 22, Santa Fe Institute, Studies in the Sciences of Complexity. Reading, MA: Addison-Wesley.

Churchland, P. S. (1995b). Feeling reasons. In: Damasio, A.R., Damasio, H., and Christen, Y. (Eds.), *Neurobiology of decision-making*. New York: Springer, pp. 181–199.

Churchland, P. S., and Sejnowski, T. (1992). *The computational brain*. Cambridge: MIT Press.

Ciompi, L. (1982). *Affektlogik. Über die Struktur der Psyche und ihre Entwicklung: Ein Beitrag zur Schizophrenie-Forschung* [The logics of affects. On the structure of the psyche and its development: A contribution to research on schizophrenia]. Stuttgart: Klett-Cotta.

Ciompi, L. (1993). Die Hypothese der Affektlogik [The hypothesis of affect logics]. *Spektrum der Wissenschaft*, Feb., pp. 76–87.

Ciompi, L. (1997). *Die emotionalen Grundlagen des Denkens: Entwurf einer fraktalen Affektlogik* [The emotional basis of thought: Outline of fractal affect logics]. Göttingen: Vandenhoeck & Ruprecht.

Clark, A. (1991). *Microcognition*. Cambridge, MA: MIT Press.

Clark, A., and Chalmers, D. (1997). The extended mind. Manuscript, found at: http://ling.uscs.edu/~chalmers

Clarke, R. (1993). Toward a credible agent-causal account of free will. *Nôus*, 27, pp. 191–203. Reprinted in: O'Conner, T. (Ed.), *Agents, causes, events.* Oxford: Oxford University Press, pp. 201–215.

Clarke, R. (1995). Freedom and determinism. *Philosophical Books*, 36, pp. 9–18.

Compton, A. H. (1935). *The freedom of man.* New Haven: Yale University Press.

Cook, K. S., and Levin, M. (1990). *The limits of rationality.* Chicago: Chicago University Press.

Crick, F. H. C. (1989). Neural Edelmanism. *Trends in Neurosciences*, 12, pp. 240–248.

Crick, F. H. C. (1994). *The astonishing hypothesis.* New York: Scribner's Sons.

Crick, F. H. C., and Koch, C. (1990). Towards a neurobiological theory of consciousness. *Seminars in the Neurosciences*, 4, pp. 263–276.

Crutchfield, J. P., Farmer, D. J., Packard, N. H., and Shaw, R. S. (1987). Chaos. *Spektrum der Wissenschaft*, Feb., pp. 78–90.

Cummings, J. L. (1985). *Clinical neuropsychiatry.* New York: Grund & Stratton.

Cummins, R. (1975). Functional analysis. *Journal of Philosophy*, 72: pp. 741–765.

Cummins, R. (1989). *Meaning and mental representation.* Cambridge, MA: MIT Press.

Damasio, A. R. (1994). *Descartes' error: Emotion, reason, and the human brain.* New York: Avon Books.

Damasio, A. R., Damasio, H., and Christen, Y. (1996) (Eds.). *Neurobiology of decision-making.* New York: Springer.

Damasio, A. R., and van Hoesen, G. W. (1983). Emotional disturbances associated with focal lesions of the limbic frontal lobe. In: Heilmann, K.M., and Satz, P. (Eds.), *Neuropsychology of human emotion.* New York: Guilford Press.

Damasio, H. (1996). Human neuroanatomy relevant to decision-making. In: Damasio, A. R., Damasio, H., and Christen, Y. (Eds.), *Neurobiology of decision-making.* New York: Springer, pp. 2–12.

Darden, L., and Cain, J. A. (1989). Selection type theories. *Philosophy of Science*, 56, pp. 106–129.

David, A. S. (1992). Frontal lobology—psychiatry's new pseudoscience. *British Journal of Psychiatry*, 161, pp. 244–248.

Davidson, D. (1970a). How is weakness of the will possible? In: Davidson, D. (1980), *Essays on actions and events.* Oxford: Clarendon Press, pp. 21–42.

Davidson, D. (1970b). Mental events. In: Davidson, D. (1980), *Essays on actions and events.* Oxford: Clarendon Press.

Davidson, D. (1973). Freedom to act. In: Davidson, D. (1980), *Essays on actions and events.* Oxford: Clarendon Press, pp. 63–82.

Davidson, D. (1980). *Essays on actions and events*. Oxford: Clarendon Press.

Davidson, R. J. (1993). Cerebral asymmetry and emotion: Conceptual and methodological conundrums. *Cognition and Emotion*, 7, pp. 115–138.

Davies, P. (1990). Chaos frees the universe. *New Scientist*, 6, pp. 48–51.

Davies, P., and Brown (1988) (Ed.). *Der Geist im Atom* [The mind in the atom]. Frankfurt: Insel.

Dawkins, R. (1971). Selective neuronal death as a possible memory mechanism. *Nature*, 229, pp. 118–119.

Dawkins, R. (1976). *The selfish gene*. Oxford: Oxford University Press.

De Sousa, R. (1987). *The rationality of emotions*. Cambridge: Cambridge University Press.

De Sousa, R. (1996). Prefrontal Kantians. A review of Descartes' error: Emotion, reason and the human brain by Antonio Damasio. *Cognition and Emotion* 10, pp. 329–333.

Deecke, L., Kornhuber, H. H., Lang, W., Lang, M., and Schreiber, H. (1985). Timing function of the frontal cortex in sequential motor learning tasks. *Human Neurobiology*, 4, pp. 143–154.

Dehaene, S., and Changeux, J. P. (1995). A simple model of prefrontal cortex function in delayed response tasks. *Journal of Cognitive Neuroscience*, 6, pp. 244–261.

Dennett, D. C. (1981). On giving libertarians what they say they want. In: Dennett, D.C., *Brainstorms*. Brighton: Harvester, pp. 286–299.

Dennett, D. C. (1984). *Elbow room: The varieties of free will worth wanting*. Cambridge, MA: MIT Press.

Dennett, D. C. (1987). *The intentional stance*. Cambridge, MA: MIT Press.

Dennett, D. C. (1991a). *Consciousness explained*. Boston: Little, Brown.

Dennett, D. C. (1991b). Real patterns. *Journal of Philosophy*, 89, pp. 27–51.

Dennett, D. C. (1995). *Darwin's dangerous idea*. New York: Basic Books.

Deutsch, D. (1985). Quantum theory, the Church-Turing principle and the universal quantum computer. *Proceedings of the Royal Society of London*. A400, pp. 97–117.

Deutsch, D. (1992). Quantum computation. *Physical World*, 5, pp. 57–61.

Devinsky, O., Putnam, F., Grafman, J., Bromfield, E., and Theodore, W. H. (1995). Contributions of anterior cingulate cortex to behavior. *Brain*, 118, pp. 279–306.

Dihle, A. (1985). *Die Vorstellung vom Willen in der Antike* [The ancient idea of the will]. Göttingen: Vandenhoeck and Ruprecht.

Ditto, W. L., and Pecora, L. M. (1993). Das Chaos meistern. [Mastering chaos]. *Spektrum der Wissenschaft*, Nov. l, pp. 46–53.

Dörner, D. (1989). Emotion, kognition und begriffsverwirrungen: Zwei Anmerkungen zur Köhler-Vorlesung von Norbert Bischof [Emotions, cognition and conceptual confusion. Two remarks on the Köhler lectures by Norbert Bischof]. *Psychologische Rundschau*, 40, pp. 206–209.

Dörner, D. (1996). Der freie Wille und die Selbstreflexion. [The free will and self-reflection]. In: von Cranach, M., and Foppa, K. (Eds.), *Freiheit des Entscheidens und Handelns, Ein problemder nomologischen psychologie*. Heidelberg: Asanger, pp. 125–150.

Doty, R. W. (1965). Philosophy and the brain. *Perspectives in Biology and Medicine*, pp. 23–24.

Double, R. (1988). Libertarianism and Rationalism. *Southern Journal of Philosophy*, 26, pp. 431–439.

Double, R. (1991). The non-reality of free will. Oxford: Oxford University Press.

Double, R. (1996). *Metaphilosophy and free will*. Oxford: Oxford University Press.

Dreher, E. (1987). *Die Willensfreiheit* [Freedom of will]. Munich: Beck.

Dretske, H. (1988). *Explaining behavior: Reasons in a world of causes*. Cambridge, MA: MIT Press.

Duke, D., and Pritchard, W. (1991) (Ed.). *Measuring chaos in the human brain*. Singapore: World Scientific.

Dummett, M. (1982). Realism. *Synthese* 52, pp. 55–112.

Dworkin, Gerald (1988). *The theory and practice of autonomy*. Cambridge: Cambridge University Press.

Earman, J. (1986). *A primer on determinism*. Dordrecht: Reidel.

Ebbeson, E. O. E. (1980). The parcellation theory and its relation to inter-specific variability in brain organization, evolutionary and ontogenetic development and neuronal plasticity. *Cell and Tissue Research*, 213, pp. 179–212.

Ebert, U. (1988). Das Vergeltungsprinzip im Strafrecht [The retaliation principle in penal law]. In: Krummacher, H. H. (Ed.), *Geisteswissenschaften—wozu?* Wiesbaden: Steiner, pp. 35–56.

Eccles, J. C. (1982). The initiation of voluntary movements by the supplementary motor area. *Archive für Psychiatrie und Nervenkrankheiten*, 231, pp. 423–441.

Eccles. J. C. (1990). A unitary hypothesis of mind-brain interaction in the cerebral cortex. *Proceedings of the Royal Society London*, B 240, pp. 433–451.

Edelman, G. (1978). *The mindful brain: Cortical organization and the group selective theory of higher brain function*. Cambridge, MA: MIT press.

Edelman, G. (1988). *Topobiology: An introduction to molecular embryology*. New York: Basic Books.

Edelman, G. (1989). *The remembered present: A biological theory of consciousness*. New York: Basic Books.

Edelman, G. (1992). *Bright air, brilliant fire*. New York: Basic Books.

Edwards, P. (1967). Determinism. In: Edwards, P. (Ed.), *Encyclopedia of philosophy*. London: Macmillan, pp. 359–373.

Eells, E. (1991). *Probabilistic causality*. Cambridge: Cambridge University Press.

Eiser, R. J. (1994). *Attitudes, chaos and the connectionist mind*. Oxford: Blackwell.

Ekman, P. (1982). *Emotion in the human face*. New York: Cambridge University Press.

Ekman, P. (1992). An argument for basic emotions. *Cognition and Emotion*, 6, pp. 169–200.

Ekman, P., Davidson, R. J., and Friesen, W. V. (1990). The Duchenne smile. Emotional Expression and brain physiology, II. *Journal of Personality and Social Psychology*, 58, pp. 342–353.

Elbert, Th., Lutzenberger, W., Rockstroh, B. Berg, P., and Cohen, R. (1992). Physical aspects of the EEG in schizophrenics. *Biological Psychiatry*, 32, pp. 595–606.

Elbert, Th., Ray, W. J., Kowalik, Z. J., Skinner, J. E., Graf, K. E., and Birbaumer, N. (1994). Chaos and Physiology. Deterministic chaos in excitable cell assemblies. *Physiological Reviews*, 74, pp. 1–47.

Eliasmith, C. (1996). The third contender: A critical examination of the dynamicist theory of cognition. *Philosophical Psychology*, 4, pp. 441–463.

Elliott, R., Frith, C. D., and Dolan, R. J. (1997). Differential neural response to positive and negative feedback in planning and guessing tasks. *Neuropsychologia*, 35, pp. 1395–1404.

Ellis, A. (1995). Critical Study. Recent work on punishment. *Philosophical Quarterly*, 45, pp. 225–233.

Engel, A. K., Roelfsma, P. R., Fires, P., Brecht, M., and Singer, W. (1997). Role of the temporal domain for response selection and perceptual binding. *Cerebral Cortex*, 7, pp. 571–582.

Engels, E. M. (1987). *Erkenntnis als Anpassung?* [Knowledge as adaptation?]. Frankfurt: Suhrkamp.

Fabian, T., and Stadler, M. (1992). Applying chaos theory to delinquent behavior in psychosocial stress situations. In: Lösel, F., Bender, D., and Bliesener, T. (Eds.), *Psychology and law*. Berlin: de Gruyter, pp. 55–61.

Farah, M. J. (1996). Is face recognition special? Evidence from neuropsychology. *Behavioral Brain Research*, 78, pp. 181–189.

Fedrowitz, J., Matejosvski, D., and Kaiser, G. (Eds.) (1994). *Neuroworlds*. Frankfurt, New York: Campus.

Feyerabend, P. (1963). Comment: 'Mental events and the brain.' *Journal of Philosophy*, 60, pp. 295–296.

Fink-Eitel, H., and Lohmann, G. (1993). *Zur Philosophie der Gefühle* [On a philosophy of emotions]. Frankfurt: Suhrkamp.

Fischer, J. M. (1982). Responsibility and control. *Journal of Philosophy*, 79, pp. 24–40.

Fischer, J. M. (1983). Incompatibilism. *Philosophical Studies*, 43, pp. 127–137.

Fischer, J. M. (1986) (Ed.). *Moral responsibility*. Ithaca: Cornell University Press.

Fischer, J. M. (1989). Recent work on God and freedom. *American Philosophical Quarterly*, 29, pp. 91–109.

Fischer, J. M. (1994). *The metaphysics of free will*. Oxford: Blackwell.

Fischer, J. M., and Ravizza, M. (1992). When the will is free. In: Tomberlin, J. E. (Ed.), *Philosophical perspectives*, Vol. 6 Atascadero, CA: Ridgeview, pp. 423–451. Reprinted in: O'Connor, T. (1995) (Ed.), *Agents, causes events*. Oxford: Oxford University Press, pp. 239–269.

Fischer, J. M., and Ravizza, M. (1993) (Eds.). *Perspectives on moral responsibility*. Ithaca, London: Cornell University Press.

Fischer, J. M., and Ravizza, M. (1994). Responsibility and history. *Midwest Studies in Philosophy*, 19, pp. 430–451.

Flanagan, O. (1991). *Varieties of moral personality: Ethics and psychological realism*. Cambridge, MA: Harvard University Press.

Florey, E., and Breidbach, O. (1993) (Eds.). *Das Gehirn—Organ der Seele?* [The brain—the soul's organ?]. Berlin: Akademie Verlag.

Fodor, J. (1974). Special sciences, or the disunity of science as a working hypothesis. *Synthese*, 28, pp. 77–115.

Fodor, J. (1984). Semantics, Wisconsin Style. *Synthese*, 59, pp. 231–250.

Fodor, J., and Pylyshyn, Z. (1988). Connectionism and cognitive architecture. A critical analysis. *Cognition*, 28, pp. 3–71.

Forth, A., and Hare, R. (1989). Contingent negative variation in psychopaths. *Psychophysiology*, 26, pp. 676–682.

Forth, W., Henschler, D., Rummel, W., and Starke, K. (1996). *Allgemeine und spezielle Pharmakologie und Toxikologie* [General and special pharmacology and toxicology]. Seventh edition, Heidelberg: Spektrum.

Foster, J. (1991). *The immaterial self: A defense of the Cartesian dualist conception of the mind*. London: Routledge.

Frank, R. (1992). *Strategie der Emotionen* [Strategy of Emotions]. Oldenbourg: Scientia Nova.

Frankfurt, H. G. (1969). Alternate possibilities and moral responsibility. *Journal of Philosophy*, 66. Reprinted in Frankfurt (1987), pp. 1–10.

Frankfurt, H. G. (1971). Freedom of the will and the concept of a person. *Journal of Philosophy*, 68, pp. 11–25. Reprinted in: Frankfurt, H. G. (1988), *The importance of what we care about*. Cambridge: Cambridge University Press, pp. 5–20.

Frankfurt, H. G. (1987). Identification and wholeheartedness. In: Schoeman, F. (Ed.), *Responsibility, character, and the emotions*. Cambridge: Cambridge University Press. Reprinted in: Frankfurt, H.G. (1998), *The importance of what we care about*. Cambridge: Cambridge University Press, pp. 159–176.

Frankfurt, H. G. (1988). *The importance of what we care about*. Cambridge: Cambridge University Press.

Frankfurt, H. G. (1992). The faintest passion. *Proceedings of the American Philosophical Association*, 66, pp. 5–16.

Frege, G. (1892). Über Sinn und Bedeutung. [n sense and meaning] *Zeitschrift für Philosophie und philosophische Kritik*, NF 100, pp. 25–50. Reprinted in: Frege, G. (1986), *Funktion, Begriff, Bedeutung*, sixth edition. Göttingen: Vandenhoeck & Ruprecht, pp. 40–65.

Freeman, W. (1991). Physiologie und Simulation der Geruchswahrnehmung. [The physiology and simulation of olfactory perception.] *Spektrum der Wissenschaft*. April, pp. 60–69.

Freman, W. (1995). *Societies of the brain*. Hillsdale, NJ: Erlbaum.

French, P. A., Uehling, T. E., and Wettstein, H. K. (1994) (Eds.). Philosophical Naturalism. *Midwest Studies in Philosophy*, 19.

Freud, S. (1891). *Zur Auffassung der aphasien. Eine kritische studie* [A critical study on aphasia]. Leipzig, Vienna: Franz Deuticke.

Freud, S. (1920/1940). Jenseits des Lustprinzips und andere Arbeiten aus den Jahren 1920–24. [Beyond the principle of pleasure and other papers from the years 1920–24.] In: *Complete Works*. 13 Vols. London: Imago.

Freund, H. J. (1987). Abnormalities of motor behavior after cortical lesions in humans. In: Mountcastle, V.B. (Series ed.), Plum, F. (Vol. ed.), *Handbook of physiology. The nervous system*. Vol. V, pp. 763–810. American Physiological Society.

Freund, H. -J. (1990). Premotor area and preparation of movement. *Rev. Neurol.*, 146, pp. 543–547.

Frey, G. (1971). Entry: *Determinismus/Indeterminismus* In: Ritter, J., and Gründer, K. (Ed.), *Historisches Wörterbuch der Philosophie*, Vol. 1, Basel: Schwabe, Col. 150–157.

Frith, C. D., Friston, K. J., Liddle, P. F., and Frackowiack, R. S. J. (1991). Willed action and prefrontal cortex in man. A study with PET. *Proceedings of the Royal Society* B, 244, pp. 241–246.

Funke, G. (1990). Kants Satz über die praktische Freiheit [Kant's word on practical freedom]. *Philosophia naturalis*, 19, pp. 40–52.

Fuster, J. M. (1989). *The prefrontal cortex: Anatomy, physiology, and neuropsychology of the frontal lobe*, second edition. New York: Raven Press.

Fuster. J. M. (1995). *Memory in the cerebral cortex*. Cambridge, MA: MIT Press.

Fuster, J. M. (1996). Frontal lobe and the cognitive foundation of behavioral action. In: Damasio, A. R., Damasio, H., and Christen, Y. (Eds.), *Neurobiology of decision-making*. New York: Springer, pp. 47–62.

Gasquoine, P. G. (1993). Alien hand sign. *Journal of Clinical and Experimental Neuropsychology*, 15, pp. 653–667.

Gazzaniga, M. (1995) (Ed.). *The cognitive neurosciences*. Cambridge, MA: MIT Press.

Gerent, W. (1993). Handlungsalternativen, determinismus und schein-Kompatibilismus. [Alternative action, determinism and apparent compatibilism]. Inaugural diss., Bielefeld.

Geuss, R. (1995). *Zeitschrift für philosophische Forschung*, 49, pp. 1–14.

Ginet, C. (1966). Might we have no choice? In: Lehrer, K., *Freedom and determinism*. New York.

Ginet, C. (1990). *On action*. Cambridge: Cambridge University Press.

Glatzel, P. M. (1995). Allgemeine systemtherapie—Überlegungen zu einer universellen Therapietheorie und ihrer Anwending auf die psychotherapeutische praxis [General Systemic Therapy—On a universal theory of therapy and its application in psychotherapeutic practice]. *Fortschritte der Neurologie und Psychiatrie*, 63, pp. 49–58.

Gleick, J. (1988). *Chaos—die ordnung des universums* [Chaos—The order of the universe]. Munich.

Glynn, I. M. (1990). Consciousness and time. *Nature*, 348, pp. 477–479.

Godfrey-Smith, P. (1988). Review of language, thought and other biological categories by Ruth Garett Millikan. *Australasian Journal of Philosophy*, 66, pp. 556–560.

Godfrey-Smith, P. (1994). A modern history theory of functions. *Noûs*, 28, pp. 344–362.

Goldberg, G. (1985). Supplementary motor area structure and function. Review and Hypothesis. *Behavioral and Brain Sciences*, 8, pp. 567–616.

Goldberg, G., and Bloom, K. K. (1990). The alien hand sign. Localization, lateralization and recovery. *American Journal of Physical Medical Rehabilitation*, 69, pp. 228–238.

Goldman-Rakic, P. (1987). Circuitry of the primate prefrontal cortex and the regulation of behavior by representational knowledge. In: Mountcastle, V., and Plum, K. F. (Eds.), *The nervous system: Higher functions of the brain*, Vol. 5, Handbook of Physiology. Washington, D.C.: American Physiological Society.

Goleman, D. (1996). *Emotional intelligence*. London: Bloomsbury.

Goller, H. (1992). *Emotionspsychologie und Leib-Seele problem* [Psychology of emotions and the mind-body problem]. Stuttgart: Kohlhammer.

Goodman, N. (1978). *Ways of worldmaking.* Indianapolis: Hackett.

Gould, S. J. (1987). The limits of adaptation. Is language a spandrel of the human brain? Paper presented to the Cognitive Science Seminar, Center for Cognitive Science, MIT, Oct.

Gould, S. J., and Lewontin, R. J. (1979). The spandrels of San Marco and the Panglossian paradigm. A critique of the adaptationist programme. *Proceedings of the Royal Society of London*, 205, pp. 281–288.

Gould, S. J., and Vrba, E. S. (1982). Exaptations: A missing term in the science of form. *Paleobiology*, 8, pp. 4–15.

Grewe, W. (1994). Freiheit und Determinismus. Zur Kritik an der Argumentation von Rheinwald [Freedom and Determinism. A critique on Rheinwald's argument]. *Zeitschrift für philosophische Forschung*, 48, pp. 117–127.

Grewendorf, G. (1995). *Sprache als Organ—Sprache als lebensform* [Language as an organ—language as a life form]. Frankfurt: Suhrkamp.

Griffiths, P. (1995). Adaptive explanations and the concept of a vestige. In: Griffiths, P. (Ed.), *Trees of life.* Kluwer, pp. 11–131.

Griffiths, P. E. (1993). Functional analysis and proper functions. *British Journal for Philosophy of Science*, 44, pp. 409–422.

Grimes, T. R. (1988). The myth of supervenience. *Pacific Philosophical Quarterly*, 69, pp. 152–160.

Grush, R., and Churchland, P. (1995). Gaps in Penrose's toilings. *Journal of Consciousness Studies*, 1, pp. 241–249.

Guttenplan, S. (1994a). An essay on mind. In: Guttenplan, S., *A companion to the philosophy of mind*, Oxford: Blackwell, pp. 1–107.

Guttenplan, S. (1994b). *A companion to the philosophy of mind.* Oxford: Blackwell.

Haaland, K. Y. (1992). Introduction to the Special Section on the emotional concomitants of brain damage. *Journal of Consulting and Clinical Psychology*, 60, pp. 327–328.

Hahlweg, K., and Hooker, C. A. (1989). *Issues in evolutionary epistemology.* Albany: State University Press of New York.

Haken, H. (1983). *Synergetik. Eine Einführung* [Synergetics. An Introduction], second edition. Berlin, New York: Springer.

Haken, H. (1991). *Synergetic computers and cognition.* Berlin, New York: Springer.

Haken, H. (1992). *Erfolgsgeheimnisse der Wahrnehmung* [Success secrets of perception]. Stuttgart: DVA.

Haken, H. (1995). *Principles of brain functioning.* Berlin, New York: Springer.

Haken, H., and Commentators (1996). Synergetic und Kognitionswissenschaften [Synergetics and Cognitive Sciences]. *Ethik und Sozialwissenschaften*, 7, pp. 587–675.

Haken, H., and Haken-Krell, M. (1989). *Entstehen von biologischer Information und Ordnung* [How biological information and order originate]. Darmstadt: Wissenschaftliche Buchgesellschaft.

Haken, H., and Stadler, M. (1990) (Eds.). *Synergetics of cognition*. Berlin, New York, Heidelberg: Springer.

Hameroff, S. (1994). Quantum coherence in microtubules. A neural basis for emergent consciousness? *Journal of Consciousness Studies*, 1, pp. 91–118.

Hameroff, S., Kaszniak, A. W., and Sott, A. S. (1996) (Eds.). *Towards a science of consciousness*. Cambridge, MA: MIT Press.

Hameroff, S., and Penrose, R. (1996). Conscious events as orchestrated space-time selections. *Journal of Consciousness Studies*, 3, pp. 36–53.

Hamlyh, D. W. (1995). Metaphysics, history of Entry in: Hondevich, J. (Ed.). *The Oxford Companion to Philosophy*. Oxford: Oxford University Press, pp. 556–559.

Hampshire, S., and Hart, H. L. A. (1958). Decision, intention, and certainty. *Mind*, 67, pp. 1–12.

Hampton, J. (1994). The failure of expected utility theory as a theory of reason. *Economics and Philosophy*, 10, pp. 95–242.

Hand, I. (1992). Verhaltenstherapie der Zwangsstörungen [Behavioral therapy for compulsive disorders]. In: Hand, I., Goodman, W.K., and Evers, U. (Eds.), *Zwangsstörungen*. Berlin: Springer, pp. 157–180.

Hansch, D. (1988). Pschosynergetik—neue Perspektiven für die Neuropsychologie? [Psycho-Synergetics—new perspectives for neuropsychology?]. *Zeitschrift für Psychologie*, 196, pp. 421–436.

Hardcastle, V. (1994). Psychology's binding problem and neurobiological solutions. *Journal of Consciousness Studies*, 1, pp. 66–90.

Hardin, C. L. (1988). *Color for philosophers*. Indianapolis: Hackett.

Hare, R. M. (1952). *The language of morals*. Oxford: Clarendon Press.

Harre, R. M., and Quinn, M. J. (1971). Psychopathy and autonomic conditioning. *Journal of Abnormal Psychology*, 77, pp. 223–235.

Harkavay, A. A. (1995). *Human will: The search for its physical basis*. Frankfurt: Lang.

Hebb, D. O., and Thompson, W. R. (1968). The social significance of animal studies. In: Lindsey, G., and Aronson, E. (Eds.), *The handbook of social psychology*, Vol. 2, second edition. Reading, MA: Addison-Wesley, pp. 729–774.

Heckhausen, H., Gollwitzer, P. M., and Weinert, F. E. (1987) (Eds.). *Jenseits des rubikon: Der Wille in den Humanwissenschaften* [The will in the humanities]. Berlin, New York: Springer.

Hedrich, R. (1993). Neuroepistemologie: Pläydoyer for eine synthetische Erkenntnistheorie [Neuro-epistemology: Plea for a synthetic theory of knowledge]. In: *Neue Realitäten, XVI, Deutscher Kongress für Philosophie*, pp. 422–429.

Hegel, G. W. F. (1807/1980). Phänomenologie des Geistes [Phenomenology of Mind]. In: Bonsiepen, W., and Heede, R. (Eds.), *Complete Works*, Vol. 9. Hamburg: Meiner.

Heidelberger, M. (1992). *Kausalität: Eine Problemübersicht* [Causality. A survey of the problems]. *Neue Hefte für Philosophie*, 32/33, pp. 130–153.

Helm, B. W. (1994). The significance of emotions. *American Philosophical Quarterly*, 31, pp. 319–331.

Hempel, C. G. (1974). *Philosophie der Naturwissenschaften* [Philosophy of Natural Science]. Munich: dtv.

Hempel, C. G., and Oppenheim, P. (1948). Studies in the logic of explanation. *Philosophy of Science*, 15, pp. 135–175.

Herrmann, T. (1996). Willensfreiheit—eine nützliche Fiktion? [Freedom of will—a useful fiction?]. In: von Cranach, M., and Foppa, K. (Eds.), *Freiheit des Entscheidens und Handelns: Ein Problem der nomologischen Psychologie*. Heidelberg: Asanger, pp. 56–69.

Hill, C. (1991). *Sensations. A defense of type materialism.* Cambridge: Cambridge University Press.

Hill, C. (1992). Van Inwagen on the consequence argument. *Analysis*, 52.2, pp. 49–55.

Ho, H. M. (1996). The biology of free will. *Journal of Consciousness Studies*, 3, pp. 231–244.

Hobart, R. E. (1934). Free will as involving determinism and inconceivable without it. *Mind*, 43, pp. 1–27.

Höffe, O. (1983). *Immanuel Kant.* Munich: Beck.

Höger, R. (1992). Chaos-Forschung und ihre Perspektiven für die Psychologie [Chaos research and its perspectives for psychology]. *Psychologische Rundschau*, 43, pp. 223–231.

Holland, J. H. (1995). *Hidden order: How adaptation builds complexity.* Reading: Addison-Wesley.

Honderich, T. (1973) (Ed.). *Essays on freedom of action.* London: Routledge.

Honderich, T. (1990a). *The consequences of determinism: A theory of determinism*, Vol. 2. Oxford: Oxford University Press.

Honderich, T. (1990b). *Mind and brain: A theory of determinism*, Vol. 1. Oxford: Oxford University Press.

Honderich, T. (1993). *How free are you? The determinism problem.* Oxford: Oxford University Press.

Hooker, C. A. (1981). Towards a general theory of reduction. *Dialogue*, 20, pp. 38–60, 201–235, 496–529.

Horgan, T. (1993). From supervenience to superdupervenience: Meeting the demands of a material world. *Mind*, 102, pp. 555–586.

Horgan, T., and Tienson, J. (1991). *Connectionism and the philosophy of mind.* Dordrecht, Boston: Kluwer.

Horn, C. (1996). Augustinus und die Entstehung des philosophischen Willensbegriffs [St. Augustine and the origin of the philosophical concept of the free will]. *Zeitschrift für philosophische Forschung*, 50, pp. 113–132.

Hornak, J., Rolls, E. T., and Wade, D. (1996). Face and voice expression identification in patients with emotional and behavioral changes following frontal lobe damage. *Neuropsychologia*, 34, pp. 247–261.

Hoyningen-Huene, P. (1994). Emergenz, Mikro- und Makrodetermination [Emergence, micro and macro determination]. In: Lübbe, W. (Ed.), *Kausalität und Zurechnung* [Causality and Ascription]. Berlin, New York: de Gruyter, pp. 165–195.

Hyder, R., Phelps, E. A., Wiggens, C. J., Labar, K. S., Blamire, A. M., and Shulman, R. G. (1997). "Willed action": A functional MRI study of the human prefrontal cortex during a sensorimotor task. *Proceedings of the National Academy of Science*, 94, pp. 6989–6994.

Illich, I. (1988). *Im Weinberg des Textes* [In the vineyard of text]. Frankfurt: Luchterhand.

Jaeger, H. (1996). Dynamische Systeme in der Kognitionswissenschaft [Dynamic systems in cognitive science]. *Kognitionswissenschaft*, 5, pp. 151–174.

Jibu, M., Hagan, S., Hameroff, S. R., Pribram, H. K., and Yasue, K. (1994). Quantum optical coherence in cytoskeletal microtubules: Implications for brain function. *BioSystems*, 32, pp. 95–209.

Johnson, M. (1987). *The body and the mind: The bodily basis of meaning, imagination, and reason.* Chicago: University of Chicago Press.

Johnson, M. (1993). *Moral imagination.* Chicago: Chicago University Press.

Johnson, M. H. (1997). *Developmental cognitive neuroscience.* Oxford: Blackwell.

Johnson, M. H., and Karmiloff-Smith, A. (1990). Can neural selectionism be applied to cognitive development and its disorders? *New Ideas in Psychology*, 10, pp. 35–46.

Jonas, H. (1981). *Macht oder Ohnmacht der Subjektivität?* [Power or impotence of subjectivity?] Frankfurt: Insel.

Jordan, P. (1932). Die Quantenmechanik und die Grundprobleme der Biologie und Psychologie. [Quantum mechanics and the fundamental problems of biology and psychology]. *Naturwissenschaften*, 20.

Jordan, P. (1934). Quantenphysikalische Bermerkungen zur Biologie und Psychologie. *Erkenntnis*, 4.

Jordan, P. (1938). Die Verstärkertheorie der Organismen in ihrem gegenwärtigen stand [The current amplifier theory of organisms]. *Naturwissenschaften*, 33, pp. 537–545.

Jordan, P. (1943). Die physik und das geheimnis des lebens [Physics and the secret of life]. Braunschweig.

Joseph, R. (1996). *Neuropsychiatry, neuropsychology, and clinical neuroscience*, second ed. Baltimore: Williams and Wilkins.

Joyce, J. (1995). Recent work: Decision theory. *Philosophical Books*, 36, pp. 225–236.

Kandel, E. R., Schwartz, J. H., and Jessel, T. M. (1996) (Eds.). *Neurowissenschaften* [Neurosciences]. Heidelberg: Spektrum.

Kane, R. (1985). *Free will and values*. Albany: State University of New York Press.

Kane, R. (1988). Libertarianism and Rationalism revisited. *Southern Journal of Philosophy*, 26, pp. 441–460.

Kane, R. (1989). Two kinds of incompatibilism. *Philosophy and Phenomenological Research*, 26, pp. 219–254.

Kane, R. (1996). *The significance of free will*. Oxford: Oxford University Press.

Kanitscheider, N. (1993). Freiheit, Determinismus und Chaos [Freedom, determinism and chaos]. *Skeptiker*, 2, pp. 39–42.

Kant, I. (1786/1983). Grundlegung zur Metaphysik der Sitten [Foundation for metaphysics of morals] In: Weischedel, W. (Ed.), *Complete Works in 10 Vols.* Darmstadt: Wissenschaftliche Buchgesellschaft, Vol. 6.

Kant, I. (1794/1983). Kritik der reinen Vernunft. [Critique of Pure Reason] In: Weischedel, W. (Ed.), *Complete works in 10 Vols.* Darmstadt: Wissenschaftliche Buchgesellschaft, Vol. 7.

Kant, I. (1796/1983). Aus Soemmerring *Über das Organ der Seele* [From Soemmerring *on the organ of the soul*]. In: Weischedel, W. (Ed.), *Complete works in 10 Vols.* Darmstadt: Wissenschaftliche Buchgesellschaft, Vol. 9.

Keil, G. (1993a). Biosemantik: Ein degenerierendes Forschungsprogramm? [Biosemantics: A degenerating research programme?] In: *Neue Realitäten— Herausforderung der Philosophie* [New realities—a challenge for philosophy]. Sixteenth German Congress for Philosophy. Berlin, pp. 86–93.

Keil, G. (1993b). *Kritik des Naturalismus*. [A critique on naturalism] Berlin, New York: de Gruyter.

Keil, G. (1996). Zu Russells these vom absterben des kausalbegriffs in den wissenschaften [On Russell's thesis that the concept of causality is no longer used in science] In: Hubig, C. H., Poser, H. (Eds.), *Cognitio humana: Dynamik des Wissens und der Werte* [Cognitio humana. The dynamics of knowledge and values]. Sixteenth German Congress for Philosophy, pp. 522–529.

Keller, I., and Heckhausen, H. (1990). Readiness potentials preceding spontaneous motor acts: voluntary vs. involuntary control. *Electroencephalography and Clinical Neurophysiology*, 76, pp. 351–361.

Kelso, J. A. (1995). *Dynamic patterns: Self-organization of brain and behavior.* Cambridge, MA: MIT Press.

Kenny, A. (1975a). Between Reason and Action. In: Kenny, A., *Will, freedom and power.* Oxford: Basil Blackwell.

Kenny, A. (1975b). *Will, freedom and power.* Oxford: Basil Blackwell.

Kim, J. (1984). Concepts of supervenience. *Philosophy and Phenomenological Research*, 68, pp. 315–326.

Kim, J. (1992). "Downward causation" in emergentism and nonreductive materialism. In: Beckermann, A., Floh, H., and Kim, J. (Eds.), *Emergence or reduction?* Berlin, New York: Springer, pp. 119–38.

Kim, J. (1993). *Supervenience and mind.* Cambridge: Cambridge University Press.

Kim, J. (1994). Entry: *Supervenience.* In: Guttenplan, S. *A Companion to the philosophy of mind.* Oxford: Blackwell, pp. 575–583.

Kim, J., and Sosa, E. (1995) (Eds.). *A companion to metaphysics.* Oxford: Blackwell.

Kischka, U., Spitzru, M., and Kammer, J. (1997). Frontal-subbortikale neuronale Schalthveise. *Fortschritte Neurologic Psychiatrie*, 65, pp. 221–231.

Kitcher, P. (1993). Function and design. *Midwest Studies in Philosophy*, 18, pp. 379–397.

Klein, M. (1990). *Determinism: Blameworthiness and deprivation.* Oxford: Clarendon Press.

Koch, G. (1994). *Kausalität, Determinismus und Zufall in der naturwissenschaftlichen Weltbeschreibung* [Causality, determinism and chance in natural scientific descriptions of the world]. Berlin: Duncker & Humblodt.

Koch, C., and Davis, J. L. (1994). *Large-scale neuronal theories of the brain.* Cambridge, MA: MIT Press.

Kolb, B., and Wishaw, I. Q. (1996). *Neuropsychologie* [Neuropsychology], fourth edition. Weinheim: Spektrum.

Kötter, R., and Meyer, N. (1992). The limbic system. A review of its empirical foundation. *Behavioral Brain Research*, 52, pp. 105–127.

Kripke, S. (1972). *Naming and necessity.* Cambridge, MA: Harvard University Press.

Kristeva-Feige, R. (1994). *Funktionelle Lokalisation motorischer Areale der Grosshirnrinde vor und während Willkürbewegungen beim Menschen*

[Functional localization of motor areas in the cortex before and during willed actions in humans]. Munich: Waxmann.

Krohn, W., and Küppers, G. (1992) (Eds.). *Emergenz: Die Entstehung von Ordnung, Organisation und Bedeutung.* [Emergence: The origin of order, organization and meaning.] Frankfurt: Suhrkamp.

Kruse, P., and Stadler, M. (1995) (Eds.). *Ambiguity in mind and nature: Multistable cognitive phenomena.* Berlin: Springer.

Kruse, P., Stadler, M., Pavlekovic, B., and Vladimir, G. (1992). Instability and cognitive order formation: Self-organization principles, psychological experiments, and psychotherapeutic interventions. In: Tschacher, W., Schiepek, G., and Brunner, E.J. (Eds.), *Self-organization and clinical psychology.* Heidelberg: Springer, pp. 102–117.

Kuhl, J. (1996). Wille, Freiheit, Verantwortung: Alte Antinomien in experimentalpsychologischer Sicht [Will, freedom, responsibility. Old antinomies viewed from an experimental psychological standpoint.] In: von Cranach, M., and Foppa, K. (1996) (Eds.), *Freiheit des Entscheidens und Handelns: Ein Problem der nomologischen Psychologie.* Heidelberg: Assanger, pp. 186–218.

Küppers, G. (1996) (Ed.). *Chaos und ordnung.* [Chaos and order]. Stuttgart: Reclam.

Kurthen, M. (1992). Ahistorical intentional content. *Journal for the General Philosophy of Science,* 25, pp. 241–259.

Kurthen, M. (1994). *Hermeneutische Kognitionswissenschaft* [Hermeneutic cognitive science]. Bonn: Djre.

Kutas, M., and van Patten, C. K. (1994). Psycholinguistics electrified. In: Gernsbacher, M.A. (Ed.), *Handbook of psycholinguistics.* New York: Academic Press, pp. 83–143.

Lapierre, D., Braun, C. M. J., and Hodgins, S. (1995). Ventral frontal deficits in psychopathy: Neuropsychological test findings. *Neuropsychologia,* 33, pp. 139–151.

Lazarus, R. S. (1982). Thoughts on the relationship between emotion and cognition. *American Psychologist,* 37, pp. 1019–1024.

Leder, M. (1995). Willensfreiheit: Zwei gute Argumente und ein schlechtes [Freedom of will: Two good arguments and one poor one]. *Zeitschrift für philosophische Forschung,* pp. 76–83.

LeDoux, J. E. (1994). Das Gedächtnis für Angst [The memory for fear]. *Spektrum der Wissenschaft,* August, pp. 78–83.

LeDoux, J. E. (1996). *The emotional brain: The mysterious underpinnings of emotional life.* New York: Simon & Schuster.

Leibniz, G. W. (1747/1979). *Monadologie* [Monadology]. Stuttgart: Reclam.

Lem, S. (1980). Die siebente Reise oder Wie Trurls Vollkommenheit zum Bösen führte. In: *Die phantastischen erzählungen.* Frankfurt: Insel.

Lenneberg, E. H. (1977). *Biologische Grundlagen der Sprache* [Biological foundations of language]. Frankfurt 1977.

Lennon, K. (1994). Entry: *Reasons and causes*. In: Guttenplan, S., *A companion to the philosophy of mind*. Oxford: Blackwell, pp. 531–535.

Leventhal, H., and Scherer, K. R. (1987). The relationship of emotion to cognition: A functional approach to a semantic controversy. *Cognition and Emotion*, 1, pp. 3–28.

Lewes, G. H. (1875). *Problems of life and mind*, Vol. 2. London: Kegan Paul, French, Turbner & Co.

Lewis, D. (1986). *On the plurality of worlds*. Oxford: Blackwell.

Lewis, D. (1989). *Die Identität von Körper und Geist* [The identity of mind and body]. Frankfurt: Klostermann.

Lewis, D. (1994). Entry: *Lewis, David: Reduction of mind*. In: Guttenplan, S., *A companion to the philosophy of mind*. Oxford: Blackford, pp. 412–431.

Libet, B., and Commentators (1985). Unconscious cerebral initiative and the role of conscious will in voluntary action. *Behavioral and Brain Sciences*, 8, pp. 529–566.

Libet, B. (1981). The experimental evidence for subjective referral of a sensory experience backwards in time. *Philosophy of Science*, 48, pp. 182–197.

Libet, B. (1993). The neural time factor in conscious and unconscious events. In: Experimental and theoretical studies of consciousness. *Ciba Foundation Symposium* 174, Chichester: Wiley, pp. 123–146.

Libet, B., Gleason, C. A., Wright, E. W., Jr., and Pearl, D. (1983). Time of conscious intention to act in relation to onset of cerebral activity [readiness potential]. *Brain*, 106, pp. 623–642.

Libet, B., Wright, E. W., Jr., Feinstein, B., and Pearl, D. (1979). Subjective referral of the timing for a conscious sensory experience. *Brain*, 102, pp. 192–224.

Liddle, P. F. (1987). The symptoms of chronic schizophrenia: A re-examination of the positive-negative dichotomy. *British Journal of Psychiatry*, 151, pp. 145–151.

Liddle, P. F. (1994). Volition and Schizophrenia. In: David, A. S., and Cutting, J. C. (Eds.), *The neuropsychology of schizophrenia*. Hillsdale, NJ: Erlbaum, pp. 39–49.

Liddle, P. F., Friston, K. J., Frith, C. D., Jones, T., Hirsch, S. R., and Frackowiak, R. S. J. (1992). Patterns of cerebral blood flow in schizophrenia. *British Journal of Psychiatry*, 160, pp. 179–189.

Liebermann, P. (1984). The biology and evolution of language. Cambridge, MA: Harvard University Press.

Lindley, R. (1986). *Autonomy*. Atlantic Highlands, NJ: Humanities Press.

Lindsley, D. B. (1951). Emotion. In: Stevens, S. S. (Ed.). *Handbook of Experimental Psychology.* New York: John Wiley, pp. 473–516.

Linke, D. B., and Kurthen, M. (1988). *Parallelität von Gehirn and Seele* [Parallelism of Brain and Soul]. Stuttgart: Enke.

Llinas, R., Ribary, U., Joliot, M., and Wang, X. J. (1994). Content and context in temporal cortical binding. In: Buzaki, R. et al., (Eds.), *Temporal coding in the brain.* Berlin, Heidelberg: Springer, pp. 251–272.

Lorenz, K. (1943). Kants Lehre vom Apriorischen im Lichte gegenwärtiger Biologie [Kant's theory of a priori in light of contemporary biology]. *Blätter für deutsche Philosophie,* 15, pp. 94–125.

Lorenz, K. (1978). *Vergleichende Verhaltensforschung* [Comparative behavioral research]. Vienna, New York: Springer.

Lorenz, K. (1984). Entry: *Identity.* In: Mittelstrass, J. (Ed.), *Enzyklopädie Philosophie und Wissenschaftstheorie* [Encyclopedia for Philosophy and Theory of Science], Vol. 2. Mannheim: Bibliographisches Institut, pp. 189–192.

Lucas, J. R. (1970). *The freedom of the will.* Oxford: Oxford University Press.

Lucas, J. R. (1993). *Responsibility.* Oxford: Clarendon Press.

Lund, J. S. (1988). Anatomical organization of macaque monkey striate visual cortex. *Annual Review of Neuroscience,* 11, pp. 253–288.

Lutzenberger, W., Elbert, T., Ray, W. J., and Birbaumer, N. (1993). The scalp distribution of the fractal dimension of the EEG and its variation with mental tasks. *Brain Topography,* 5, pp. 27–34.

Lyons, W. (1980). *Emotion.* London: University Press.

Lyons, W. (1990). Intentionality and modern philosophical psychology, I. The modern reduction of intentionality. *Philosophical Psychology,* 3, pp. 247–269.

Lyons, W. (1991). Intentionality and modern philosophical psychology, II. The return to representation. *Philosophical Psychology,* 4, pp. 83–102.

Lyons, W. (1992). Intentionality and modern philosophical psychology, III. The appeal to teleology. *Philosophical Psychology,* 5, pp. 309–326.

Maar, C., Pöppel, E., and Christaller, T. (1996) (Eds.). *Die Technik auf dem Weg zur Seele* [Technology on its way to the soul]. Reinbek: Rororo.

MacDonald, C. (1989). *Mind-body identity theories.* London: Routledge.

MacDonald, C., and MacDonald, G. (1995) (Eds.). *Connectionism.* Oxford: Basil Blackwell.

Machleidt, W., Gutjahr, L., and Mügge, A. (1989). *Grundgefühle* [Basic Feelings]. New York: Springer.

Mackor, A. R. (1995). Intentional psychology is a biological discipline. *Poznan Studies in the Philosophy of the Sciences and the Humanities,* 45, pp. 329–348.

MacLean, P. D. (1970). The triune concept of the brain and behavior. In: Boag, T. J., and Campbell, D. (Eds.), *The Neurosciences: Second study program.* New York: Rockefeller University Press, pp. 336–349.

MacLean, P. D. (1990). *The triune brain in evolution.* New York: Plenum Press.

Mainzer, K. (1994). Aufgaben, Ziel und Grenzen der Neurophilosophie [Tasks, goals and limits of neurophilosophy] In: Fedrowitz, J., Matejosvski, D., and Kaiser, D. (Ed.), *Neuro worlds.* Frankfurt, New York: Campus, pp. 131–151.

Mainzer, K. (1995). *Computer—Neue Flügel des Geistes?* [Computers—New wings for the mind?]. Berlin, New York: de Gruyter.

Mandelbrot, B. B. (1977). *The fractal geometry of nature.* New York: Freeman.

Margenau, H. (1967). Quantum mechanics, free will and determinism. *Journal of Philosophy,* 64, pp. 714–725.

Marquard, O. (1981). *Abschied vom Prinzipiellen* [Departing from principles]. Stuttgart: Reclam.

Maturana, H. R. (1985). *Erkennen: Die Organisation und Verkörperung von Wirklichkeit.* [Knowledge: The organization and embodiment of reality]. Braunschweig: Vieweg.

Maturana, H., and Varela, F. J. (1984). *El árbol del conocimiento.*

Mayr, E. (1991). *Eine neue Philosophie der Biologie* [A new philosophy of biology]. Munich: Pieper.

McCall, S. (1994). A model of the universe. Oxford: Clarendon Press.

McGinn, C. (1989). *Mental content.* Oxford: Basil Blackwell.

McKay, D. (1967/1978). Freedom of Action in a Mechanistic Universe. The twenty-first Arthur Stanley Eddington Memorial Lecture delivered at Cambridge University 17. Nov. 1967.

Mele, A. (1992). History and personal autonomy. *Canadian Journal of Philosophy,* 23, pp. 271–280.

Mele, A. (1995). *Autonomous agents.* Oxford University Press.

Merricks, T. (1995). Supervenience and mind. *Philosophical Books,* 36, pp. 156–164.

Metzinger, T. (1985). *Neuere Beiträge zur Diskussion des Leib-Seele-Problems* [Recent contributions to the discussion on the mind-body problem]. Frankfurt, New York: Peter Lang.

Metzinger, T. (1993). *Subjekt und Selbstmodell* [Subject and Self-model]. Paderborn: Mentis.

Metzinger, T. (1995) (Ed.). *Bewusstsein* [Consciousness]. Paderborn: Mentis.

Miller, G. A., Galanter, E., and Pribram, K. H. (1960). *Plans and the structure of behavior.* New York: Holt, Rinehart & Winston.

Millikan, R. G. (1984). *Language, thought and other biological categories.* Cambridge, MA: MIT Press.

Millikan, R. G. (1991). Speaking up for Darwin. In: Loewer, B., and Georges, R. (Eds.), *Meaning in mind: Fodor and his critics.* Oxford: Blackwell, pp. 151–164.

Millikan, R. G. (1993a). *White queen psychology.* Cambridge, MA: MIT Press.

Millikan, R. G. (1993b). Mentalese orthography. In: Dahlbom, B. (Ed.), *Dennett and his critics.* Oxford: Blackwell, pp. 97–123.

Millikan, R. G., and Commentators (1998). A common structure for concepts of individuals, stuffs, and real kinds: More mama, more milk and more mouse. *Behavior and Brain Sciences.*

Mittelstrass, J. (1987). Der arme Wille: Zur Leidensgeschichte des Willens in der Philosophie [The poor will. How the will has suffered in philosophy] In: Heckhausen, H., Gollwitzer, P. M., and Weinert, F. E. (Eds.), *Jenserts des Rubikon: Der Wille in den Human Wissenschaften.* Berlin, New York: Springer, pp. 33–48.

Moore, G. E. (1912/1970). *Principia ethica.* Stuttgart: Reclam.

Moreno, A., Fernandez, J., and Etxeberria, A. (1997). Computational Darwinism as a basis for cognition. *Revue Internationale de Systémique,* 6, pp. 205–221.

Müller, U. (1996). Philosophische Zergliederung des Sichtbaren und Unsichtbaren am Menschen: Kants Irrtum und die Folgen für das Verhältnis von Philosophie und kognitiver Neurowissenschaft [Separating the visible from the invisible in humans: Kant's error and the consequences for the relationship between philosophy and cognitive neuroscience]. Manuscript for a lecture at the seventeenth German Congress for Philosophie in Leipzig.

Mumford, M. (1992). On the computational architecture of the neocortex, II: The role of cortico-cortical loops. *Biological Cybernetics,* 66, pp. 241–251.

Munn, A. I. (1962). *Free will and determinism.* London: MacGibbon and Kee.

Nagel, E. (1961). The structure of science. New York: Harcourt, Brace.

Nagel, T. (1976). Moral Luck. *Proceedings of the Aristotelian Society,* Supplement, Vol. 50, 137–151.

Nagel, T. (1987). *What does it all mean?* New York: Oxford University Press.

Nahm, F. K. D., Tranel, D., Damasio, H., and Damasio, A. R. (1993). Crossmodal associations and the human amygdala. *Neuropsychologia,* 31, pp. 727–744.

Nathan, N. M. L. (1992). *Will and world.* Oxford: Oxford University Press.

Neander, K. (1991a). Functions as selected effects. *Philosophy of Science,* 58, pp. 168–184.

Neander, K. (1991b). The teleological notion of "function." *Australasian Journal of Philosophy,* 69, pp. 454–468.

Nesse, R. M. (1989). Evolutionary explanations of emotions. *Human Nature,* 1, pp. 261–289.

Nisbett, R., and Ross, L. (1980). *Human inference: Strategies and shortcomings of social judgment.* Englewood Cliffs, N.J.: Prentice Hall.

Nørretranders, T. (1994). *Spüre die Welt* [Feel the world]. Reinbek: Rowohlt.

Northoff, G. (1995). Ethische Probleme bei Hirngewebstransplantationen [Ethical problems of transplanting brain tissue] *Ethik der Medizin*, 7, p. 87–98.

Northoff, G. (1997a). Neuropsychiatrie und Neurophilosophie [Neuropsychiatry and Neurophilosophy]. In: Northoff, G., *Neuropsychiatrie und Neurophilosophie*. Paderborn: Mentis, pp. 9–35.

Northoff, G. (1997b). *Neuropsychiatrie und Neurophilosophie* [Neuropsychiatry and Neurophilosophy]. Paderborn: Mentis.

Nowell-Smith, P. H. (1948). Free will and moral responsibility. *Mind*, 57, pp. 45–61.

Nowell-Smith, P. H. (1954). *Ethics*. Harmondsworth.

Nozick, R. (1969). Newcomb's problem and two principles of choices. In: Rescher, N. et al. (Ed.), *Essays in honor of Carl G. Hempel*. Dordrecht: Reidel, pp. 114–146.

Nozick, R. (1981). Choice and indeterminism. In: Nozick, R., *Philosophical explanations*. Cambridge, MA: MIT Press. Reprinted in: O'Connor, T. (Ed.), *Agents, causes, events*. Oxford: Oxford University Press, pp. 101–114.

Nüse, R., Groeben, N., Freitag, B., and Schreier, M. (1991). *Über die Erfindungen des Radikalen Konstruktivismus* [On the inventions in radical constructivism]. Weinheim: Deutscher Studienverlag.

Oakley, J. (1992). *Morality and the emotions*. London: Routledge.

Oatley, K., Johnson-Laird, P. (1987). Towards a cognitive theory of emotions. *Cognition and Emotion*, 1, pp. 29–50.

O'Connor, T. (1995a) (Ed.). *Agents, causes, events*. Oxford: Oxford University Press.

O'Connor, T. (1995b). Agent causation. In: O'Connor, T. (Ed.), *Agents, causes, events*. Oxford: Oxford University Press, pp. 173–200.

Oeser, E., Seitelberger, F. (1988). *Gehirn, Bewusstsein und Erkenntnis* [Brain, consciousness and knowledge]. Darmstadt: Wissenschaftliche Buchgesellschaft.

O'Leary-Hawthorne, J. O., and Pettit, P. (1996). Strategies for free will compatibilists. *Analysis*, 56.4, pp. 191–201.

Oshana, M. A. (1994). Autonomy naturalized. *Midwest Studies in Philosophy*, 14, pp. 76–94.

O'Shaughnessy, B. (1980). *The will: A dual aspect theory*, 2 Vols. Cambridge: Cambridge University Press.

Ott, E., Grebogi, C., and Yorke, J. A. (1990). Controlling chaos. *Physical Review Letters*, 64, p. 1196.

Panksepp, J., and Commentators (1982). Toward a general psychobiological theory of emotions. *The Behavioral and Brain Sciences*, 3, pp. 407–467.

Papez, J. W. (1937). A proposed mechanism of emotion. *Archives of Neurology and Psychiatry*, 38, pp. 725–743.

Papineau, D. (1987). *Reality and representation*. Oxford: Blackwell.

Papineau, D. (1993). *Philosophical naturalism*. Oxford: Blackwell.

Papineau, D., Steward, H., Godfrey-Smith, P., and Tye M. (1996). Book symposium on *Philosophical Naturalism*. *Philosophy and Phenomenological Research*, 56, pp. 657–697.

Pasemann, F. (1996). Repräsentation ohne Repräsentation: Überlegungen zu einer Neurodynamik modularer kognitiver Systeme [Representation without representations. Thoughts on the neurodynamics of modular cognitive systems]. In: Rusch, G., Schmidt, S. J., and Breidbach, O. (Eds.), *Interne Repräsentationer*. Frankfurt: Suhrkamp, pp. 42–91.

Paslack, R. (1991). *Urgeschichte der Selbstorganisation* [Prehistory of self-organization]. Munich: Vieweg.

Passingham, R. E. (1993). *The frontal lobes and voluntary action*. Oxford: Oxford University Press.

Patzig, G. (1994). *Philosophische Anmerkungen zu Willensfreiheit, Verantwortung, Schuld* [Philosophical remarks on free will, responsibility, and guilt] In: Patzig, G., *Gesammelte Schriften I: Grundlagen der Ethik* [Collected Papers I, Foundations of Ethics]. Göttingen: Wallstein, pp. 190–208.

Pauen, M. (1997). Der Rigorismus der Freiheit: Wille, Determinismus und der Begriff der Person. [The rigorism of freedom: The will, determinism and the concept of person]. Manuscript.

Peitgen, H.-O., Jürgens, H., and Saupe, D. (1992). *Bausteine des Chaos: Fraktale* [Components of chaos. Fractals]. Stuttgart: Klett-Cotta.

Penrose, R. (1989). *The Emperor's new mind: Concering computers, minds, and the laws of physics*. Oxford: Oxford University Press.

Penrose, R. (1994a). *Shadows of mind*: A preview of his new book. *Journal of Consciousness Studies*, 1, p. 17–24.

Penrose, R. (1994b). Mechanisms, microtubules and the mind. *Journal of Consciousness Studies*, 1, pp. 241–249.

Penrose, R. (1994c). *Shadows of mind*. Oxford: Oxford University Press.

Penrose, R., and commentators (1990). Précis of The Emperor's new mind: Concerning computers, minds and the laws of physics. *Behavioral and Brain Sciences*, 13, pp. 643–705.

Penrose, R., and Hameroff, S. (1995). What Gaps? *Journal of Consciousness Studies*, 2, pp. 99–112.

Phelps, E. A., Hyder, F., Blamire, A. M., and Schulman, R. G. (1997). FMRI of the prefrontal cortex during overt verbal fluency. *Neuroreport*, 8, pp. 561–565.

Piatelli-Palmarini, M. (1989). Evolution, selection and cognition. From "learning" to parameter setting in biology and the study of language. *Cognition*, 31, pp. 1–44.

Pieper, A. (1985). *Ethili und Moral*. München: Beck.

Pinker, S., and Prince, A. (1988). On language and connectionism: Analysis of a parallel distributed processing model of language acquisition. *Cognition*, 28, pp. 73–193.

Pinker, S. (1996). *Der Sprachinstinkt* [The Language Instinct]. Munich: Kindler.

Pinker, S., Bloom, O., and Commentaries (1990). Natural language and natural selection. *Behavioral and Brain Sciences*, 13, pp. 707–784.

Planck, M. (1936/1978). Vom Wesen der Willensfreiheit. [On the essence of free will]. In: Pothast, U. (Ed.), *Seminar: Freies Handeln und Determinismus*. Frankfurt: Suhrkamp, pp. 272–293.

Plato (1987). *Phaedo*. Stuttgart: Reclam.

Plato (1990). *Collected works* (German version). Darmstadt: Wissenschaftliche Buchgesellschaft.

Plutchik, R. (1980). *Emotion: A psychoevolutionary synthesis*. New York: Harper & Row.

Pöppel, E. (1985). *Die Grenzen des Bewusstseins* [The limits of consciousness] Munich: dtv.

Popper, K. (1950). Indeterminism in quantum physics and in classical physics. *British Journal for the Philosophy of Science*, 1, pp. 117–133.

Popper, K. R. (1972) *Objective knowledge*. Oxford: Clarendon Press.

Popper, K. R. (1982). *The open universe*. Totowa, NJ: Rowman and Littlefield.

Popper, K. R., and Eccles, J. C. (1977). *The self and its brain*. London: Springer.

Port, R., and van Gelder, T. (1995) (Ed.). *Mind as motion*. Cambridge, MA: MIT Press.

Posner, M. I., and Raichle, M. E. (1996). *Bilder des Geistes: Hirnforscher auf den Spuren des Denkens* [Pictures of the mind: Brain researchers seeking thought] Heidelberg: Spektrum.

Pothast, U. (1978) (Ed.). *Seminar: Freies Handeln und Determinismus* [Seminar: Voluntary action and determinism]. Frankfurt: Suhrkamp.

Pothast, U. (1980). *Die Unzulänglichkeit der Freiheitsbeweise* [The insufficiency of proofs of freedom]. Frankfurt: Suhrkamp.

Power, M., and Dalgleish, T. (1996). *Cognition and emotion*. Hove, East Sussex: Psychology Press.

Prauss, G. (1983). *Kant über Freiheit als Autonomie* [Kant on freedom as a utonomy]. Frankfurt.

Preiss, G., and Forster, H. (1994). Neurodidaktik. Thoeretische und praktische Beiträge: Symposium in Malerserschloss in Heitersheim [Neuro-Didactics. Theoretical and practical contributions. Symposium in Malerser Castle in Heitersheim], 13–15 October 1994.

Pribram, K. H. (1965). Freud's project: An open, biologically based model for psychoanalysis. In: Greenfield, N. S., and Lewis, W. C. (Eds.), *Psychoanalysis and current biological thought*. Madison, Milwaukee: University of Wisconsin Press, pp. 81–92.

Prince, A., and Smolensky, P. (1997). Optimality. From neural networks to universal grammar. *Nature*, 275, pp. 1604–1610.

Prinz, W. (1996). Freiheit oder Wissenschaft? [Freedom or Science?]. In: von Cranach, M., and Foppa, K. (Eds.), *Freiheitdes Entscheidens und Handelns: Ein Problem del Nomologischer Psychologie*, Heidelberg: Asanger, pp. 86–103.

Putnam, H. (1967). Psychological predicates. Retitled: The nature of mental states. In: Putnam, H., *Mind, Language and Reality: Philosophical Papers*, Vol. 2. Cambridge. Cambridge University Press, pp. 429–440.

Putnam, H. (1975). The meaning of meaning. In: Gunderson, K. (Ed.), *Minnesota Studies in the Philosophy of Science*. Minneapolis: University of Minnesota Press, vol. 7, pp. 131–193.

Putnam, H. (1981). *Reason, truth and history*. Cambridge: Cambridge University Press.

Putnam, H. (1982). Why reason can't be naturalized. *Synthese*, 52, pp. 3–23.

Putnam, H. (1992a). *Renewing philosophy*. Cambridge: Harvard University Press.

Putnam, H. (1992b). *Vernonft, Wahrksit und gischichk*. Frankfurt: Suhrkamp.

Quante, M. (1993). Mentale Verursachung: Die Krisis des nicht-reduktiven Physikalismus [Mental Causation: The crisis of nonreductive physicalism]. *Zeitschrift für philosophische Forschung*, 47, pp. 615–628.

Quante, M. (1997). Personal autonomy and the structure of the will. In: Kotkavirta, J. (Ed.), *Right, morality, ethical life: Studies in G.W.F. Hegel's Philosophy of Right*. Jyväskyla, pp. 45–74.

Raleigh, M., McGuire, M. M., Melega, W., Cherry, S., Huang, S.-C., and Phelps, M. (1996). Neural mechanism supporting successful decisions in Simians. In: Damasio, A. R., Damasio, H., and Christen, Y. (Eds.), *Neurobiology of decision-making*. New York: Springer, pp. 62–68.

Ramsey, W., Stich, S. P., and Garon, J. (1991). Connectionism, eliminativism and the future of folk psychology. In: Ramsey, W., Stich, S. P., and Rumelhart, D. E. (Eds.), *Philosophy and connectionist theory*. Hillsdale, N.J.: Erlbaum, pp. 199–228.

Ravn, I. (1995) (Ed.). *Chaos, Quarks und schwarze Löcher* [Chaos, quarks and black holes]. Munich: Kunstmann.

Rheinwald, R. (1990). Zur Frage der Vereinbarkeit von Freiheit und Determinismus [On the question of whether freedom and determinism are compatible]. *Zeitschrift für philosophische Forschung*, 44. pp. 194–219.

Richards, J., and von Glaserfeld, E. (1984). Die Kontrolle von Wahrnehmung und die Konstruktion von Realität: Erkenntnistheoretische Aspekte des Rückkoppelungs-Kontroll-Systems [Controlling perception and constructing reality: Epistemological aspects of feedback-control systems]. *Delfin*, 3, pp. 4–25.

Richards, N. (1986). Luck and desert. *Mind*, 95, pp. 198–201.

Rickert, H. (1921). *System der Philosophie. Erster Teil: Allgemeine Grundlegung der Philosophie* [The system of philosophy. Part One: General Foundations of Philosophy]. Tübingen.

Riedl, R. (1980). *Biologie der Erkenntnis* [Biology of knowledge], second edition. Hamburg: Parey.

Riedl, R., and Delpos, M. (Eds.). *Die evolutionäre Erkenntnistheorie im Spiegel der Wissenschaften* [Evolutionary epistemology as mirrored by science]. Vienna: WWW Universitätsverlag.

Ritter, H., Martinetz, T., and Schulten, K. (1990). *Neuronale Netze. Eine Einführung in die Neuroinformatik selbstorganisierender Netzwerke* [Neuronal nets: An introduction to neuro-computer science of self-organizing networks]. Bonn: Addison-Wesley.

Rockland, K. S. (1993) (Ed.). Special issue of *Cerebral Cortex*, 3.

Rojas, R. (1993). *Theorie der neuronalen Netze: Eine systematische Einführung* [Theory of neuronal nets. A systematic introduction]. Berlin, New York: Springer.

Rolls, E. T., Hornak, J., Wade, D., and McGrath, J. (1994). Emotion related learning in patients with social and emotional changes associated with frontal lobe damage. *Journal of Neurology, Neurosurgery and Psychiatry*, 57, pp. 1518–1524.

Rosenberg, A. (1992). Causation, probability and the monarchy. *American Philosophical Quarterly*, 29, pp. 305–318.

Röska-Hardy, L. (1995). Denken, Handeln und Erklärung nach Gründen [Thinking, acting and explaining by reasons]. *Deutsche Zeitschrift für Philosophie*, 43, pp. 259–270.

Rost, W. (1990). *Emotionen: Elixiere des Lebens* [Emotions: Life's fountain of youth]. Berlin, New York: Springer.

Roth, G. (1994). *Das Gehirn und seine Wirklichkeit* [The brain and its reality]. Frankfurt: Suhrkamp.

Rowe, W. (1991). *Thomas Reid on freedom and morality*. Ithaca: Cornell University Press.

Rowe, W. (1994). Two concepts of freedom. *Proceedings of the American Philosophical Association*, 61, pp. 43–64. Reprinted in: O'Connor, T. (Ed.), *Agents, causes, events*. Oxford: Oxford University Press, 151–171.

Rumelhart, D. E., and McClelland, J. L. (1986) (Ed.). *Parallel distributed processing*, 2 Vols. Cambridge, MA: MIT Press.

Rungaldier, E. (1996). *Was sind Handlungen?* [What are actions?]. Stuttgart: Kohlhammer.

Rusch, G., Schmidt, S. J., and Breidbach, O. (1996) (Eds.). *Interne Repräsentationen* [Internal representations]. Frankfurt: Suhrkamp.

Sabini, J., and Silver, M. (1987). Emotions, responsibility and character. In: Schoeman, F. (Ed.) *Responsibility, character, and emotions*. Cambridge: Cambridge University Press, pp. 165–175.

Saver, J. L., and Damasio, A. R. (1991). Preserved access and processing of social knowledge in a patient with acquired sociopathy due to ventromedial frontal damage. *Neuropsychologia*, 29, pp. 1241–1249.

Scanlon, T. M. (1988). The significance of choice. In: McMurrin, S. M. (Ed.), *The Tanner Lectures on human values*, Vol. 7. Salt Lake City: University of Utah Press.

Schachter, S., and Singer, J. E. (1962). Cognitive, social, and physiological determinants of emotional state. *Psychological Review*, 69, pp. 379–399.

Schaffner, K. (1967). Approaches to reduction. *Philosophy of Science*, 34, pp. 137–147.

Schedlowski, M., and Thewes, U. (1996). *Psychoneuroimmunologie* [Psychoneural Immunology]. Heidelberg: Spektrum.

Scheerer, E. (1996). Orality, literacy, and cognitive modeling. In: Velichkovsky, B. (Ed.), *Communicating meaning*. Hillsdale, NJ: Erlbaum, pp. 211–256.

Scherer, K. J. (1993). Neuroscience projections to current debates in emotion psychology. *Cognition and Emotion*, 7, pp. 1–42.

Schiepek, G. (1996). Der Appeal der Chaos for schring für die Psychologie. In: Küppers (Ed.), pp. 353–338.

Schlesinger, G. (1974). The unpredictability of free choices. *British Journal for the Philosophy of Science*, 25, pp. 209–211.

Schlick, M. (1930/1978). Wann its der Mensch verantwortlich? [When is a person responsible?] In: M. Schlick: *Fragen der Ethik* [Ethical Questions], chapter 7. Reprinted in Pothast, U. (1978), *Seminar: Freies Handeln und Determinismus*. Frankfurt: Suhrkamp, pp. 157–168.

Schmidt, S. J. (1987) (Ed.). *Der Diskurs des radikalen Konstruktivismus* [The discourse on radical constructivism]. Frankfurt: Suhrkamp.

Schmitz, H. (1996). *Physiologischer Neukantianismus und evolutionäre Erkenntnistheorie* [Physiological Neukantianism and evolutionary epistemology]. Frankfurt, New York: Peter Lang.

Schnädelbach, H. (1987). Vermutungen über die Willensfreiheit [Conjectures about free will]. In: H. Schnädelbach: *Vernunft und Geschichte* [Reason and History]. Frankfurt: Suhrkamp (stw), pp. 96–124.

Schneider, F. (1997). Funktionelle Kernspintomographie von Emotionen bei Gesunden und schizophrenen Patienten [Functional magnetic resonance imaging of emotions in healthy subjects and schizophrenic patients]. *Nervenarzt*, 67, Suppl. 1, p. 200.

Schneider, F., Wciss, U., Hessler, C., Muller-Gartner, H. W., et al. (1999). Subcortical correlates of differential classical conditioning of aversive emotional reactions in social phobia. *Biological Psychiatry*, 45, pp. 863–871.

Schoeman, F. (1987) (Ed.). *Responsibility, character, and the emotions.* Cambridge: Cambridge University Press.

Schönrich, G., and Kato, Y. (1996). *Kant in der Diskussion in der Moderne* [Kant's role in the discussion about Modern Times]. Frankfurt: Suhrkamp.

Schreiber, H.-L. (1994). Rechtliche Grundlagen der psychiatrischen Begutachtung [Legal basis for psychiatric appraisals]. In: Venzlaf, U., and Foerster, K. (Eds.), *Psychiatrische Begutachtung*. Stuttgart: Fischer, pp. 3–82.

Schroeter, F. (1993). Kants Theorie der formalen Bestimmung des Willens [Kant's theory of formally defining the will]. *Zeitschrift für philosophische Forschung*, 47, pp. 388–407.

Schünemann, B. (1997). Willensfreiheit und Recht [Freedom of Will and Justice]. Lecture at the third international congress of the society for analytical philosophy: "Rationality, Realism, Revision," Munich.

Schütt, H. P. (1996). *Die Adoption des "Vaters der modernen Philosophie"* [Adopting the "father of modern philosophy"]. Frankfurt: Klostermann.

Searle, J. R. (1983). *Intentionality*. Cambridge: Cambridge University Press.

Searle, J. R. (1984). *Minds, brains and science*. Cambridge, MA: Harvard University Press.

Searle, J. R. (1992). *The rediscovery of mind*. Cambridge, MA: MIT Press.

Searle, J. R., and Commentaries (1990). Consciousness, explanatory inversion and cognitive science. *Behavioral and Brain Sciences*, 13, pp. 585–642.

Seebass, G. (1992). *Wollen* [Volition]. Frankfurt/M.: Klostermann.

Seebass, G. (1993). Freiheit und Determinismus [Freedom and determinism]. *Zeitschrift für philosophische Forschung*, 47, pp. 1–22, 223–245.

Seidenberg, M. S. (1997). Language acquisition and use: learning and applying probabilistic constraints. *Nature*, 275, pp. 1599–1603.

Seiffert, J. (1989). *Das Leib-Seele-Problem und die gegenwärtige Philosophische diskussion* [The mind-body problem and its current philosophical debate]. Darmstadt: Wissenschaftliche Buchgesellschaft.

Sejnowski, T. J., and Rosenberg, C. R. (1987). Parallel networks that learn to pronounce English text. *Complex systems*, 1, pp. 145–168.

Shallice, T. (1982). Specific impairments of learning. *Philosophical transactions of the Royal Society of London*, B 268, pp. 199–209.

Shallice, T. (1988). *From neuropsychology to mental structure*. Cambridge: Cambridge University Press.

Shatz, D. (1986). Free will and the structure of motivation. *Midwest Studies in Philosophy*, 10, pp. 451–482.

Shatz, D. (1988). Compatibilism, values and "could have done otherwise." *Philosophical topics*, 16, pp. 151–200.

Singer, W. (1994). Putative functions of temporal correlation in neocortical processing. In: Koch, C., and Davis, J. (Eds.), *Large-scale neuronal theories of the brain*. Cambridge, MA: MIT Press, pp. 201–237.

Singer, W., and Gray, C. (1995). Visual feature integration and the temporal correlation hypothesis. *Annual Revue of Neuroscience*, 18, pp. 555–586.

Skarda, C., Freeman, W., and Commentaries (1987). How the brain makes chaos in order to make sense of the world. *Behavioral and Brain Sciences*, 10, pp. 1612–195.

Slote, M. A. (1980). Understanding free will. *Journal of Philosophy*, 77(1), pp. 36–151.

Slote, M. A. (1982). Selective necessity and the free will problem. *Journal of Philosophy*, 79, pp. 5–24.

Smart, J. J. C. (1961). Free-will, praise and blame. *Mind*, 70, pp. 291–306.

Smolensky, P., and Commentaries (1988). On the proper treatment of connectionism. *Behavioral and Brain Sciences*, 11, pp. 1–74.

Smythies, J. R., and Beloff, J. (1989) (Eds.). *The case for dualism*. Charlottesville: University Press of Virginia.

Spence, S., and Commentaries (1996). Free will in the light of neuropsychiatry. *Philosophy, Psychiatry and Psychology*, 3, pp. 75–100.

Spence, S. A., Brooks, D. J., Hirsch, S. R., Liddle, P. F., Meehan, J., and Grasby, P. M. (1997). A PET study of voluntary movement in schizophrenic patients experiencing passivity phenomena (delusions of alien control). *Brain*, 120, pp. 1997–2011.

Sperry, R. W. (1980). Mind-brain-interaction: Mentalism, yes; dualism, no. *Neuroscience*, 5, pp. 195–206.

Sperry, R. W. (1986). Discussion: Macro- versus micro-determinism. *Philosophy of Science*, 53, pp. 265–270.

Spitzer, M. (1996). *Geist im Netz* [Mind in the network]. Heidelberg: Spektrum.

Spitzer, M. (1997). *Neuronale Netzwerke und* Psychopathologie [Neuronal networks and psycho-pathology]. *Nervenarzt*, 68, pp. 21–37.

Sporns, O., and Tonini, G. (1994) (Eds.). Selectionism and the brain. New York: Academic Press (also as Vol. 37 of the *International Review of Neurobiology*).

Springer, S. P., and Deutsch, G. (1995). *Rechtes gehirn, linkes gehirn* [Left brain, right brain], third edition. Heidelberg: Spektrum.

Sproat, R. (1995). Computational interpretations of neurolinguistic observations. In: Gazzaniga, M. (Ed.), *The cognitive neurosciences.* Cambridge, MA: MIT Press, pp. 931–942.

Stadler, M., Kruse, P., and Carmsin, H. O. (1996). Erleben und Verhalten in der Polarität von Chaos und Ordnung [Experience and behavior between the poles of chaos and order]. In: Küppers, G. (Ed.), *Chaos und Ordnung.* Stuttgart: Reclam, pp. 323–352.

Steels, L., and Brooks, R. (1995) (Eds.). *The artificial life route to artificial intelligence: Building embodied, situated agents.* Hillsdale, NJ: Erlbaum.

Steinvorth, U. (1987). *Freiheitstheorien in der Neuzeit* [Theory of freedom in modern times]. Darmstadt: Wissenschaftliche Buchgesellschaft.

Steinvorth, U. (1995). Zum Problem der Willensfreiheit [The problem of free will]. *Zeitschrift für philosophische Forschung,* 49, pp. 398–415.

Stekeler-Weithofer, P. (1990). Wille und Willkür bei Kant [The will and free will in Kant's work]. *Kant Studien,* 81, pp. 30–320.

Stephan, A. (1992). Emergence: A systematic view of its historical facets. In: Beckermann, A., Flohr, H., and Kim, J. (Eds.), *Emergence or reduction?* Berlin, New York: Springer, pp. 25–48.

Stephan, A. (1996). Ordner, Sklaven und andere Systemgeister [Orderlies, slaves and other ghosts in the system]. *Ethik und Sozialwissenschaften,* 7, pp. 642–643.

Stephan, A. (1999). *Emergenz: Von der Unvorhersagbarkeit zur Selbstorganization* [Emergence: From unpredictability to self-organization]. Dresden-Munich: Dresden University Press.

Stephan, A., and Beckermann, A. (1994). Emergenz [Emergence]. *Information Philosophie,* 3, pp. 46–51.

Stephens, G. L., and Graham, G. (1994). Self-consciousness, mental agency, and the clinical psychopathology of thought insertion. *Psychology, Psychiatry and Philosophy,* 1, pp. 1–10.

Stich, S. (1983). *The fragmentation of reason.* Cambridge, MA: MIT Press.

Stöckler, M. (1992). Entry "Reduction" in: Gründer, K., and Ritter, J., *Historisches Wörterbuch der Philosophie* [Historical dictionary for philosophy], Vol. 8. Basel: Schwabe, col. 378–383.

Strawson, G. (1986). *Freedom and belief.* Oxford: Oxford University Press.

Strawson, G. (1989). Consciousness, free will and the unimportance of determinism. *Inquiry,* 32, pp. 3–27.

Strawson, P. F. (1962). Freedom and Resentment. *Proceedings of the British Academy,* 48, pp. 187–211.

Streminger, G. (1992). *Gottes Güte und die Übel der Welt: Das theodizeeproblem* [God's Goodness and the Evil in the World: The theodicy problem]. Tübingen: Mohr.

Strube, G., et al. (1996). *Wörterbuch der Kognitionswissenschaft* [Dictionary for Cognitive Science]. Stuttgart: Klett-Cotta.

Stuhlmann-Laeisz, R. (1983). *Das Sein-Sollen-Problem: Eine modallogische Studie* [The description-norm problem: A modal logical study]. Stuttgart-Bad Cannstatt: Fromman-Holzbog.

Sugden, R. (1991). Rational choice: A survey of contributions from economics and philosophy. *The Economic Journal*, 101, pp. 751–785.

Sulloway, F. J. (1982). *Freud: Biologe der Seele. Jenseits der psycho-analytischen Legende* [Freud: The soul's biologist. Beyond the psycho-analytical legend]. Cologne: Hohenheim.

Swinburne, R. (1995). Die Hypothese, des es einen Gott gibt [The hypothesis that God exists]. *Information Philosophie*, 2, pp. 32–39.

Swinburne, R. (1997). *The evolution of the soul*, second ed. Oxford: Clarendon.

Taylor, R. (1974). *Metaphysics*. Englewood Cliffs: Prentice Hall.

Taylor, R. (1982). Agent and patient. Is there a distinction? *Erkenntnis*, 18, pp. 223–232.

Tennant, N. (1995). Entry *anti-realism*. In: Kim, J., and Sosa., E. (Eds.), *A companion to metaphysics*. Oxford: Blackwell, pp. 14–18.

Tetens, H. (1991). Lösen die Naturwissenschaften das Leib-Seele-Problem? *Information Philosophie*, 3, pp. 5–13.

Tetens, H. (1994). *Geist, Gehirn, Maschine* [Mind, brain, machine]. Stuttgart: Reclam.

Thalberg, I. (1967). Do we cause our actions? *Analysis*, 27, pp. 196–201.

Thelen, E. (1993). Self organization in developmental processes. Can system approaches work? In: Johnson, M. (Ed.), *Brain development and cognition*. Oxford: Blackwell, pp. 555–591.

Thelen, E., and Smith, L. B. (1994). *A dynamic system approach to the development of cognition and action*. Cambridge, MA: MIT Press.

Thomas, H., and Leiber, T. (1994). Determinismus und Chaos in der Physik. [Determinism and chaos in physics] In: Mainzer, K., and Schirrmacher, W. (Eds.), *Quanten, Chaos und Dämonen* [Quantum, chaos and demons]. Mannheim: Bibliographisches Institut.

Thompson, E. (1994). *Colour vision: A study in cognitive science and the philosophy of perception*. London: Routledge.

Thorp, J. (1980). *Free will: A defense against neurophysiological determinism*. London: Routledge.

Tomkins, S. S. (1982). Affect, imagery and consciousness, Vol. 3: *Cognition and affect*. New York: Springer.

Tooby, J., and Cosmides, L. (1995). *Mapping the evolved functional organization of mind and brain*. In: Gazzaniga, M. (Ed.), *The cognitive neurosciences*, Cambridge, MA: MIT Press, pp. 1185–1190.

Toulmin, S. (1972). Human understanding. Oxford.

Townsend, J. T., and Busemeyer, J. (1995). Dynamic representation of decision making. In: Port, and Gelder (1995), pp. 101–120.

Tugendhat, E. (1987). Der Begriff der Willensfreiheit [The concept of free will]. In: Cramer, K., Fulda, H.F., Horstmann, R.P., and Pothast, U. (Eds.), *Theorie der Subjektivität* [Theory of subjectivity]. Frankfurt: Suhrkamp, pp. 373–382.

Van Gelder, T. (1990). Compositionality: A Connectionist variation on a classical theme. *Cognitive Science*, 14, pp. 355–385.

Van Gelder, T. (1993). Beyond symbolic: Prolegomena to a Kama-Sutra of Compositionality. In: Honvar, V., and Uhr, L. (Eds.), *Symbol processing and connectionist models in AI and cognition: Steps towards integration*. New York: Academic Press.

Van Gelder, T. (1995). What might cognition be if not computation? *Journal of Philosophy*, 91, pp. 345–381.

Van Gelder, T., and Port, R. F. (1995). It's about time: An overview of the dynamical approach to cognition. In: Port, R., and Van Gelder, T. (Eds.), *Mind as Motion*. Cambridge, MA: MIT Press, pp. 1–43.

Van Inwagen, P. (1975). The Incompatibility of Free Will and Determinism. *Philosophical Studies*, 27, pp. 185–199.

Van Inwagen, P. (1986). *An Essay on Free Will*, second ed. Oxford: Clarendon Press.

Van Inwagen, P. (1989). When is the will free? In: Tomberlin, J.E. (Ed.), *Philosophical perspectives*, Vol. 3. Atascadero, CA: Ridgeview, pp. 399–422. Reprinted in: O'Connor, T. (Ed.), *Agents, causes, events*. Oxford: Oxford University Press, pp. 219–238.

Van Inwagen, P. (1994). When the will is not free. *Philosophical Studies*, 75, pp. 95–114.

Varela, F. J. (1982). Biologie der Freiheit [Biology of freedom]. *Psychologie heute*, 9, pp. 83–93.

Varela, F. J. (1985). *Kognitionswissenschaft* [Cognitive Science]. Frankfurt: Suhrkamp.

Varela, F. J. (1997). Neurophenomenology: A methodological remedy for the hard problem. *Journal of Consciousness Studies*, 3, pp. 330–349.

Varela, F. J., and Thompson, E. (1991). *Der Mittlere Weg der Erkenntnis* [The middle way of knowledge]. Bern/Munich/Vienna: Scherz.

Vaitl, D. (1995). Interozeption: Ein neues interdisziplinäres Forschungsfeld [Interoception. A new interdisciplinary field of research]. *Psychologische Rundschau*, 3, pp. 171–185.

Venzlaff, U., and Foerster, K. (1994) (Eds.). *Psychiatrische Begutachtung*. [Psychiatric appraisal], second edition. Stuttgart: Fischer.

Vogeley, K. (1995). *Repräsentation und Identität* [Representation and identity]. Berlin: Duncker und Humblodt.

Vollmer, G. (1975). Evolutionäre Erkenntnistheorie [Evolutionary epistemology]. Stuttgart: Hirzel.

Vollmer, G. (1984). *Was können wir wissen? Die Natur der Erkenntnis* [What can we know? The nature of knowledge]. Stuttgart: Hirzel.

Vollmer, G. (1992a). Das Ganze und seine Teile. Holismus, Emergenz, Erklärung und Reduktion. [The whole and its parts. Holism, emergence, explanation and reduction]. In: Deppert, W., Kliemt, H., Lohff, B., and Schaefer, J. (Eds.), *Wissenschaftstheorien in der medizin*. Berlin, New York: de Gruyter.

Vollmer, G. (1992b). Ist evolutive Selbstorganistion zu Leben und Bewusstsein doch denkbar? [Is evolutionary self organization for life and consciousness conceivable after all?] *Fichte-Studien*, 4, pp. 53–67.

Vollmer, G. (1994). Erfahrung und Hypothese—Einführung in die Wissenschaftstheorie [Experience and Hypothesis—Introduction to the theory of science]. Lectures.

Vollmer, G. (1995). *Biophilosophie* [Bio-philosophy]. Stuttgart: Reclam.

Von Cranach, M., and Foppa, K. (1996) (Eds.). *Freiheit des Entscheidens und Handelns. Ein problem der nomologischen Psychologie* [Freedom of decision and action. A problem of nomological psychology]. Heidelberg: Asanger.

Von Foerster, H. (1985). *Sicht und Einsicht* [Sight and Insight]. Braunschweig: Vieweg.

Von Glasenapp, H. (1992). *Die fünf Weltreligionen* [Five world religions], eleventh edition. Munich: Diedelrichs.

Von Glasersfeld, E. (1987). *Wissen, Sprache und Wirklichkeit* [Knowledge, language and reality]. Braunschweig: Vieweg.

Von Weizäcker, V. (1950). *Der Gestaltkreis* [The Gestalt circle]. Stuttgart: Thieme.

Von Wright, G. H. (1974a). *Causality and determinism.* New York: Columbia University Press.

Von Wright, G. H. (1974b). *Erklären und Verstehen* [Explaining and understanding]. Königstein/Ts.: Athenäum.

Wagner, S., and Warner, R. (1993) (Eds.). *Naturalism.* South Bend: Notre Dame University Press.

Waldrop, M. M. (1993). *Inseln im Chaos: Die Erforschung komplexer Systeme* [Islands in the midst of chaos: Researching complex systems]. Reinbek: Rowohlt.

Waller, B. N. (1988). *Freedom without responsibility.* Philadelphia: Temple University Press.

Waller, B. N. (1993). Natural autonomy and alternative possibilities. *American Philosophical Quarterly*, 30, pp. 73–81.

Waller, B. N. (1995). Authenticity naturalized. *Behavior and Philosophy*, 23, pp. 21–28.

Walter, H. (1993). Chaos, physiology and free will. A piece of naturalized philosophy. *Third International Colloquium of Cognitive Science*, San Sebastian, pp. 187–190.

Walter, H. (1996a). Die Freiheit des Deterministen. Chaos und Neurophilosophie [The determinist's freedom. Chaos and neurophilosophy]. *Zeitschrift für philosophische Forschung*, 50, pp. 364–385.

Walter, H. (1996b). Minimale Neurophilosophie. [Minimal neurophilosophy]. In: Hubig, Ch., and Poser, H. (Eds.), *Cognitio humana: Dynamic des Wissens und der Werte* [Cognitio humana. Dynamics of knowledge and values]. Seventeenth German Congress for Philosophy, pp. 1515–1522.

Walter, H. (1996c). Körperlose Gefühle? [Bodiless Emotions?] *Ethik und Sozialwissenschaften*, 7, pp. 346–350.

Walter, H. (1996d). Die Neurobiologie menschlicher Autonomie [The neurobiology of human anatomy]. *Nervenarzt*, 67, Suppl. 1, p. 19.

Walter, H. (1997a). Authentizität und emotive Neurowissenschaft [Authenticity and emotive neuroscience]. *Philosophia naturalis*, 34, pp. 147–174.

Walter, H. (1997b). Neuroimaging and philosophy of mind. In: Northoff, G. (Ed.), *Neuropsychiatrie und Neurophilosophie*. Paderborn: Mentis, pp. 193–222.

Walter, H. (1997c). Proper functions in der Klemme? [Proper functions in trouble?] In: Meggele, and Steinacker, P. (Eds.), *Analyomen 2. Proceedings of the 2nd Conference "Perspectives in Analytical Philosophy."* Berlin, New York: de Gruyter, pp. 186–193.

Walter, H. (1998). No cognition without emotion. In: Machleidt, W., Haltenhof, H., and Garlipp, P. (Eds.), *Ist die schizophrenie eine affektive Erkrankung?* [Is schizophrenia an affective disorder?]

Warner, R., and Szubka, T. (1994) (Eds.). *The mind-body problem*. Oxford: Basil-Blackwell.

Watson, G. (1982). Free agency. In: Watson, G. (Ed.), *Free will*. Oxford: Oxford University Press, pp. 96–110.

Watson, G. (1987). Free action and free will. *Mind*, 49, pp. 145–172.

Watson, G. (1992a). Entry: *Freedom and determinism*. In: Becker, L.C., and Becker, C.B. (Eds.), *Encyclopedia of ethics*. New York, London: Garland, pp. 365–388.

Watson, G. (1992b). Review of Freedom within Reason. *Philosophical Review*, 101.

Watson, G. (1995). Entry: *Free will*. In: Kim, J., and Sosa, E. (Eds.), *A companion to metaphysics*. Oxford: Blackwell, pp. 175–182.

Watzlawick, P. (1975) (Ed.). *Die Erfundene Wirklichkeit* [Invented Reality]. Hamburg: Piper.

Weatherford, R. (1991). *The implications of determinism*. London: Routledge.

Wesson, R. (1993). *Chaos, Zufall und Auslese in der natur* [Chaos, chance and selection in nature]. Frankfurt: Insel.

Whyte, J. (1993). Purpose and content. *British Journal for the Philosophy of Science*, 44, pp. 45–60.

Wiesendanger, H. (1987). Mit Leib und Seele [With body and soul]. Frankfurt, New York: Lang.

Wiggins, D. (1973). Towards a reasonable libertarianism. In: Honderich, T. (Ed.), *Essays on freedom of action*. London: Routledge, pp. 31–62.

Wiggins D. (1993). Locke, Butler and the stream of consciousness. In: Noonan, H. (Ed.), *Personal identity*. Dartmouth.

Williams, B. (1976). Moral luck. *Proceedings of the Aristotelian Society*, Supplement vol. 50, 115–135.

Wilson, E. (1979). Free will and determinism. In: Wilson, E.: *The mental as physical*. London: Routledge, pp. 243–271.

Wolf, S. (1980). Asymmetrical freedom. *Journal of Philosophy*, 77, pp. 151–166.

Wolf, S. (1990). *Freedom within reason*. Oxford: Oxford University Press.

Wright, L. (1973). Functions. *The Philosophical Review*, 82, pp. 139–168.

Wright, R. (1994). *The moral animal: The new science of evolutionary psychology*. Pantheon Books.

Young, J. Z. (1964). *A model of the brain*. Oxford: Clarendon Press.

Young, J. Z. (1987). *Philosophy and the brain*. Oxford: Oxford University Press.

Zanone, P. G., and Kelso, J. A. S. (1992). Evolution of behavioral attractors with learning: Nonequilibrium phase transitions. *Journal of Experimental Psychology*, 18, pp. 403–421.

Zeki, S. (1993). *A vision of the brain*. Oxford: Blackwell.

Zilles, K. (1994). Vom Seelenorgan zum neuronalen System—historische und gegenwärtige Konzepte zur Lokalisation von Hirnfunktionen [From the soul's organ to a neuronal system—historical and contemporary concepts for localizing brain functions] In: Fedrowitz, J., Matejosvski, D., and Kaiser, G. (Eds.), *Neuroworlds*. Frankfurt, New York: Campus, pp. 177–207.

Zimmer, D. E. (1988). *Die Vernunft der Gefühle* [The Rationality of Emotions], third edition. Munich: Piper.

Index